Fungal Diseases: From Infections to Prevention

Fungal Diseases: From Infections to Prevention

Zoe Parker

AMERICAN
MEDICAL PUBLISHERS
www.americanmedicalpublishers.com

AMERICAN
MEDICAL PUBLISHERS
www.americanmedicalpublishers.com

Cataloging-in-publication Data

Fungal diseases : from infections to prevention / Zoe Parker.
p. cm.
Includes bibliographical references and index.
ISBN 979-8-88740-127-0
1. Mycoses. 2. Mycoses--Prevention. 3. Mycoses--Etiology. 4. Infection.
5. Medical mycology. I. Parker, Zoe.
RC117 .F86 2023
616.969--dc23

American Medical Publishers,
41 Flatbush Avenue,
1st Floor, New York,
NY 11217, USA

ISBN 979-8-88740-127-0 (Hardback)

Contents

Preface

A disease caused by fungus is called fungal infection or mycosis. Fungal infections are divided into three categories depending on the part of body they affect. They are classified as superficial, subcutaneous, and systemic. Superficial fungal infections are benign infections which affect the skin, scalp and nails. They are caused by dermatophytes or Candida albicans. Subcutaneous infections such as eumycetoma and chromoblastomycosis target the tissues in and under the skin. Systemic fungal infections are more fatal and include cryptococcosis, histoplasmosis, pneumocystis pneumonia, aspergillosis, and mucormycosis. These fungal infections can be caused by fungi such as yeasts, molds, and fungi that can be both a mold and yeast. The line of treatment is based on the nature of the fungal infection, and usually requires topical or systemic antifungal medicines. Prevention of fungal infections involves wearing clean clothes and practicing good hygiene. This book, with its detailed analyses and data, will prove immensely beneficial to researchers and students involved in the study of fungal diseases. It is a collective contribution of a renowned group of international experts. This book strives to provide a fair idea about the fungal infections as well as their prevention.

Significant researches are present in this book. Intensive efforts have been employed by authors to make this book an outstanding discourse. This book contains the enlightening chapters which have been written on the basis of significant researches done by the experts.

Finally, I would also like to thank all the members involved in this book for being a team and meeting all the deadlines for the submission of their respective works. I would also like to thank my friends and family for being supportive in my efforts.

Zoe Parker

Fungal Disease: An Overview

Fungal infections or mycoses are the great neglected diseases of medical history.[1] There are numerous histories of viral, bacterial and protozoan infections, for all times and all places, but very few studies of those caused by fungi. Why? It cannot be because of prevalence. Historical sources and contemporary epidemiological investigations show that fungal infections were and are ubiquitous in human and animal populations. Everyone in Britain and the United States in the last half a century would have heard of, if not suffered from, athlete's foot or thrush. In the first half of the twentieth century, children feared the school nurse finding ringworm on their scalp and having to endure, not only the pains of X-ray depilation or having their shaven head painted with gentian violet, but also exclusion from school and the shame of being stigmatised as 'unclean'.[2]

It seems that medical historians have followed the agenda of the medical profession in showing relatively little interest in conditions, such as the majority of cases of mycoses, that do not lead to 'illness' as such, but cause inflammation, irritation and discomfort. Medical history remains dominated by studies of diseases that had, or continue to have, a high profile within medicine, or have attracted government interest and investment because they cause significant morbidity or mortality. Yet, the majority experience of ill health was, and is, of self-limiting and self-treated conditions, where sufferers did not, and do not, consult a doctor and become 'patients'. In their efforts to recover 'the patient's view', medical historians have ignored the minor illnesses, injuries and infections that were, and remain, outside of the medical gaze.[3]

But medical historians have also largely ignored the ailments brought on by medical advances, and here too the history of fungal infections can be instructive. The grand narrative of Western medicine in the twentieth century was one of 'progress', evidenced by greater, scientifically based knowledge of the aetiology and pathology of disease, more accurate diagnostics, improved management of symptoms and pain, more effective treatments, innovations in surgery, improved health care, falling mortality rates and greater longevity.[4] Those telling this story recognised that progress was not unalloyed, yet amongst doctors such was the step change in their effectiveness and efficiency that problems, like the development of antibiotic resistance, were discounted or seen as something that would be solved by further scientific and technological advances.[5] However, medical professionals soon realised that therapeutic and technological advances often led to intractable problems; for example, the practice of managing the adverse effects of one drug with another could lead to patients taking more medicines to manage side effects than for their primary illness. Such practices were criticised in the 1960s, but for our narrative of fungal infections Ivan Illich's book *Medical Nemesis*, first published in 1975, is most relevant.[6] Illich made *iatrogenesis* – doctor induced disease – central to his critique of modern medicine, claiming that around 10% of all clinical encounters were for such conditions. He argued that the cures of modern medicine were often worse than the disease – if indeed there was a disease in the first place, as Illich also attacked the medicalisation of everyday life, anticipating the burgeoning of risk-defined conditions that emerged in the last quarter of the twentieth century.[7]

Thrush, the most prevalent opportunistic mycosis of the twentieth century, exemplifies these trends. In the 1940s and 1950s, the emergence of resistant bacteria was only one side effect of the new drugs. More important then was the development of so-called 'superinfections', also caused by antibiotics as they removed not just disease-causing bacteria but many others, and altered the normal microbial flora of the body. These changes opened the body to opportunistic infection by other bacteria, such as *Staphylococcus aureus*, and by fungi, especially *Candida*. This fungus had previously only affected the 'external' mucus membranes in the mouth and genitalia, but emerged in the 1950s as a rare, but serious, internal and systemic infection, where fungi grew on major organs, such as the heart. It was not just patients on antibiotics who were vulnerable. There were a growing number of patients whose immune systems were weakened or immunocompromised. Initially, this situation developed as a side effect of steroids and other similar treatments, but then such states were deliberately produced by doctors to aid the acceptance of transplanted organs, or as a by-product of new cancer therapies. In 1987, John W. Rippon, a leading American medical mycologist, reflected on the situation.

> The mycology of human infections in the 1980s is the mycology of the soil, rotting vegetables, shower curtains, toilet bowls, leaf piles, wilted flowers and dung heaps. Organisms literally come out of the walls to infect immunosuppressed patients. Technical medical and surgical expertise is such that we can pass around hearts, lungs, and livers only to be thwarted by a *Fusarium* from a rotting plum.[8]

Rippon was pointing to a larger truth about human fungal infections, namely, that their prevalence has been linked to specific ecological conditions and interactions, not only within the body, but also within the wider social and physical environment. At the time Rippon wrote, the United States, and soon the Western world, was gripped by a popular health panic about fungal disease. Some fringe doctors promoted the view that *Candida* infection was responsible for all manner of 'modern' ailments, including chronic fatigue syndrome (CFS) and inflammatory bowel disease (IBD), in what they styled as 'the yeast connection'.[9]

In this book, we discuss the changing medical and public profile of fungal infections in the period 1850–2000. We consider four sets of diseases: ringworm and athlete's foot (dermatophytosis); thrush or candidiasis (infection with *Candida albicans*); endemic, geographically specific infections in North America (coccidioidomycosis, blastomycosis and histoplasmosis) and mycotoxins; and aspergillosis (infection with *Aspergillus fumigatus*). We discuss each disease in relation to developing medical knowledge and practices, and to social changes associated with 'modernity'. Thus, mass schooling provided ideal conditions for the spread of ringworm of the scalp in children, and the rise of college sports and improvement of personal hygiene led to the spread of athlete's foot. Antibiotics seemed to open the body to more serious *Candida* infections, as did new methods to treat cancers and the development of transplantation. Regional fungal infections in North America came to the fore due to the economic development of certain regions, where population movement brought in non-immune groups who were vulnerable to endemic mycoses. Fungal toxins or mycotoxins were discovered as by-products of modern food storage and distribution technologies. Lastly, the rapid development and deployment of new medical technologies, such as intensive care and immunosuppression in the last quarter of the twentieth century, increased the incidence of aspergillosis and other systemic mycoses.

In understanding and managing infectious diseases, scientists and doctors have long argued for thinking about them in terms of the metaphor of 'seed and soil', where the 'seed' is the infectious organism or pathogen: that is, virus, bacteria, fungi, protozoa (single cell) or metazoan (multicellular); and the 'soil' is the human body and its environs.[10] Thus, for someone with the common cold, the notion of 'seed and soil' ensures that we go beyond focusing only on infection by the virus (the seed) and consider the sufferer (the soil). This means looking at the conditions in which the person was exposed to the virus, the quantity and quality of the virus reaching the body, the nature of the body's specific immune response and the overall health of the individual. We all know that we do not 'catch a cold' every time we are exposed to the virus and that some people suffer longer and more serious illness than others do. Some variations are individual, but epidemiological studies have always shown patterns of exposure, susceptibility, sickness and recovery by age, gender, class, occupation, ethnicity and other socio-cultural variables. For example, in their history of pulmonary tuberculosis, René and Jean Dubos systematically use the notion of 'seed and soil' to discuss the disease at all levels, from biological factors influencing the susceptibility of cells and tissues, through to the socio-economic and technological variables that have shaped global trends in morbidity and mortality.[11] In this book, we frame our history of fungal infections in terms of 'seed and soil'; hence, our 'seeds' are specific fungal pathogens and we interpret 'soils' widely to include the human body, social relations and structures, and the medical, material and technological environment.

Fungi

Fungi and how they cause diseases are not well known, so it will be useful here to give a brief introduction to the nature of the 'seeds' of mycoses. Our account is part historical and part current.

Mycology is the branch of science that studies fungi and until the 1960s, it was a part of botany, at which time its subject matter was moved to the animal kingdom. Since then, fungi have been placed in their own kingdom, with the other four being plants, animals, protozoa and monera (bacteria).[12] Current estimates are that there are well over 100,000 species of fungi and many more are still to be classified, let alone discovered. Some fungi are large and multicellular, like toadstools. However, most species are microscopic, single cell organisms and are best known as industrial agents (yeast fungi in the production of bread and beer) and as medical agents (*Penicillia* spp. remain the source of the world's mostly widely used antibiotic). The larger fungi develop as microscopic filaments called hyphae, which branch and grow into networks or colonies called mycelia, whereas smaller fungi, such as yeasts, are single cell microorganisms.

Many writers divide fungi into 'good' and 'bad', judged by their impact on human existence; fungi themselves, of course, are just filling niches that allow them to multiply and survive. In popular writing, the 'good' fungi are those used in industrial processes or medicine, such as yeasts and penicillins mentioned above, plus those that can be eaten, break down waste or work in plant roots to fix nitrogen. The 'bad' fungi are those that produce diseases in plants, animals and humans. In terms of impact on humanity, fungi do most harm as causes of crop diseases and amongst farm animals, but they are also a threat to homes, where their ability to breakdown organic matter is seen most strikingly in the dry rot fungus which can destroy wooden structures very rapidly. Most fungi are saprophytic, that is, they obtain their nutrients from breaking down organic matter, normally dead tissues, and absorbing the products to 'feed' their metabolism. They mostly live on or within the material on which they are feeding. A small number of fungi, and of course the ones that concern medical mycologists, derive their nutrients from infecting living tissue, either by destroying it, or through establishing a symbiotic relationship that affects human tissues and their functioning.

Following long-established Linnaean principles, the classification of fungi was mainly by their reproductive and sexual characteristics. Thus, the 1911 *Encyclopaedia Britannica* divided fungi into three groups: the *Basidiomycota,* which produce club-like fruit bodies that spread spores (e.g. mushrooms); the *Ascomycota*, which produce fruit bodies on special pods or sac structures (e.g. baker's yeast, penicillin and most human fungal pathogens); and the *Phycomycetes* that reproduce sexually by spores joining (e.g. black bread mould). These classifications held for most of the twentieth century, though with many refinements and revisions with individual groups, genera and species. Certain fungi proved very difficult to classify as they had different forms in different stages of their life cycle. In the final decades of the century, the whole basis of ordering fungi changed as the new types of analysis of their DNA (their genome or genotype) revealed different relationships from those of their form and function (phenotype). The fluidity of understanding of the nature and classifications of fungi was evident with the microorganism known currently as *Pneumocystis jiroveci*. Through the 1980s, this organism was regarded as a protozoan and named *Pneumocystis carinii*, when it was the subject of extensive research as it was a major cause of pneumonia and death in HIV/AIDS sufferers.[13] Indeed, *Pneumocystis carinii* pneumonia (PCP) was an early marker of the epidemic and allegedly responsible for the deaths of celebrities such as Freddie Mercury. The redesignation of the organism as a fungus was first made in 1988, based on work using the new techniques of DNA sequencing, though this remained controversial until the late 1990s when the reclassification was finally accepted.[14]

Fungal diseases

Geoffrey Ainsworth, who has written most extensively on the history of fungal diseases, argues that fungi are amongst the oldest recognised causes of infection in humans.[15] Hippocrates seemingly wrote on 'aphthae' (sores in the mouth) in 500 BC, which modern mycologists have identified as thrush. Two millennia later, ringworm infection was present on the skin and in the hair of the subjects of Old Masters' paintings. In the modern medical era, the first systematic writings on fungi as a source of human disease were by the Hungarian born, Paris-based physician and microscopist David Gruby in 1842–1844. At the time, fungi were understood to be the sources of a number of diseases and attracted considerable scientific interest. In the 1830s, the Italian entomologist Agostino Bassi published claims that the devastating muscardine disease of silkworms was due to a microscopic fungus *Tritirachium shiotae*, which was eventually renamed in his honour as *Beauveria bassiana*.[16] Bassi was a major influence on Louis Pasteur, both in his work on the silkworm diseases of *pébrine* and *flacherie* in the 1860s and on the idea that living microorganisms might cause infectious diseases. The work of Bassi and Pasteur showed that fungal infections were, and in fact still are, the cause of economic problems in agriculture and related industries.[17] Ainsworth goes on to make the point that most 'mycologists' in Britain and the United States work as plant pathologists, with a disciplinary allegiance to botany, and that medical mycologists were and remain quite a small minority, with a quite different orientation.

In medicine in the 1830s, and in keeping with the then fashionable focus on pathological anatomy and lesions, distinctive and specific fungal infections of the skin, such as favus and ringworm, were well recognised. Classifications or nosologies of skin diseases were produced in the early nineteenth century, most influentially in Thomas Bateman's *A Practical Synopsis of Cutaneous Diseases According to the Arrangement of Dr Willan* (1813) and an atlas *The Delineations of Cutaneous Disease* in 1817.[18] Many authors followed the French physician Jean Louis Alibert in using extensive colour illustrations and some copied the wax models (*les moulages*) that he collected at the Hôpital Saint-Louis in Paris.[19] The use of colour illustrations continued with photography, as in Charles-Philippe Lallier's *Leçons cliniques sur les teignes*, published in 1878.[20]

The contagious and infectious aspects of fungal disease meant that, from the 1860s, doctors and scientists regarded them as 'germ diseases'.[21] Early historians of germ theories of disease certainly traced the familiar lineage from van Leeuwenhoek through Bassi to Pasteur, and the natural philosophers and medical men who used microscopy and culturing to study fungi. David Gruby first linked specific fungi to favus, sycosis and ringworm infections of the human scalp in the 1840s. For the latter, he first described the clinical condition of tinea tonsurans (scalp ringworm), though the terms 'herpes tonsurans' and 'teigne tondante' also enjoyed currency.[22] In the 1850s, botanists and dermatologists agreed on *Trichophyton* – literally hair-fungus due to its shape seen through microscopes – as the main ringworm germ and, in line with the wider switch to naming diseases by their causes rather than their signs and symptoms, in France tinea tonsurans became 'trichophytie'. As we discuss in Chapter 1, these developments were followed by leading dermatologists, such as William Tilbury Fox and Thomas M'Call Anderson, but most doctors and dermatologists remained focused on morbid anatomy and nosologies based on signs and lesions.

Fungus theories of infectious disease were popular in the 1840s and the best known was the 'cholera fungus'.[23] In a paper read to the Microscopical Committee of the Bristol Literary and Philosophical Institution in 1849, 'fungoid' bodies were reported in the faeces of cholera sufferers.[24] The authors emphasised analogies between the growth and decay of fungi, and the rise and fall of zymotic diseases in individuals and in populations over epidemic periods. However, given that contemporaries thought that fungi were the 'appointed executioners and nimble scavengers of nature', any such organisms were understood by contemporary doctors to be the consequences rather than the causes of cholera. Medical views on the causal role of living organisms in disease waxed and waned from the 1840s to the 1880s, until bacterial germs were accepted as major pathogens.[25] At this time, bacteria were termed as the 'Schizomycetes', literally the splitting fungi, so named because they reproduced by the division of cells, and were believed to be a type of fungi because of their microscopic form and physiological function as saprophytes.

One of the first British textbooks on the new science of germs was German Sims Woodhead and Arthur Hare's *Pathological Mycology* published in 1885.[26] However, this was the only time 'mycology' was used in this context; the German term *Bacteriologie* soon took over. In the new manuals and textbooks on 'bacteriology' and 'microbiology', fungi as causes of infection were, at best, described briefly and typically in a final chapter or appendix. For example, Muir's and Ritchie's influential *Manual of Bacteriology*, published in 1899, had a chapter entitled 'Non-Pathogenic Micro-organisms – Fungi', and presented them as likely laboratory contaminants rather than pathogens. The authors discussed *Mucor* spp., *Oidium* spp., *Aspergillus niger, Penicillium glaucum*, plus yeasts, and ended with the comment, 'Certain fungi closely related to the above are pathogenic agents.' Readers were referred to Anton De Bary's *Comparative Morphology and Biology of the Fungi, Mycetozoa and Bacteria*, first published in 1886, for further details.[27]

In the twentieth century, fungi were recognised as causing three types of disease in humans and animals. First, there were infections where fungi develop parasitically in the tissues of the host, at (literally) three levels: superficial mycoses, like athlete's foot, where infection is limited to the outermost layers of the skin, nails and hair; subcutaneous mycoses, like the tropical disease of Madura foot (mycetoma), where the growth extends to the underlying layers of the skin and perhaps into bone; and systemic mycoses, like aspergillosis, where infection spreads through internal organs and tissues.

Second, there were fungal poisons, either toxins in the fungi themselves, as with poisonous toadstools, or toxins produced by the growth of fungi on foodstuffs, as with aflatoxins (produced by *Aspergillus flavus*). Third, there were allergic reactions to fungal spores and moulds, which range from mild to acute, depending on the dose and susceptibility of the host; thus, fungi are a common cause of asthma. There was a fourth type of disease that was 'discovered' in the 1980s and remains highly contested – 'fungal overgrowth'. As we show in Chapter 3, this condition has been widely dismissed by the medical profession as a fiction, yet it had wide currency with the public and was linked to CFS and other 'diseases of modernity'. In the cultural climate in North America and Europe, where lifestyle was increasingly regarded as a cause, as well as a solution, to ill health, books such as William G. Crook's *The Yeast Connection* (1983), which attributed various chronic conditions to the overgrowth of *C. albicans*, became a best seller and spawned many imitators. Crook also had the cure: dietary and lifestyle changes, plus a course of antifungal antibiotics, which was surprising given his pedigree in 'alternative medicine'.

The history of medical mycology

The multi-faceted career of medical mycology's leading historian Geoffrey Ainsworth exemplifies the diverse and changing character of the field in the twentieth century. He studied pharmacy at University College, Nottingham, and then pursued a dual career in plant pathology and medical mycology.[28] He first worked on the virus diseases of plants at Britain's two leading botanical institutions, the Rothamsted Experimental Station and the Experimental and Research Station in Cheshunt. He spent the Second World War at the Imperial Mycological Institute at Kew, developing abstracting services on all aspects of mycology. After the war, he moved to the pharmaceutical industry, as head of the mycological department of the Wellcome Research Laboratories at Beckenham, Kent. There he led work on the antibiotics produced by fungi, such as streptomycin and penicillin. He then moved, first, to the London School of Hygiene and Tropical Medicine and later to the University of the South West (later the University of Exeter), before returning to the now Commonwealth Mycological Institute, where he stayed until his retirement in 1968. Ainsworth published widely on all aspects of fungi. His major works were *Dictionary of the Fungi* (1943), *British Smut Fungi* (1950) with Kathleen Sampson, *Medical Mycology* (1952), and the multi-volume *The Fungi: An Advanced Treatise* (1965–1973) with A. S. Sussman and F. K. Sparrow.

Towards the end of his career, Ainsworth developed an interest in the history of mycology and published three books that have been immensely valuable in the research and writing of this book: *Introduction to the History of Mycology* (1976), *Introduction to the History of Plant Pathology* (1981) and *Introduction to the History of Medical and Veterinary Mycology* (1987).[29] In his preface to the latter volume, he sets out his approach and the scope of the topic.

> Although possessing deep, if slender roots that can be traced back to ancient times, medical and veterinary mycology is essentially a development of the twentieth century, especially the last fifty years during which time several mycoses at first considered to be rarities have been shown to affect millions of men, women, and children and their domesticated animals.... Here the attempt made to sketch in

> the historical background, by illustrating the approaches to a series of basic problems, is limited to what might be described as the 'natural history' of human and animal mycoses.[30]

While we agree with Ainsworth on the point that the development of medical mycology was a phenomenon of the twentieth century, our work differs in two ways. First, we do not take the specialism of medical mycology as given, or historically constant, rather as a social institution that had to be created and sustained. Second, we do not set out a lineage of ideas, but rather discuss changing knowledges in specific institutional and social settings, and also explore practices and meanings.[31]

The history of medical mycology in the United States in the twentieth century has been described in great detail in a monograph by Ana Victoria Espinel-Ingroff published in 2006.[32] Her narrative is comprehensive and wonderfully rich in characters and institutional detail. It focuses on training and mapping the professional networks that have shaped medical mycology across the country. At the same time, the author tells the story of discoveries in the understanding and management of the main fungal infections that affect Americans. It is history informed by disciplinary politics, as Espinel-Ingroff's reference point is what she sees as a crisis in medical mycology in the United States. On the one hand, the importance of mycoses has grown with their increased prevalence and the arrival of effective antifungal drugs. Yet, on the other hand, the field seems to be fragmenting, being drawn at one end to molecular approaches and basic biology, and at the other to applied clinical research, leading to the neglect of the old, middle ground of taxonomy, aetiology, physiology and pathogenesis.

Woven into Espinel-Ingroff's history narrative is a narrative of developments in the field in the twentieth century, with five periods defining her chapters. The discussion of the 'Era of Discovery (1894–1919)' explores how work on fungi followed that in bacteriology in seeking the causal organisms of specific infections and the understanding of basic fungal biology. The 'Formative Years (1920–1949)' are characterised by the establishment of training programmes, laboratory services and epidemiological studies of common diseases, such as athlete's foot and thrush, or the then very rare systemic mycoses. The period 1950–1969, the 'Advent of Antifungal and Immunosuppressive Therapies', was dominated by drug discoveries (nystatin, amphotericin B, griseofulvin) and the increased incidence of severe opportunistic systemic fungal infections that were linked to antibiotics and immunosuppressive therapies. The 'Years of Expansion (1970–1979)' are portrayed as the apogee of medical mycology, seen in the establishment of services to deal with the increased incidence of infections, basic research to underpin clinical innovations and the recognition of the specialty by the American Society for Microbiology (ASM). Finally, the 'Era of Transition (1980–1996)' saw continued increase in the incidence of opportunistic infections in cancer and transplant patients, and amongst AIDS patients, but also the fragmentation and relative neglect of the specialism.

What few histories there are of fungal infections are largely embedded in accounts of the development of the specialty of medical mycology, but there are a number of books and journal articles on specific infections. There is only one monograph on a disease discussed in this book, Thomas Daniel and Gerald L. Baum's *Drama and Discovery: The Story of Histoplasmosis*.[33] Their narrative follows the emergence of the disease from social changes in its endemic areas and the research networks in which new understandings of its epidemiology, aetiology, pathology and treatment developed. It is typical of much work on the history of mycoses, as with Ainsworth and Espinel-Ingroff, in being written by medical mycologists, but is quite different and richer as it explores the social as well as medical history of histoplasmosis.[34] There are no book length histories of coccidioidomycosis and blastomycosis comparable to *Drama and Discovery*, but there are very useful practitioner histories, for example, Jan Hirschmann's account of the early history of coccidioidomycosis in America.[35]

Yet, as we have indicated, 'biographies' of mycoses written by medical historians are rare. Aspergillosis has no thoroughgoing histories.[36] Ringworm has few historians in Britain and the United States, and even reflections by practitioners are rare.[37] It has only excited attention in Israel, in relation to the controversy of the long-term effects on children of X-ray treatment of the scalp and popular representations of the practice as the 'Ringworm Holocaust'.[38] It is also surprising that historians of medicine in the United States, who have thoroughly investigated popular medications and health activism, have missed athlete's foot, a condition that plagued not only the athletes but the country's youth, soldiers and miners.

Mycoses and medical history

In this book, we aim to do more than provide a narrative of a group of neglected infections. Our study also gives new perspectives on the history of twentieth-century medicine on a number of fronts: specialisation; minor illnesses and self-treatment; and 'orphan diseases'. Firstly, we present an account of an area of medicine – medical mycology – that for most of the twentieth century was small and marginal, and where practitioners struggled to establish an area of specialist work. The development of specialisms and specialisation has long interested historians of medicine.[39] George Rosen's study of ophthalmology was path breaking and work since then has linked the division of labour to many factors within medicine and outside. George Weisz, in the most recent and comprehensive study on the topic, finds that 'divide and conquer' best explains the overall process in medicine, as these terms '[express] a fundamental intellectual strategy', whereby medical professionals were, in a matter of a century, divided into 'smaller and more manageable groups based on common attributes' and conquered by 'organization based on a novel kind of expertise'.[40]

Most histories of specialisation and specialisms are of successful enterprises and can be teleological, charting the seemingly inevitable journey to the present division of labour in medicine. Our narrative of medical mycology runs against this grain, though it does not present medical mycology as a failed specialism, rather one, as Espinel-Ingroff's work makes clear, the position and status of which was always problematic. For most of the twentieth century, it was small, institutionally fragmented and dispersed geographically. Its practitioners tried to 'divide' themselves off from other specialisms but were relatively unsuccessful because their services were never in sufficient demand to form a critical mass either numerically or politically. Thus, we challenge the accepted, though often implicit, view that specialisation was an inevitable path in twentieth-century medicine, where it becomes ever more populated with full-time 'mono-specialists'; that is, clinicians and scientists who worked on a single disease or group of diseases, a particular organ or organ system, specific technologies or a restricted patient group, say, by age or sex. Our research on the doctors and researchers who treated and studied fungal infections shows a different, and perhaps equally common, pattern of work: clinicians and scientists making a living as working in and combining a number of specialisms.[41]

We suggest that it is useful to think about twentieth-century medicine generally in terms of the doctors, and other health workers for that matter, developing careers in a number of 'specialist practices'. Historians of medicine often overlook the fact that doctors and medical scientists had to 'make a living', and that in less wealthy times, when health was a lower priority in private and state budgets, this was done by earning where they could and what they could.[42] In this context, 'medical mycology' was an area of 'specialist practice' for certain botanists, dermatologists, bacteriologists, hospital physicians and surgeons, infectious disease doctors, microbiologists, general practitioners or, of course, combinations of these. Typically, 'specialist practice' was in cognate areas; hence, the first 'medical mycologists' were mostly botanists, or those who created the specialism of dermatology. Nevertheless, in the late nineteenth century few doctors were able to work full-time on skin diseases, so dermatologists were often general practitioners, who functioned as part-time specialists, part-time in hospital outpatient clinics.

Secondly, and as noted already, fungal infections represent the overwhelming experience of illness, then and now, like the common colds, sickness and diarrhoea, and sore throats that are self-limiting, self-treated or treated after one short consultation with a general practitioner.[43] Research in the 1980s revealed that on average only one in 20 'symptom episodes' led to a medical consultation, a pattern that was termed the 'iceberg of illness'.[44] If that was the position in a country with a National Health Service, offering care that was 'free at the point of delivery', the proportion would almost certainly be lower in pay-for-service medical and healthcare systems, then and now. There are few studies, except for the era of 'bedside medicine', of the everyday experience of illness, and of decisions on when and how to self-treat, and when and how to seek medical consultation and become a patient.[45] That said, our focus is on the *medical* history of mycoses – a sufferer's history would be quite different and, in fact, very difficult to research. However, we do try to capture sufferers' agency, for example, in our discussion of the proliferation of proprietary remedies for athlete's foot and thrush.

Thirdly, and at the other end of the scale of prevalence, systemic fungal infections have been classified as 'orphan diseases'; that is, those too rare to attract the attention of research agencies or the interest of many clinicians and researchers.[46] The term originated in the United States and the Orphan Drug Act, 1983, promoted by the National Organization for Rare Disorders and the Federal Drugs Agency (FDA). In the United States 'orphan diseases' are those with a prevalence of less than 2,000 cases per year. By the end of the twentieth century, the rise in the incidence of mycoses meant that this designation only applied to the geographically localised infections and the rarer types of hospital acquired or nosocomial infections. Yet, for most of the twentieth century, opportunistic, invasive mycoses were rare and medical mycologists and other interested parties bemoaned their neglect. In part, this was because such infections were seen as 'diseases of the diseased' and affected patients who were seriously ill and close to death. In fact, doctors spoke of these patients receiving 'salvage therapies', where ethical standards were different and there was scope of experiment and the non-standard use of standard drugs. Interestingly, when invasive mycoses ceased to be 'rare', they attracted the attention of many surgical and medical specialists, and researchers in pharmaceutical companies, who sought to transfer their successes with mass market, external antifungals to invasive, systemic disease. Indeed, the story of medical mycology in the second half of the twentieth century is dominated by the development of new antifungal antibiotics, principally polyenes (e.g. nystatin and amphotericin B), azoles (e.g. clotrimazole and ketoconazole), triazoles (e.g. fluconazole and itraconazole) and echinocandins (e.g. caspofungin), targeted at the 'seeds' of infection.

The book

We discuss our four sets of infection in five chapters: two on ringworm (dermatophytosis), and one each on thrush, the geographically specific mycoses and mycotoxins, and aspergillosis. We present histories of each disease group and while our approach is essentially thematic, there is an overall movement through time. Thus, the first chapter on ringworm begins in the mid-nineteenth century and ends around 1910, while the final chapter on aspergillosis is mainly about changes in the last quarter of the twentieth century. Our narrative moves between Britain and the United States following the changing locations where medical and social interest and activity was greatest. We are neither comprehensive nor comparative in our discussion of medical mycology in these two national contexts. However, we use the fact that work on fungal infections in the twentieth century, as demonstrated by the work of the International Society for Human and Animal Mycology (ISHAM), was dominated by an Anglo-American axis, though this is not to diminish in any way activities in other countries, which we discuss as appropriate.

Our first chapter frames ringworm as a disease of schools and schoolchildren. The disease had been reported previously in orphanages and similar institutions, but its incidence and profile increased with the arrival of mass schooling, which provided ideal conditions for its spread, both through increased opportunities for contagion (seeding) and the exposure of poor children (weakened soil). We look at responses to the problem, one of which was special schools for the isolation and treatment of sufferers, and which became sites for the use of the new X-ray technologies, not to kill the seeds of infection, but to alter the soil by removing hair, the locus of infection. In the second chapter, we move from head to toe, from Britain to the United States, and focus on athlete's foot. Concern over ringworm infection of the feet, along with infection of the crotch, armpit and similar areas of the body, began in the 1920s, principally amongst sportsmen and women. Athlete's foot was described as a perverse consequence of the nation's attempt to improve the health and fitness of its youth, especially with the burgeoning of college sports and improved hygiene facilities. The infection was met with the tools of modern public health propaganda, being presented in some instances as equivalent to a sexually transmitted disease, and by new methods of treatment produced by the pharmaceutical industry, first in a rash of proprietary medicines and then antifungal antibiotics.

Thrush, the subject of our third chapter, was regarded at the start of the twentieth century as a disease of weak children, but moved in the medical and public view to a genital infection, principally of women and was linked mainly to alterations in the body due to pregnancy and lifestyle changes.[47] We then discuss how, in the second half of the twentieth century, thrush was linked in different ways to the development of antibiotics. It was soon recognised as a side effect of penicillin therapy, while the search for new and better bacterial antibiotics led to the discovery of nystatin – the first modern antifungal antibiotic, which soon became a specific treatment for thrush. Systemic *C. albicans* infection, known as invasive candidiasis, became, paradoxically, more prevalent in patients taking bacterial antibiotics, but also in those with cancers, transplants and inflammatory conditions. This problem was met by a search for new antifungal drugs, with successes improving the institutional position of medical mycology. We end the chapter with a discussion of 'The Yeast Connection' phenomenon.

In Chapter 4, we discuss the regionally specific fungal infections in the United States that came to the fore as a consequence of the economic development of certain regions in the South and Midwest, where population movement brought in non-immune groups who were vulnerable to endemic mycoses. The forms of economic development were also important, as new methods of production and types of industrial and domestic construction created new environmental conditions, and in some cases literally transformed and transported fungi-laden soil dust. In the same vein, we show how new technologies of food production, transportation and storage produced a new class of hazardous compounds – mycotoxins. In our final chapter, we discuss aspergillosis, the most serious of the invasive mycoses that have emerged from new medical technologies, such as intensive care and immunosuppression. An important theme here is iatrogenesis, as attempts to control aspergillosis exemplified the now routine issue in modern medicine of balancing the benefits and adverse effects of primary treatment, with secondary and tertiary interventions.

1

School Settings and Ringworm

Education is a near universally recognised 'good' across histories of the modern world, with more and better quality schooling seen as a progressive social reform and a marker of a modern, civilised society. However, the introduction of mass schooling in Britain and America was the product of a social and political struggle which was not easily won.[1] Few disagreed that education improved the minds of pupils, but many people argued that it was not always good for their bodies; indeed, schools became great centres of contagion. Epidemics of major childhood infections such as measles, diphtheria and chickenpox periodically affected institutions and in some cases led to school closures.[2] Less recognised then, as now, was that schools were sites of exchange of endemic, social diseases, from serious, typically fatal infections, such as tuberculosis, through to endemic conditions, such as ringworm, which had mild symptoms but carried severe social stigma. The term 'ringworm' is very old and comes from the circular patches of peeled, inflamed skin that characterises the infection. In medicine at least, no one understood it to be associated with worms of any description.

In the early part of the nineteenth century, ringworm was well recognised by doctors and the public as an inflammation of the scalp, associated with reddening of the skin, itching, circles of peeling skin and hair loss. In children it was also popularly known as 'scald-head', a term derived from 'scaled' and 'scabby' rather than burns, and in medicine as a form of porrigo – skin complaints associated with the production of pustules. The naming and classification of skin diseases had been hugely contested from the 1790s until the publication of a system proposed by the English physician Robert Willans, who worked at the Carey Street Public Dispensary in London.[3] However, by the 1830s, when serious medical attention first focused on ringworm, the debate had settled to become one between those who saw the condition as localised in the skin and those who also looked to constitutional, internal factors. Both sides agreed that it was contagious and prevalent in children, especially the poor, who lived in crowded conditions and in orphanages, boarding schools and other institutions. The exciting cause was mostly talked about as a 'fungus', but susceptibility was explained in terms of the child having immature skin, a weak general constitution, dirty skin and poor hygiene, or all of these.

The role of 'seed and soil' in the causes, pathology, treatment and prevention of ringworm was debated throughout the nineteenth century and beyond. In this chapter, we tell the story of how and why the understanding of doctors and the public about the nature of ringworm changed in the period 1830–1910, focusing on the disease in school children. We first set the story of ringworm in the context of the emergence of dermatology, a specialism that grew largely in outpatient and dispensary settings. At this time, fungal diseases generally were understood mostly to affect the skin and outer membranes of the body, which was the domain of surgeons and later the new specialists in dermatology. We discuss the role of dermatologists in the development and spread of germ theories of skin diseases, showing that they were pioneers amongst clinicians in working with these ideas and changing to antiseptic practices. Our narrative then turns to the problem of ringworm in school children and attempts to manage the disease for sufferers and their families, and we show that the social consequences and stigma of the infection were far worse than the disease itself. Finally, we analyse new treatments, especially the use of X-rays, and school medical inspections, where children worried about the nurse finding both nits and ringworm.

'Scald-head'

Robert Willans, London's leading skin specialist in the late eighteenth and early nineteenth centuries, reported that in his career he had seen children from over 200 schools and colleges in London affected by ringworm. While its effects on the physical body were localised and relatively mild, on personal development they were serious, as Samuel Plumbe, Willan's successor, explained in 1835.[4]

> In the earlier periods of the lives of children there is no disease, no species of deviation from sound health, if we except scrofula, which operates so perniciously on the future prospects of the individual, as ring-worm, if of long continuance. The moment an unfortunate child

> is found by the schoolmaster or the schoolmistress with a spot on the head, the latter, very properly (not merely for interest's sake, but as a duty to the parents of all the other children), sends the child home, refuses to readmit until thoroughly cured. The consequence of this is, to the unfortunate child, a loss of time at that period of life when it can be least afforded, the period of early education.[5]

It was not only children who suffered, their teachers did too. Plumbe observed that the disease was 'destructive of the best instructors of children, for the conductors of establishments of previously high character and reputation found their pupils drop off in large numbers, and many good schools have been utterly ruined by it'.[6]

There are no figures for the incidence of ringworm in the nineteenth century, but every indication is that it was very prevalent.[7] There were, for instance, a huge number of proprietary ointments, lotions and potions sold by local chemists and self-treatment advice was proffered in popular health manuals and advertisements. The 1790 edition of William Buchan's *Domestic Medicine* recommended 'keeping the head very clean, cutting off the hair, combing and brushing away the scabs, & c.', plus the use of ointments.[8] Mrs Beeton offered several treatment regimes in her *Book of Household Management*, including the application of sulphur and treacle, creosote, or calomel.[9] There were numerous reports of cases and treatments in national and regional medical journals, for all types of infection.[10] At many sites on the body, the characteristic rings were hidden by clothing and hard to see, which meant that sufferers and doctors found it difficult to distinguish ringworm from other inflammatory afflictions, such as favus, eczema, psoriasis and impetigo. Surgeons considered therapy relatively straightforward on any part of the body except the scalp, where ringworm was typically persistent. Although the disease affected all ages, medical discussion focused on children and on their scalps.[11] It was the most visible form of the disease, both medically and socially, as infected children were stigmatised as unclean and their parents regarded as uncaring.

In Britain, ringworm first attracted national medical and public attention in 1835, following reports of its high prevalence at Christ's Hospital School, one of London's foremost public schools, which included amongst its old boys Charles Lamb and Samuel Taylor Coleridge.[12] In this outbreak there were two issues: firstly, the infection was often said to be an indicator of poor management by the governors and staff, as well as damaging to the reputation of the school; and secondly, if children were excluded for weeks on end, their education was suffering and the school was losing income.[13] An editorial in the *Lancet* complained that the governors had been negligent in not drawing upon the expertise of doctors, especially those who had dealt successfully with other serious outbreaks at the London Orphan Asylum and the Royal Naval School.[14] A committee of Christ's governors was appointed to look into the problem and they invited Plumbe to advise them. His report nicely illustrates medical thinking on the affliction at the time in terms of exciting causes (contagion) and predisposing causes (general health and cleanliness). As was typical of the fractious character of skin specialists at this time, he was dismissive of Robert Willans – who he saw as no better than a nostrum monger – and of the French dermatologists. His view of the nature of ringworm was that it was both constitutional and contagious:

> The simple circular contagious ringworm is not, as has been supposed by many, produced only by infection or contagion. It arises in a very large portion of cases from the same sources as other diseases of the skin, such as improper diet, producing constipation of the bowels; restraint of the due and healthy exercise of children; repletion from over feeding, or from merely a single indulgence of sweet-meats or cakes, producing acidity. Yet thus originating it is quite as contagious as that which has spread directly in a family, from child to child, by contact, where no derangement of the stomach or system can be traced or suspected.[15]

Plumbe advised surveillance to control the spread of the disease by examining boys on entry, washing bedding regularly and isolating those infected. This might involve moving those suffering to separate rooms, or simply making them wear protective caps or headwear. He also wanted pupils to have improved diets, both in quantity and in quality. He linked this to the danger of scurvy, writing that 'the almost entire privation of vegetables tends to produce, if it be not the sole cause of the eruptive diseases'.[16] Plumbe was a 'skin doctor' before the era of specialisation, so it would be anachronistic to characterise him as a dermatologist; indeed, that term did not gain currency until the 1880s, but he does represent the common situation in the nineteenth century where surgeons had known areas of specialist expertise.[17]

Dermatology and fungus theories of skin diseases

Historians of nineteenth century British clinical medicine have highlighted that key national characteristic of resistance to specialism in hospital practice amongst elite physicians and surgeons and the celebration of the virtues of the generalist.[18] 'The narrow specialism of dermatology', as it was termed in 1874, was one of a number of organ- or technique-based specialist areas that drew the wrath of critics.[19] For example, a reviewer of Mapother's *Diseases of the Skin*, published in 1875, was severe on the author's expertise and his claims to special competence.

> It is, indeed, but too true that the great body of specialists is composed largely of those who are intellectually quite incapable of comprehending all the departments for the healing arts. They succeed only by limiting their sphere of action; they triumphantly paddle in pools who would not live a moment in the stream. With the exception of ophthalmologists, specialists cannot, as a rule, be said to be amongst the best educated of the profession; and worse than all, the exclusive practice of some small speciality tends to perpetuate and increase ignorance, if it do not also deprave professional morals.[20]

However, Edward Dillon Mapother was no exclusive practitioner.[21] He had been Medical Officer of Health for Dublin in the 1860s, wrote extensively on medical education, and was appointed Professor of Anatomy and Physiology at the Royal College of Surgeons of Ireland, eventually becoming its president. He had special interests in syphilis and gout, as well as in skin diseases.

Why was so much scorn poured on specialists? One explanation was the rivalry between surgeons and physicians, though this was complicated by the emergence of another divide between general practitioners and consultants.[22] Both consultant surgeons and physicians attacked specialisation, but many practitioners had niches with particular diseases, and combined general and specialist work. The case of the emergent specialism of dermatology is instructive.[23] It grew from surgical practice after the mid-nineteenth century, with specialist journals being published from the 1870s. The diagnosis and treatment of skin diseases had been a large and important part of surgeons' work and hence income. The future of general surgery seemed to lie in two directions: on the one hand extending the number and range of operations, while on the other hand becoming more 'medical'. For example, in the treatment of syphilis, the cauterisation or excision of primary lesions on the skin was regarded as ineffectual and surgeons relied more upon constitutional treatment with mercury.[24] Treating syphilis may have been a good source of income for surgeons, but sufferers were stigmatised and this rubbed off on surgeons. In fact, the term 'quack', widely applied to so-called specialists, was a contraction of 'quacksalver', or quicksilver, one of the most widely used specific treatments for syphilis.

Specialist practice in skin diseases was largely in hospital outpatient departments and dispensaries, the first of which, the Royal London and Westminster Infirmary for the Treatment of Cutaneous Diseases, was opened in 1819.[25] In the capital, a Hospital for Diseases of the Skin (later the Blackfriars Skin Hospital) followed in 1841, with satellite dispensaries opening in 1843, 1844, 1850, 1851 and 1857.[26] A new era in skin hospitals began in 1863 with the opening of the St John's Hospital for Disease of the Skin, followed by many more such institutions.[27] John Laws Milton founded St John's initially with the support of leading figures on diseases of the skin, such as Erasmus Wilson, William Tilbury Fox and J. Mill Frodsham.[28] The new skin hospitals had few beds and their dispensary work directly challenged the businesses of local general practitioners and elite consultants. In response, many voluntary hospitals set up 'skin departments', promising the best of all worlds: specialist, accessible care without hospitalisation, available in general hospitals where other specialist and general consultants were available.

Erasmus Wilson was Britain's leading authority on diseases of the skin and he founded the short-lived *Journal of Cutaneous Medicine* in 1867.[29] He was a polymath and populariser, who published books on the skin, food and Egyptology, and is best known for funding the transportation of Cleopatra's Needle to London in 1878. Wilson popularised the term 'dermatology', first lecturing on the subject in 1840, and publishing *On Diseases of the Skin: Practical and Theoretical Treatise* in 1842. His private practice and investments were so successful that in 1869 he donated monies to the Royal College of Surgeons to establish a professorship of dermatology, which he held from 1869 to 1878, giving an annual series of lectures. In his own clinical practice, Wilson saw no conflict between generalism and specialism, but he was opposed to the exclusive specialist practice of others. Although trained as a surgeon, he claimed that almost all skin diseases were internal and constitutional in origin, which required medical as much as external surgical or topical treatments. Thus, skin diseases needed to be diagnosed and treated by someone who understood the workings of the whole body, not just its outer layer. He was an opponent of contagious germ or fungal explanations of skin conditions, believing that any such matter present was a 'secondary or adventitious product' rather an exciting cause.[30]

In the 1860s, two teaching hospitals, University College Hospital and the Glasgow Western Infirmary, established dermatology departments, and appointed two men who made ringworm a model for germ theories of skin disease: Thomas M'Call (sometimes McCall) Anderson and Tilbury Fox.[31] M'Call Anderson published *On the Parasitic Affections of the Skin* in 1861 and Tilbury Fox published his *Skin Diseases of Parasitic Origin* two years later.[32] Like Wilson, Tilbury Fox opposed specialisms, whereas M'Call Anderson argued that this was how progress was being made in medicine in France and Germany and that Britain should follow.[33] Yet M'Call Anderson was another example of someone who combined general and specialist practice. He became Professor of Clinical Medicine at the Glasgow Western Infirmary and then Regius Professor in 1904, and his obituary celebrated how he maintained specialist work and writing on skin diseases, along with clinical teaching and running a large private practice. Tilbury Fox and M'Call Anderson united against Wilson's claim that fungi had no causal role in skin diseases. Given his dominant position, it is unsurprising that Wilson represented what was termed the 'British school of dermatology' that saw most skin diseases to be of internal, constitutional origin – mostly forms of eczema – which required internal remedies.

Fungus germs

From the 1850s, ringworm was regarded as a fungus disease. This made it an early candidate to be a germ disease when debates about the causes of infectious and contagious diseases turned to microorganisms in the 1870s.[34] Some histories of germ theories of disease, anticipating the closure on bacterial causes in the 1880s, have ignored the many types of entity – animal, vegetable and mineral – that were candidates to be disease germs in 1860s and 1870s. Good examples of such openness were the views of Samuel Wilks, the leading London physician. In his Address in Medicine at the British Medical Association (BMA) in June 1872, he spoke variously of disease being caused by 'vegetable germs', 'a fungus', 'specific organic particles' and 'a virus'.[35] Wilks also made the point that the 'seeds' of disease, its germs, needed to find suitable 'soil'. Ringworm was one of his examples and he placed it, no doubt surprisingly for modern readers, alongside cancer as a disease that grew and spread within the body.

> A ringworm grows and grows wherever the soil is propitious; the itch insect spreads over the body and the hydatid often swells until its

> host is destroyed. Cancer-cells divide and propagate until they have killed their victim which has supplied them with nourishment; and the germs of small-pox will do the same.[36]

Another key issue with fungi (the collective botanical name at the time was the *Mycetes*) was whether they were made up of fixed species, or were they so simple that their biology was shaped by the conditions in which they grew. Moreover, if there were fixed species, how could these be differentiated when their forms and modes of reproduction were so variable.

The same question was important in germ theories of diseases, not least with bacterial versions. The scientific name for bacteria at this time was the *Schizomycetes*, literally, 'fission fungi'.[37] Being surgeons by training, dermatologists were early adopters of antiseptics, if not converts to germ theories of putrefaction and inflammation, and through the promotional activities of Joseph Lister had early and consistent exposure to new ideas on germs. The standard chemical antiseptic, carbolic acid, was tried as a fungicide with ringworm and other skin infections, along with sulphurous acid, acetic acid, iodine and mercuric chloride.[38] However, the lengthy applications of such caustic substances meant that the treatment was often worse than the cure.

The books of Tilbury Fox and M'Call Anderson, which many read as suggesting that almost all skin diseases were of fungal origin, prompted debates that anticipated many of the issues that divided opinion over bacterial germ theories of disease in the last quarter of the nineteenth century.[39] First, there was the question of whether any fungi found in diseased skin were necessary causes of disease or just concomitants.[40] Second, doctors asked whether fungi, when present, could only develop on dead tissue, acting as saprophytes; or whether they could actually invade and colonise living tissue, as infective agents or *contagium viva*. It was in this vein that the cholera fungus controversy in the late 1840s and 1850s had been framed.[41] Third, if fungi were agents of disease, was there one pathogenic fungus that produced different diseases because its effects and form depended on the tissue on which it grew: that is, it was pleomorphic (*pleo* – many + *morphic* – form). Or, did distinct species of pathogenic fungi produce different diseases? In his volume, Tilbury Fox argued that all pathogenic fungi were forms of *Tinea* – the ringworm fungus – which he made 'the generic term for parasitic affections of the surface', echoing the views of the Ernst Hallier in Germany on the pleomorphic character of fungi.[42] Against this, M'Call Anderson maintained that different fungi caused distinct and specific diseases, and that they could do so in both dead and living tissue. He classed fungal infections as 'vegetable parasitic affections', placing them alongside animal parasitic ones, such as scabies, and those caused by 'poisons' or 'viruses', such as syphilis.

The impact of bacteriology on the management of skin diseases was to shift treatments to be anti-germ.[43] As noted above, doctors recommended germ-killing antiseptics, but also tried to break the passage of germs by 'isolating' the infected area, by covering it with a dressing or grease of some type. The ringworm caps worn by children combined all of these. The exclusion of infected children from school became more common and there were some suggestions of isolating families in their homes. At the same time, most doctors continued to recommend measures that aimed to strengthen the bodily 'soil' against the 'seeds' of disease. Although it would be wrong to make too much of the conjunction, the Dermatological Society of London was founded in 1882, the very same year in which Koch announced his discovery of the *Tubercle bacillus*, which could also infect the skin and was associated with leprosy and lupus.[44] From this time, leading dermatologists associated particular germs with specific skin diseases.[45]

Ringworm in schools – ringworm schools

Outbreaks of ringworm in schools, workhouse and other institutions were reported throughout the mid-Victorian period, but they attracted little medical or public attention. However, things changed after the introduction of mass schooling following the 1870 Education Act and Tilbury Fox was called upon in 1875 for advice on control and prevention by the government.[46] School attendance had revealed both the 'verminous condition' of many children and created 'nurseries of ringworm' as classroom and playgrounds were ideal for spreading infection.[47] Ringworm was one of a number of health problems that were taken up by medical officers of health, and later school medical officers.[48] The *Lancet* established a Commission on the Sanitary Condition of Our Public Schools, which released a report in 1875, calling for improvements in buildings, dietary and welfare, plus measures to control infectious diseases, especially scabies, scarlet fever and ringworm.[49] There was broad medical agreement that children with ringworm should be excluded from school, though there was disagreement on remedial action: some doctors recommended shaving the head and wearing a cap, others preferred the vigorous application of disinfectant ointments and lotions. When children who had been excluded could return was, in fact, more of an issue than when to exclude them.[50] Capped and shaved ringworm children represented popular fears of contagion, though doctors often played down the link with dirt and insanitary environments, claiming ringworm was simply a 'catching', germ disease. Indeed, Robert Liveing, a leading authority on dermatology, noted in 1879 that 'gutter children' tended to be exempt from infection, despite being filthy and unkempt. Why? Because they did not attend school, nor did they ever brush their hair, so they were never exposed to the germs.[51]

The leading medical authority on ringworm in the latter part of the nineteenth century was Herbert Alder Smith, who spent his whole career as a medical officer at Christ's Hospital School at Newgate in London.[52] His book, *Ringworm: its diagnosis and treatment*, went through four editions between 1880 and 1897.[53] Alder Smith took the view that ringworm was a local infection that had no impact on general health; hence, it should be treated locally, with general remedies only used as an adjunct. He only saw the bodily 'soil' in terms of age and diet, making the familiar point that the disease was rarely present after puberty and that children who disliked fat, along with those who were ill-nourished, seemed more vulnerable. He gained a readership in part because of his experience and in part because he offered a novel treatment. He claimed that he had identified 'nature's method of effecting a cure', a type of inflammation he termed 'kerion' which led to hair loss.[54] To produce a localised 'kerion' reaction artificially, he applied drops of croton oil, a widely used counter-irritant, to individual hair follicles to make them 'tender, swollen, red and infiltrated'; the aim was to produce 'a speedy and certain cure' by depilation.[55]

However, this was one was amongst hundreds, possibly thousands, of formulae that doctors prescribed for ringworm, with new treatments being regularly reported in medical journals.[56] On hairless parts of the body, such as the hands and face, ringworm was readily treatable, with school children finding ordinary writing ink very effective, probably because it contained, 'gallic acid and tannin (derived from vegetable galls), ferrous sulphate, mucilage, and haematoxylin (derived from logwood)'. However, ringworm on the scalp was often unmoveable, hence the attraction of shaving and chemical depilation. In addition to medical remedies, ringworm was included in the conditions cured by the huge number of proprietary or popular remedies sold by chemists and available from many sources. For example, advertised in the Manchester press in 1889 was the 'Health Restorer Ointment', which was said to be the 'Best, Safest and Speediest Cure in the World for Burns, Scalds, Ulcer, Chilblains, Itch, Ringworm, Scabbed Heads, Eczema, and all Skin

Diseases', whilst 'Old Doctor Townsend's blood purifying 'Old American Sarsaparilla' offered cleansing from within.[57] Londoners could try 'Cook's Antiseptic Soap', which had been endorsed in the *Lancet* in May 1888, and 'Grasshopper Ointment', which also cured 'Bad Legs, House-Maids Knee, Ulcerated Joints, Carbuncles, Poisoned Hands, Tumours, Cancers and Abscesses'.[58]

The main impact of germ ideas and practices was in public health, with a switch to policies that focused on individuals as carriers of pathogens and practices of disinfection, isolation and notification.[59] With regard to infectious diseases overall, this change particularly affected children, who were by far the majority of patients in the new isolation hospitals and whose health was targeted by school medical inspections.[60] A prominent example of the new concerns and approaches was in 1891, when the Poor Law North Surrey Board School in Anerley called in a top London dermatologist to advise on dealing with the large number of children with persistent ringworm.[61] Joseph Payne found 23 out of 45 children had been in isolation for over a year and five had suffered for over four years. He found no fault in the 'thorough, scientific and conscientious' response of the teachers, the medical officer or the managers.[62] He made recommendations, but the problem persisted. Two years later, in May 1893, the school turned to another London specialist, Dr Alfred Eddowes. He found 47 cases and, while agreeing that the medical officer was highly competent, he nevertheless recommended that he took overall control, as with ringworm 'detail' was all important.[63] He visited once a fortnight over four months, after which he claimed to have cured 25 children and improved the remainder; eventual eradication seemed inevitable.[64]

Policies for ringworm were developed along similar lines to diphtheria and scarlet fever, although it was much less serious, because of its impact on sufferers and their families. It became, quite literally, a social disease. Infected children were given special status and treatment because they seemed manifestly 'unclean' and stigmatised by other children and their families, and by neighbours. In addition, teachers and doctors expressed concerns about the consequences of exclusion for the individual, their family and the future mental fitness of the nation. Abraham and Eddowes explained the issues in 1894.

> Now that school attendance is compulsory and that the well-cared-for children of poor but respectable families often have to associate at school with those of the dirtiest and most careless classes of the community it is a moral duty that all reasonable precautions should be

> insisted on by the authorities in order to minimise the risk of infection from the diseased to the healthy. A skin disease also, contracted at school, may be taken home to the brothers and sisters.[65]

Malcolm Morris, a leading dermatologist and syphilologist, while unwavering on the need for the strict exclusion of affected children, called for a survey to determine the extent of the problem, suggesting that there should be special ringworm schools where excluded children could continue their education.[66]

Ringworm was targeted by London's Metropolitan Asylums Board (MAB) when, in 1897, it included specific measures in its plans for a variety of special institutions 'to eradicate the physical taints of pauperism and to place them on a fairer level of health for the race of life'.[67] Ringworm was included alongside contagious diseases of the eye, convalescence and open air treatment, mental defectives, the physically disabled, and 'young offenders'.[68] The first, and as it turned out, temporary special institution for ringworm was the Bridge School in Witham, Essex, started in 1901. It was replaced by the Downs Ringworm School (also known as Banstead Road School) in Sutton, Surrey, in February 1903. Here children were housed in blocks of 70 beds, attended lessons within the institution, and were treated by the daily bathing of their scalp, intensive applications of lotions and the extraction of diseased hairs.[69] In the first ten months, 618 children were admitted, of whom 208 were discharged, 153 'cured' and the remainder recalled by local Poor Law Guardians.[70]

Children sent to special schools were the exception; most children with ringworm were excluded from school and treated at home. Some doctors thought exclusion unnecessary and unproductive, as very few parents were able to keep infected children away from their siblings, or from playing with other children after school. Phineas Abraham, surgeon at the Hospital of the Skin at Blackfriars, London, argued in 1900 that when a child's head was 'kept greasy with germicidal ointments and always covered with a closely fitted cap', they should be allowed to attend school.[71] Everyone who wrote on the subject agreed that the ringworm caused more social than physical suffering. Infected children had no pain (other than from itching and the caustic lotions), no general illness, and there were no permanent effects on the skin or hair. Their suffering was 'exclusion from school and, to a great extent, banishment from society'.[72] Parents endured some degree of stigma and had to manage their child's isolation.[73] Also, while doctors accepted that all social classes were vulnerable and that 'dirt' as such was not a factor, ringworm was far less common amongst the well-to-do, because they were allegedly 'less ignorant and gave greater care to their offspring'.

Doctors' confidence in their ability to prevent and treat the condition grew as they increasingly believed that they knew their enemy.[74] The French dermatologist, Raimond Sabouraud, who had trained at the Institut Pasteur, was a leading doctor at the famous Hôpital Saint-Louis in Paris, and published major works on the biology of ringworm organisms. In 1886, the Saint-Louis had opened its 'L'ecole des teigneux', or 'ringworm school', colloquially known as a school for the scabby children. A decade later it opened 'le laboratoire municipal des teignes de la Ville de Paris'.[75] Sabouraud was the first director and his institution became famous for adapting bacteriological methods to working with fungi in the laboratory and for work on *les teignes* – 'ringworm'.[76] He identified three groups of causal organisms, promising closure to the uncertainty over whether there was one ringworm fungus or many, and the degree to which species were pleomorphic.[77] His publications were well received, but it was above all his demonstrations and displays at the 1896 International Congress of Dermatology in London that were decisive in enrolling others to his standpoints.[78] In 1897 Herbert Aldersmith (he changed his name from Alder Smith in the 1890s) wrote that Sabouraud's 'new views have completely revolutionised all older ones, and necessitated the separate description of the different forms of ringworm, and their microscopic appearances'.[79]

A key finding was distinguishing between ectothrix infections that affected the outside of the hair (e.g. *Microsporon* spp.) and endothrix ones that invaded the hair shaft (e.g. *Trichophyton* spp.) There was some dissent in Britain, notably from two leading London dermatologists, Thomas Colcott Fox and Frank Blaxall, of the Westminster Hospital, who maintained that *Trichophyton* and *Microsporon* were not in separate families, and from Leslie Roberts who emphasised physiological over morphological differences.[80] Nonetheless, Sabouraud's classification framed medical work on ringworm for the next decade, not least in epidemiological surveys of the incidence of the different organisms.[81] For example, a survey in 1903 found that over 90% of ringworm cases in London hospitals were due to *Microsporon audouinii* and *Microsporon canis*, the latter found in dogs, which compared with 60% in Metropolitan Asylums Board school children.[82] In Paris the main species were *M. audouinii* and *T. mentagrophytes*, the latter having a reservoir in dogs, cats and other animals.

Medical interest in ringworm in the United States was much less pronounced than in Britain.[83] The schooling system was more fragmented, being organised at state and local level across a vast area. While education was regarded as very important and widely available, compulsory schooling in all states arrived around 1900, three decades after Britain.[84] There was no dedicated American medical publication on ringworm until 1921, when John P. Turner's booklet *Ringworm and its successful treatment* was published.[85] Turner was a medical inspector of public schools in Philadelphia, though he wrote as a general practitioner recommending the application of simple chemicals and cleanliness. There were few articles in American medical journals on ringworm, though cases were discussed at dermatological meetings, along with scabies, pediculosis and impetigo, but as problems of individual hygiene rather than being associated with age or class. The main problem was with *M. canis*, perhaps reflecting the closeness of humans to pets and other animals, even in urban settings in America at this time.

However, medical and public responses to the related fungal disease of favus were quite different. By the turn of the century, favus had been linked to the fungus *Achorion schoenleinii* and had been found to be the most common skin infection amongst immigrants from Europe. Favus was characterised as a 'loathsome disease' and, after trachoma, a contagious eye infection, was the second largest cause of immigrants being rejected, or sent to isolation for treatment after inspections at Ellis Island.[86] Howard Markel has discussed why trachoma attracted so much attention given its low incidence and the same argument applies to favus; namely, that it was an easily recognised condition that was made a marker of the person being 'unclean' and hence 'unfit' for acceptance into the United States.[87] In American cities, school children with ringworm were sometimes excluded, but there were no special institutions as there were in Paris and London.[88]

'The X-ray Revolution'

In the 1900s, Raimond Sabouraud's reputation as the world's leading authority on ringworm was taken to a new level when he pioneered the X-ray treatment of infected scalps.[89] At this time, X-rays were one of the technological wonders of the age as 'skiagraphs' revealed the body's internal structure. They promised not just the transformation of medicine but also wider social and cultural progress.[90] Sabouraud's innovation, first reported in 1904, used X-rays not to kill fungi, but to produce depilation. The rationale was to remove the *nidus* of infection and allow germicides or fungicides easier penetration into hair follicles. As noted already, depilation was an accepted as an effective means of treating ringworm; indeed, Aldersmith had written in 1897 that,

> In fact, my chief experiments during the last few years have been an effort to discover something that will always cause disease hairs to fall out from patches of ringworm, for I fully believe that this troublesome disease will in time be cured by this method and not by the discovery of new parasiticides.[91]

However, attempts to achieve this by chemical and mechanical means had proved fraught with difficulties, not least because the inflammation and skin damage meant that the treatment was irritating and opened the skin to other infections.

The potential of X-rays for the treatment of skin diseases had been explored from the very beginning of their introduction into medicine in the mid-1890s. The ability to 'see' inside the body excited contemporaries and has interested historians, but in many hospitals their main use, along with the Finsen lamp, was for the topical treatment of skin diseases.[92] Around 1900, the potency of X-rays was double-edged: they could reveal the inner structure of the body and cure certain diseases, but they could also maim and kill if too high a dose was given. The most immediate and visible damage caused by X-rays was to the skin. Indeed, it was this experience that led doctors to explore their use as counter-irritants, germicides and fungicides. However, experimental studies quickly showed that X-rays did not readily destroy bacteria or fungi. Hair loss was noticed after incidental exposures and X-rays were said to have cosmetic as well as medical possibilities. Indeed, a report in the *Lancet* even suggested that exposure to X-rays might be a more convenient method of removing a beard than conventional shaving![93] The systematic application of X-rays for depilation was first reported in 1897 by Leopold Freund, who worked at the Medizinische Universität Wien.[94] He used X-rays for cosmetic procedures, removing surplus hair and unsightly features, such as hairy moles. The problem with such work was controlling the dose received by the patient. If the dose was too large, it could lead to permanent hair loss and skin damage. There is no evidence of similar experimentation amongst British and American dermatologists; however, they did keep up with the new applications developed by doctors in continental Europe.

Freund and Schiff in Vienna were probably the first to try X-rays to treat ringworm cases, but the treatment was, and still is, identified with Sabouraud.[95] He had recognised the therapeutic value of depilation and had tried thallium acetate, otherwise used as a rat poison, but this produced severe side-effects. X-ray depilation, therefore, promised to be safer. Sabouraud's key innovations, which he developed in collaboration with Henri Noiré and Maurice Pignot, were methods and materials to control the dosage of X-rays received by patients, which were lower than with skiagraphs.[96] His first invention was a generator with controllable output that allowed variation in the intensity of X-rays emitted; the second was developing a chemical that changed colour on exposure to X-rays in a graded way that enabled monitoring of the dose a patient received.[97] The latter was crucial to avoid X-ray burns.

The X-ray therapy developed by Sabouraud was cumbersome. It required the patient to remain very still for up to 40 minutes, which was difficult to achieve with children, and much more so if many sessions (the contemporary term was 'séances') were required. Sabouraud claimed that five sessions on different parts of the scalp were safe; most doctors concurred, though one British doctor wrote that this was 'criminal'.[98] With large areas of infection there were two problems: first, the convex form of the skull meant that it was difficult to ensure even exposure; and second, it was imperative to avoid overlapping exposures that would produce burns or permanent baldness. The clinical picture reported by Sabouraud was that X-rays produced reddening of the skin and hair loss in 12–14 days.[99] He wrote that once the fungi had been carried away with the hair, the doctor's task was to ensure that the treated areas did not become re-infected, which meant instructing patients on the conscientious and thorough application of fungicidal lotions. Hair started to re-grow after six to eight weeks, but did so only slowly, allowing for the long-term application of fungicidals (Figures 1.1 and 1.2).

Despite the laborious procedure, X-rays had two advantages when judged against fungicides alone and other treatments: they brought treatment times down from years to months and produced permanent cures.[100] Sabouraud reported a 100% increase in his cure rates, including many that had previously been intractable; and all this reduced costs eightfold, from 2,000 to 260 francs per patient.

In Britain, X-ray treatment was taken up in the outpatient departments of voluntary hospitals and in some of the new radiotherapy clinics. The first, very positive results were published in 1905.[101] The leading dermatologist, Malcolm Morris, confidently claimed that X-rays would mark, the beginning of a new era in the treatment of an affection which has previously been one of the stumbling blocks of medical practice. It was fitting that we should owe the means of easy victory over a peculiarly rebellious disease to the distinguished man [Sabouraud] who has done so much to dissipate the darkness in which till lately its origin was enshrouded.[102]

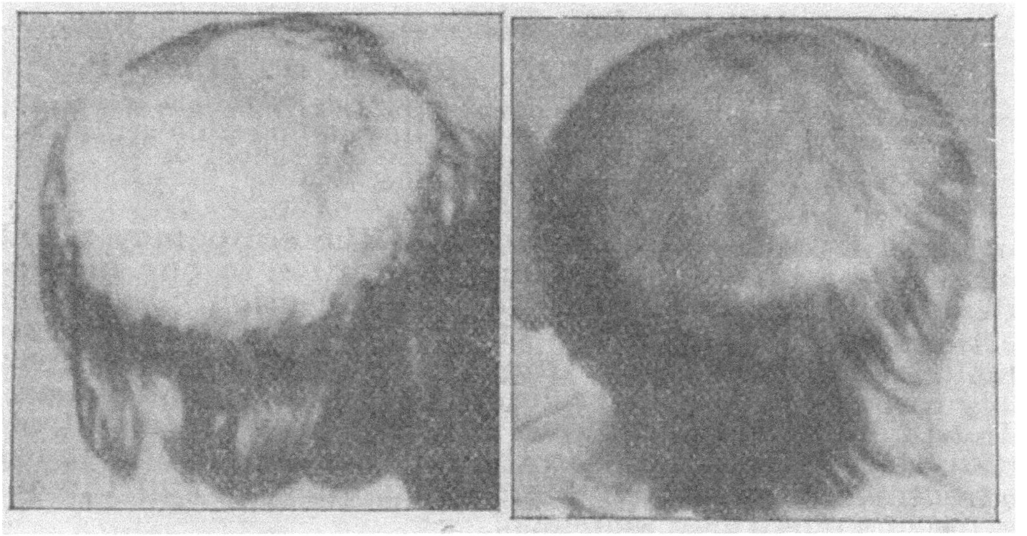

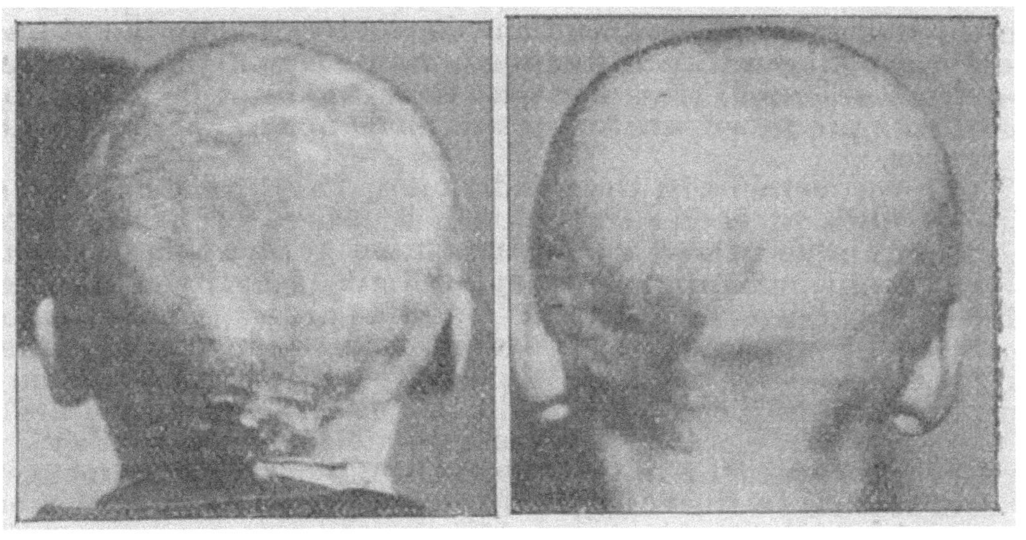

Figures 1.1 and 1.2 Photographs of X-ray depilation treatment of ringworm of the scalp.[103] *British Medical Journal*, 1905, ii: 14.

The number of published reports of success grew. These were typically of a small number of cases, with doctors cautioning that time was needed to assess whether the cures were permanent. John MacLeod, physician at Charing Cross Hospital and the Victoria Hospital for Children, did not regard X-rays as a panacea.

> It is a treatment, however, which is by no means easy; first there are the difficulties of the technique, second there is the all-important local treatment with the parasiticide remedies, and, third, there is the care which is requisite to avoid mishaps.... The immediate dangers of the treatment... can, as a rule, be avoided, but with regard to the ultimate dangers, if there be any, sufficient time has not yet elapsed to disclose them. It has been suggested that the exposure of the scalp to the rays might have some harmful effect on the underlying brain. Certainly in an infant or a child under 3 years of age, where the scalp is thin and the fontanelles have not closed, one would be timid about submitting the scalp to the X-rays, but with regard to older children no misfortune of that nature has, as far as we are aware, been recorded.[104]

In fact, British dermatologists struggled to obtain results as good as those reported by Sabouraud; yet, even a 50% cure rate was regarded as outstanding compared to other methods.[105] Better results were anticipated once doctors developed mastery of the equipment and pastilles, and when patient compliance could be improved[106] (see Figure 1.3).

The first systematic use of X-ray treatment in Britain was at the ringworm schools of the MAB; indeed, their success reportedly improved turnover so much that the Bridge School at Witham closed in 1908, saving £500 per year, when the remaining children were transferred to the Downs School.[107] Treatment there was directed by Thomas Colcott Fox, with day-to-day matters in the hands of the school's medical officer Dr Sale. Within a year they reported 400 cures.[108] The doctors enjoyed access to a large number of cases and developed facilities for treating many children at once (see Figure 1.4). They were treating pauper children, who were in triple isolation: in a special institution, within the Poor Law, and away from parents, hence, there were no problems with consent, and compliance with young children was largely a matter of discipline. Colcott Fox and Sale conducted a large 'trial', but as was typical for the time there were no controls. Unsurprisingly, when they published their results there was no discussion of the ethics of this 'trial', only wonder at its success.[109] Indeed, the London County

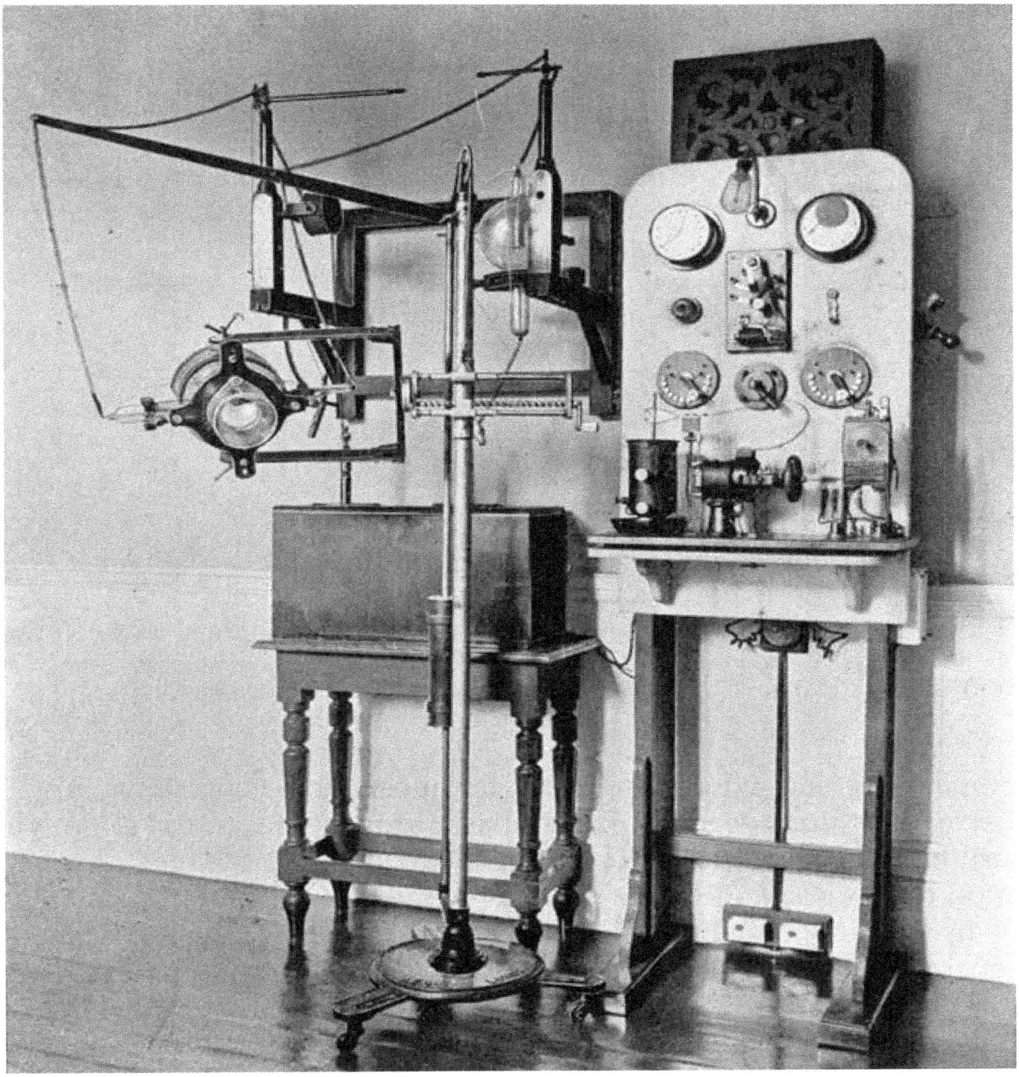

Figure 1.3 X-ray apparatus. Suitable for treatment of ringworm and other cutaneous affections.[110] This figure © 2013 Wellcome Images is used under Creative Commons Attribution – Non-commercial

Council's Board of Education was so impressed that in 1907 it considered a scheme to provide free X-ray treatment for the capital's children at hospitals and special centres.

The Board's scheme was to be part of a larger plan of school medical inspection and treatment for pupils in elementary schools, that aimed to deal with a range of health problems: bad teeth, poor vision,

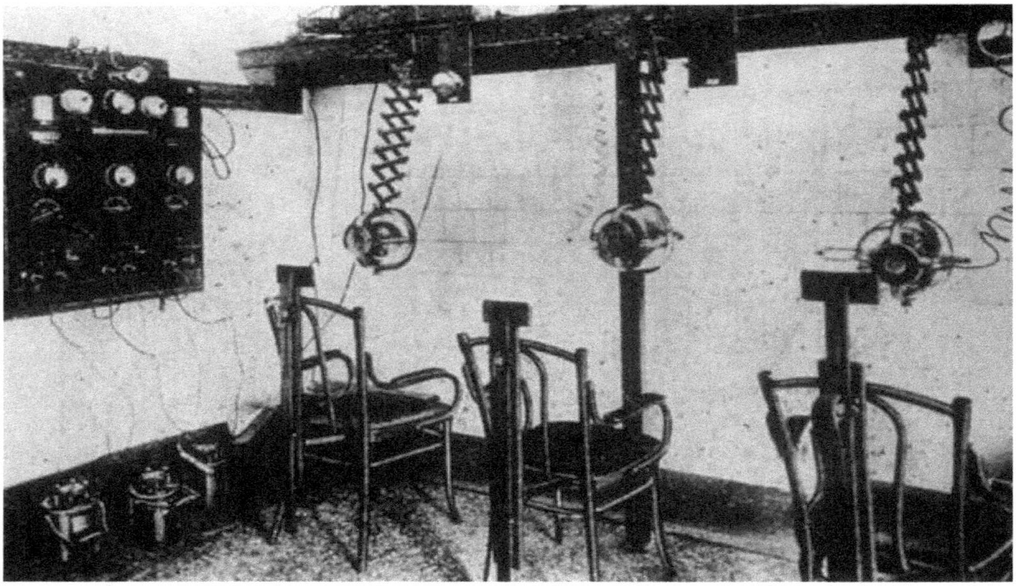

Figure 1.4 Radiotherapy room for ringworm. 1905. This figure is used courtesy of The Royal London Hospital Archives, Wellcome Images, 'This image is used under Creative Commons Attribution-NonCommercial-NoDerivs

suppurating ears and adenoids, tuberculosis and general debility.[111] These 'conditions' were seen as threats at three levels: to the long-term health and educational development of the child; to the efficient operation of schools; and to the progress of the race. Ringworm was taken up by the school medical service because they saw it being neglected by general practitioners, hospitals, public health authorities and parents. Proposals were considered in 1908 by a sub-Committee of the London County Council (LCC), which had replaced the MAB, which recommended that school clinics deal only with teeth defects, eye defects, skin diseases ('chiefly parasitic, such as, ringworm, scabies, pediculosis & c.') and ear defects.[112] In 1909, this became policy and because of the anticipated high demand, ringworm treatment was contracted out to London voluntary hospitals, with children compelled to attend if ringworm was identified at school medical inspections.[113] Other cities and large towns introduced similar schemes while outside of urban areas, where there were fewer or less well-resourced voluntary hospitals, older treatment regimes persisted.[114]

The official endorsement of X-ray treatment brought prompt criticism. Dr Dawson Turner, who worked in the Electrical Department at the

Edinburgh Royal Infirmary and described himself as an 'old worker with X-rays', who had suffered permanent injury from exposures, wrote to the *Times* in March 1909, with what turned out to be a prescient caution.

> The deleterious effects of continuous exposures to X-rays in the case of adults are only too well known to X-ray operators and it is probable that delicate cells of the growing brain of a child may be injuriously affected by much short exposures, though the evidence of impairment of function may not become noticeable until development is complete. No helpless child should have the chief centre of its nervous system exposed to the X-rays without the express consent of its parent, obtained after the possible risks of the treatment have been fully explained.[115]

His plea was answered in a report by two directors of London hospital electro-therapeutic departments. They stated that ordinary precautions had ensured no ill effects in their patients, nor did they expect any from other controlled uses of X-rays.[116] However, the use of X-rays was resisted by some parents, though this was as much about distrust of hospitals and dislike of compulsion, as it was about worries over radiation. Mr Harris, a jeweller from Rotherhithe, on being instructed to take his daughter to Guy's Hospital, wrote back to the LCC's Child Care Branch stating he did not have 'much faith in those places' and that his wife, who was a trained nurse, was treating the child.[117] Walter Longley asserted his independence in similar vein, saying that his boys were already being treated with sassafras oil and that his family would not trouble the LCC, nor the London ratepayer.[118] Henry Carter wrote that the instruction to take his children to the Evelina Hospital was 'insulting to my wife and self'.[119]

Armed with X-rays and with the backing of the LCC administration, dermatologists and school medical offices were optimistic about the future control of ringworm.[120] Nonetheless, in 1909, the *Lancet* set up an enquiry to address 'the grave prevalence' and 'the disastrous influence' ringworm was having on the education of children.[121] The *Lancet* Commission on Ringworm, consisting of 'two thoroughly competent dermatologists' (who remained anonymous), reported on 1 January 1910. They dealt almost exclusively with the situation in London.[122] The authors opened in eugenic terms, stating that ringworm was more prevalent in the 'less educated classes' and that those affected were 'really representatives of lower grades of civilisation', where infestation with internal and external parasites was a marker of being left behind by social progress. The authors endorsed X-ray treatment administered by dermatologists and radiotherapists, along with a positive assessment of the capacity of existing facilities to cope with the scheme of mass treatment that the LCC was contemplating. However, they were ambivalent about whether to use voluntary and local authority hospitals, or to recommend the creation of special treatment centres, but whatever was decided they were certain it would be cost-effective.

The Commission's report took seriously public concerns about the safety of X-rays, noting that in early years there had been accidents leading to permanent baldness and ulcers. However, burns were said to be a thing of the past as exposures were now well managed. With regard to brain damage, the authors wrote that the experience of thousands of cases, over many years, showed no evidence of any effects and that 'It is incumbent now on those who imagine that harm does follow the application of X-rays to produce the grounds for the view.'[123] Against this backdrop, many parents allowed their children to be treated with X-rays but, as mentioned above, others refused. The manufacturers of popular alternatives, especially antiseptic creams like 'Germolene' and 'Zambuk' – 'The Balm that Benefits the Bairns', also offered their products as direct alternatives to X-rays.[124] However, some medical officers raised the stakes. For example, Dr Bostock Hill, the Medical Officer of Health for Warwickshire, claimed in 1911 that he instructed parents that 'they would be dealt with under the Children's Act for cruelty . . . or the case would be referred to the N.S.P.C.C' [National Society for the Protection of Children], if they refused to allow their children to be treated.[125]

Ernest Dore, a dermatologist at the Evelina Hospital for Sick Children, made a telling observation in his review of X-ray treatment in 1911, a year after the publication of the *Lancet* Commission report.[126] He returned to the issue of stigma, arguing that before X-ray treatments a diagnosis of ringworm was far worse than any physical suffering.

> A trivial complaint as regards the health of the child, tinea tonsurans brings in its train so long a category of ills that I have more than once heard long-suffering mothers say that they dreaded scarlet fever or pneumonia less. The disorganisation of the home that ensues from the isolation of the sufferers; the anxiety of the parents lest other children in the family should become infected; the complications with medical men and schoolmasters; the social ostracism; the loss of schooling; the wearisome process of constantly rubbing on

> ointments with little apparent result except the production of sore heads in the children and sore hearts in the parents, these are some of the difficulties which have to be faced under the old *régime*.[127]

Given the reactions of children, family, friends, neighbours, teachers and doctors to ringworm, and its position as a marker of 'low civilisation' and social danger, it is clear why a disease that never killed or caused permanent injury attracted such high-profile medical and public attention. Indeed, Dore wanted to up the stakes further, hinting at the possibility of stamping out the disease if compulsion was used: either in prevention, 'such as the wearing of some kind of head gear, like the muzzle in the prophylaxis of rabies', or with X-ray treatment.

A national picture of ringworm in school children was represented in the Reports of the Medical Officer to the Board of Education, Dr George Newman; the first of which was for 1908.[128] The prevalence of ringworm was around 1% amongst children inspected in school, much lower than other 'defects', which were: vision (10%), hearing (3–5%), adenoids and enlarged tonsils (6–8%), tooth decay (40%) and unclean bodies or heads (30–40%).[129] The main issue with ringworm was exclusion and its effects on a child's education; plus, from an administrative perspective, the impact of long absences on a school's grant income. Although prevalence was low, it still meant that, on average, 3,000 children were absent every day, with a typical absence duration of nine weeks.[130] Nationally, the longest average exclusion reported of 29 weeks was in Somerset. This finding was seen as surprising for a rural county with few large towns and low population density, and was attributed to poor inspection regimes causing early cases to be missed. Although impetigo, by this time associated with *Staphylococcus aureus* infection, was the most prevalent skin disease found in inspections, ringworm was taken much more seriously.[131] Dr Ritchie, the School Medical Officer for Manchester, reported that inspections in 1913 had revealed the following: impetigo – 353, ringworm – 187, scabies – 39 and other skin diseases – 110.[132] However, cases reported by doctors and parents led to 2,003 notifications of ringworm in the city, with up to 1,500 children under supervision at any time. The Manchester containment regime was strict, '... no cases of ringworm of the scalp are allowed to attend school unless the hair over and around the patches is cut and a washable cap worn.... Children affected with ringworm of the body are not allowed to attend school.'[133] In the same year, a ringworm school was established in Edinburgh for long-term absentees, including one boy who allegedly had been excluded for four years.[134]

In his annual reports, Newman began to report improvements, particularly in areas where X-ray treatment was available. In London, new cases fell from 5,573 in 1913 to 4,449 a year later, while in Beckenham in Kent, new cases had fallen from 133 in 1911 to just 48 in 1914.[135] However, nationally, the provision of special services was patchy. Only one third of education authorities had made special provision for ringworm treatment and in many areas, especially outside of cities and large towns, there was still no access to X-ray treatment at all. In addition, many general practitioners chose to continue to recommend topical fungicides and left treatment to 'unreliable' parents.[136]

The decline of ringworm

In Britain, doctors reported that the incidence of ringworm of the scalp in school children fell during the First World War, but increased afterwards because of the shortage of school nurses, many of whom continued to work with casualties and invalids.[137] However, this was a minor peak as the incidence fell steadily over the inter-war period. In London, the number of new cases had reduced from 6,214 in 1911, to 3,983 in 1920. The number dropped further, to 513 in 1930 and by 1936 they was just 89.[138] As early as 1925, the district medical officer for Beckenham reported no new cases, while in Ilford, ringworm was also said to have been 'abolished'.[139] In his 26th and final report, for the year 1933, George Newman observed with satisfaction that 'Ringworm is steadily disappearing.'[140] This situation was reflected in treatment facilities, the number of which was reduced from 150 clinics in 1923 to 80 in 1938. The London ringworm school, which had moved to the Goldie Leigh Cottage Children's Homes, Woolwich, in 1914, took fewer and fewer residential cases, and became instead a centre for day treatment with X-rays.[141]

Doctors attributed the decline in the reported incidence of ringworm, in the words of Norman Walker in 1929, not so much to the character of the infection, but to 'the value of cooperation between the scientist, the clinician, and the organiser'.[142] Success was said to have come from school inspection spotting early cases, which were followed up by effective treatments such as X-rays. The provision and use of X-rays was variable across the country. In the early 1930s only 20% of diagnosed cases in England were receiving X-rays. The rates of use varied: London was the highest and rural counties were several times lower[143] (Table 1.1).

Table 1.1 Cases of ringworm in England and Wales treated by X-ray or other methods, 1933

England	By X-rays	Otherwise	X-ray treatment as percentage of total
Counties	149	2058	6.8
County boroughs	540	2040	20.9
Boroughs	120	597	16.7
Urban districts	22	90	19.6
London	160	18	89.9
Wales			
Counties	20	88	18.5
County boroughs	52	19	73.2
Boroughs	0	24	0.0
Urban districts	7	29	19.4

Chemical and mechanical methods of depilation continued to be used and there was particular interest again in the 1930s in giving thallium acetate.[144] Some doctors, particularly in the United States, argued that thallium treatment was safer than X-rays; however, critics termed it 'A Dangerous Drug' because the margin between achieving effective epilation and poisoning was very small.[145] During the inter-war period, dermatologists on both sides of the Atlantic showed less interest in ringworm of the scalp, reflecting lower incidence and relatively stable therapeutic regimes.[146] Their new areas of interest were ringworm in athletes, college students, soldiers and miners.

Ringworm, although no doubt a common human infection for centuries, only gained serious medical and public attention in the second half of the nineteenth century, and then in a specific social group and setting: school children and schooling. The aggregation of children in crowded classrooms for hours at a time seemed to provide ideal conditions for contagion. None the less, it was as a social rather than physical disease that ringworm gained medical and public attention. Ringworm epidemics were one of the unintended consequences of the progressive reform of mass schooling, which revealed changing social attitudes to markers of disease and the growing stigmatisation of the palpably 'unclean'. While historians such as Nancy Tomes have detailed public responses to the threat of invisible germs, we have revealed the reactions, some similar and others unique, to conditions where the germs were highly visible. Perhaps, the 'gospel of germs' won converts more readily for diseases such as ringworm, favus and trachoma, where the physical and social manifestations of infection were obvious and reinforcing.

From 1905, ringworm was also seen as a pathology that could be remedied by medical progress, and not just any new technology, but by the medical icon of the age, X-rays. The use of X-ray depilation was an innovation that was taken up rapidly, in large measure because it promised so much, but also because the necessary equipment was becoming more readily available and there were opportunities for clinical and organisational innovations. In Britain, major public bodies such as the LCC, having been persuaded to create special ringworm institutions, subsequently invested in the new technologies of treatment. This all seemed to pay off, as the reported incidence of ringworm of the scalp in children declined rapidly in the inter-war period.[147] There was debate about the causes of the fall. Was it due to medical inspection regimes and new treatments, or to social factors, such as more bathrooms, better medicated shampoos, the fashion for shorter hair and grooming with hair creams? 'Brylcreem' was introduced in 1928 and marketed for better 'bounce' in styling and control of dandruff, then said to be caused by a yeast fungus *Pityrosporon*. Whatever the specific reasons, all factors responsible for the decline were seen by contemporary commentators to be due to medical and social progress.

2

Hygiene, Fitness and Athlete's Foot

In May 1939, a review of the American yearbook of dermatology and syphilology observed:

> As usual they make a prominent feature of an introductory article on some branch of therapeutics, and this year they deal with the treatment of the deeper fungous infections of the skin, including ringworm of the scalp and bearded regions, and the comparatively rare fungous affections of the subcutaneous tissues. As a matter of fact this subject is not of great practical importance in the British Isles, especially in England, where the incidence of ringworm of the scalp has been reduced to quite a trivial number of cases per annum, and ringworm of the beard has become an actual rarity. No doubt the state of affairs is otherwise in the United States, where the standard of living, both among the large negro population and also to a lesser extent among the more recent immigrants from Central Europe, is such that these infections are much commoner; moreover, a considerable area of the U.S.A. boasts a subtropical climate in which parasitic fungi are far more active than in the temperate zones.[1]

While this statement rightly reflects on improvements in Britain, its perception of ringworm in the United States was wrong. Across the Atlantic, it was not a problem amongst immigrants and African Americans; rather it had been framed as a public health menace in the affluent classes, especially amongst those who frequented swimming pools, and college students and, of course, athletes. While its prevalence had seemingly shifted up the social scale and from children to adults, its principal site of infection had moved too, from head to toe, with 'athlete's foot' being one of the most common and most talked about diseases in America in the 1930s.[2]

Manufacturers of popular remedies gave ringworm of the foot the name 'athlete's foot' and this was adopted by the public, but in medicine the infection was known as tinea pedis. It was seen as new disease, or in modern parlance an emerging infection, having been first described by Arthur Whitfield, a dermatologist at King's College Hospital, London in 1908.[3] Nonetheless, it was in the United States that tinea pedis became an epidemic, seemingly spread by modern lifestyles and hygiene practices, and encouraged by modern socks and shoes, which made infection liable to chronicity by keeping the feet moist and warm. It is perhaps surprising, given the unhygienic conditions of previous centuries and the ubiquity of ringworm of the scalp, that the feet of Europeans and Americans had been seemingly free of ringworm infection until the mid-twentieth century. Nonetheless, there was a clear understanding in the inter-war years that tinea pedis was new disease and one linked to modernity. One consequence of the growth of medical attention to tinea pedis was the stimulus it gave to the specialism of medical mycology, with investment in diagnostic services, research on the conditions in which mycoses spread and their treatment. In turn, this led to the creation of a cadre of medical mycologists, who identified more fungal infections in specific social groups and the general population.

We begin this chapter with a discussion of the development of medical mycology, especially in the United States, which led the world in the creation of centres of expertise, training and research. We then discuss the movement of medical and public concern about ringworm from children's heads to athlete's toes. In the 1940s, the condition was also recognised as a problem amongst soldiers and miners, and was seen in terms of greater exposure to new pathogenic species of fungi and the increased vulnerability of the human soil in tropical and specific work conditions. While orthodox medicine approached tinea pedis as something that was difficult to treat and needed to be prevented, proprietary medicine companies peddled remedies that filled the therapeutic vacuum with numerous 'certain cures'. We follow the controversies around popular and medical treatments, and the emergence in the late 1950s of medically approved, clinically trialled antifungal drugs, modelled on the antibiotics developed for bacterial infections. The most important of these was griseofulvin, which promised to be effective and safe with topical and oral administration. This was followed in the 1970s with a range of azole drugs. These antifungals accelerated the disappearance of athlete's foot as a medical, if not public term, thereby divorcing ringworm from its locus of infection or site of contagion, making it a type of dermatophytosis, literally, skin fungal infection.

Medical mycology: 'An Orphan Science'[4]

Glenn S. Bulmer has recently characterised the manner in which work on human fungal diseases developed in the inter-war period as the result of the movement and coalescence of specialists: 'botany types came forth and usually joined Departments of Microbiology &/or Immunology – two subjects that most had never taken in school'.[5] He may have had in mind the founders of the first specialist medical mycology laboratory in the United States, which opened in 1926 at the Columbia-Presbyterian Medical Center (C-PMC). One leading light was the botanist was Bernard O. Dodge, who then worked at the New York Botanical Gardens.[6] He was known for his work on genetics and for introducing T. H. Morgan to *Neurospora*, an organism that became a widely used experimental model in genetics.[7] Dodge was interested in fungal diseases in humans and animals, and between 1928 and 1939 he was a consultant in mycology at the C-PMC, while at the same time lecturing on dermatology at the College of Physicians and Surgeons. The other founder as a clinician, the dermatologist J. Gardner Hopkins, who worked at the C-PMC's Vanderbilt Clinic; previously he had worked on a cure for the plague with Hans Zinsser in Serbia during the First World War.[8] Indeed, his research spanned infectious diseases, especially syphilis and moniliasis. In the 1920s and 1930s it was mainly 'botany types', with the ability to identify types of fungi, who dominated the new field, which was principally concerned with diagnosis, requiring microscopy and culturing skills, combined with taxonomy. In 1926, Hopkins hired Rhoda W. Benham – a botanist by training – to undertake mycological diagnoses, and went on to develop a research laboratory from this base.[9] His initiative was aided by a grant of $50,000 from the Rockefeller Foundation in 1929, which eventually enabled Columbia to develop the first specialist training in human fungal diseases in 1935.

Hopkins's laboratory became an influential research centre, producing key figures such as Chester W. Emmons (1900–1985), the first medical mycologist employed by the National Institutes of Health (NIH) in Bethesda.[10] Emmons took his PhD with Robert A. Harper in the Botany Department at Columbia on the subject of mildew, before working with Dodge and publishing two articles on dermatophytes in *Archives of Dermatology and Syphilis*. Neither author was medically qualified. Emmons stated later that when he sought a reference to move to Hopkins's laboratory, Harper had asked, 'Why do you want to study those abortive and uninteresting medical fungi?'[11] Indeed, Emmons referred to medical mycology as 'an orphan science' as it was never taught by mycologists, whose main interest, outside of taxonomy, reproduction and other purely biological matters, was in plant pathology. In his first medical publications, Emmons proposed redefining the genera of the main fungal causes of skin infection: *Microsporum*, *Trichophyton* and *Epidermophyton*. His approach was to use their morphologies, rather than their pathological effects, pioneering what became the preferred method of standardising diagnoses and avoiding the variability and inconsistency of clinical criteria.[12] Emmons then worked with Arturo Carrión in Puerto Rica on chromoblastomycosis, publishing in the *Puerto Rico Journal of Public Health and Tropical Medicine*. In the event, the move to fungal diseases turned out well, as his appointment at NIH was as principal mycologist. He stayed for 30 years, becoming recognised as one of 'founding fathers' of medical mycology in the United States.

The first monograph in the field was Harry Jacobson's *Fungous Diseases: A Clinico-Mycology Text* published in 1932. The author was a dermatologist in Los Angeles and he presented ten chapters on 'dermomycoses, moniliasis, maduromycoses, sporotrichoses, blastomycoses, actinomycoses, coccidioides, toruloses and aspergilloses'.[13] A review in *Archives of Dermatology* concluded that the book was 'useful' and, perhaps surprisingly, observed that 'the mycologic aspects of the subject are better handled than the clinical aspects'. The second monograph was published from Harvard, where there had been instruction since 1924, and it was this course that was written up in 1935 by Carroll W. Dodge, a botanist who was no relation of Bernard O. Dodge.[14] The book was compiled at the suggestion of Roland Thaxter, who was medically trained, but had switched to botany, eventually becoming professor of cryptogamic botany at Harvard. Carroll Dodge's *Medical Mycology: Fungous Diseases of Man and Other Animals* was the first use of 'medical mycology' in a book title. Here, and in later works, the primary focus was on fungi and their identification, with little on the pathology of the infections they caused. Before publication, Dodge had moved to become professor of botany at Washington University and continued to research fungal diseases in Central America, before moving to Lichenology after 1950.

Writing the *New England Journal of Medicine* in August 1936, Jacob H. Swartz, of the Department of Cryptogamic Botany at Harvard University, maintained that,

> Mycology is no longer a mysterious subject known only to a few. It has been proved to be a part of medicine just as bacteriology, physiology and so forth. Some knowledge of mycology is necessary for a better understanding of disease.[15]

He was contributing to a discussion on fungi and internal medicine, where the focus was not on skin diseases, but on systemic infections and allergy, with an emphasis on the importance of predisposition – the human soil – as a factor with infection. Many contributors stressed the role of the laboratory in confirming clinical diagnoses; though Swartz worried that since the 'mystery' of fungi had been largely solved, clinicians were no longer turning to the laboratory and were relying solely on clinical signs. The 'orphan science' had been adopted by doctors, but it was not being nurtured. Swartz closed the discussion demanding the creation of a mycological department in every medical school and hospital, stating that 'Mycology at present is in chaos' and calling for the field to be 'simplified and made useful to all branches of medicine'.[16] Arthur Greenwood, a dermatologist at Massachusetts General Hospital, suggested the way forward was to create more people trained to work between clinicians and mycologists.[17] One factor fuelling the demand for more medical mycologists, reflected in the discussion prompted by Swartz, was recognition of geographically localised foci of fungal disease, which we examine in Chapter 4. Meanwhile, athlete's foot or tinea pedis was emerging as a dominate concern for dermatologists and nascent medical mycologists.

Athlete's foot

Infection in areas other than the scalp came to the fore in the First World War, when ringworm of the groin ('dhobi itch') was found to be prevalent amongst American and British troops in France.[18] Some doctors thought that damp and crowded conditions of the Western Front increased susceptibility and were ideal for contagion; others believed a new fungus had been brought to Europe and the Americas by troops returning from the tropics.[19] The bacteriological facilities available to the military medical services meant that specific pathogens were identified, using the methods developed by Sabouraud in the 1900s. Most cases were of *Trichophyton interdigitalis*, but there were increasing reports of *Trichophyton rubrum*, though at this time there was little interest in the epidemiology of types of infection.[20] Rather, discussion focused on the observation that, paradoxically, tinea pedis was a disease of hygiene. In the British military, the highest rates of infection were found amongst officers, who through bathing regularly opened themselves to infection through contact and softening of the skin. Also, tightly laced, ankle-high army boots, worn in hot, damp environments, for long periods without changes of socks, were understood to provide ideal conditions for tinea pedis to flourish.[21]

In the United States too, ringworm of the feet was 'discovered' as a malady of soldiers in the First World War. Two West Coast American doctors, Oliver Ormsby and James Mitchell, put ringworm of the feet on the medical map in the United States in 1916, in an article on infection of the hands and feet.[22] The alleged first use of the term 'athlete's foot' was in December 1928, in an article in the *Literary Digest*, prompted by reports from Dr Charles F. Pabst, of Greenpoint Hospital Brooklyn.[23] Pabst claimed that the condition was already well-known in the United States, with an estimated ten million sufferers, three quarters of whom were unaware of the infection. The article stated that the problem was of recent origin, but that 'at least half the adult population suffer from this malady at some time'. However, the term athlete's foot took hold, not as a disease of the masses, but one of the America's affluent classes, who could now afford to enjoy leisure activities and modern hygiene facilities. Pabst, perhaps revealing his limited social circle and awareness, claimed that 'almost everyone who uses a swimming-pool, golf club, athletic club, or any place where there is a common dressing room, has the infection on his feet'.[24] Further medical recognition came in May 1929, when three doctors, working at the University of California student health service, published data that showed tinea pedis was endemic amongst students.[25] They wrote that many students arrived at college with the infection: 53% of males and 15% of females, and the incidence rose to 85% in those final year students who took gymnasium classes. In a follow up study, the doctors showed at the end of their first year, the incidence amongst freshmen had risen from 53% to 78%, but was only 2% higher in female students.[26] The sex differences suggested to contemporaries four factors in the emergence of tinea pedis: the new male enthusiasm for using gymnasia, swimming baths and other sports facilities; the poor facilities for changing and showering at these locations; male indifference to personal hygiene; and the types of socks and shoes worn for sport and after, where the lighter, open shoes of women militated against infection taking hold. Athlete's foot was also possibly a consequence of public sanitary facilities, where the sexes, social classes, races and different ages mingled, and where anyone might be a 'carrier'.

Awareness of the problem grew quickly. The link between tinea pedis and athletes was evident in 1931 when the *Los Angeles Times* termed it the 'gymnasium malady'.[27] In the same year, W. L. Gould, a physician from Albany, New York State, reported to the United States Public Health Service that possibly 50% of all adults suffered from tinea pedis and that its incidence was particularly high in the states bordering the

Gulf of Mexico and in California, due to heat and humidity.[28] At the 1932 Olympic Games in Los Angeles, special antiseptic footbaths were provided to prevent infection.[29] By the mid-1930s there was recognition that it was not just students and athletes who were vulnerable. J. H. Swartz wrote of 'the addiction of our generation to the frequenting of gymnasiums (*sic*), baths and locker rooms . . . and the tendency to exercise violently and perspiring in unsterilizable socks and body clothing'. He went on to wonder if the Romans were similarly affected?[30] Dermatologists also saw tinea pedis as threat to the family, through cross-infection in the home, where baths and showers were becoming more common.[31] However, Ayu Majima has shown that ringworm amongst the poor – even tinea pedis – was never described with the neologism of athlete's foot and sufferers remained stigmatised.[32]

Doctors prescribed a variety of remedies for tinea pedis, but because of mixed results, their advice was mainly that prevention was better than cure. Thus, anyone visiting a swimming baths and showering in public facilities was told to disinfect their feet where possible, to avoid walking on floors in bare feet, to dry their feet and toes after bathing, never to share towels or clothing, and to wash socks at high temperatures. The main remedies were topical antifungal creams. The standbys were Whitfield's ointment (the active ingredients were 5% salicylic acid and 3% benzoic acid in petroleum jelly) and Castellani's carbol-fuchsin paint. However, the variable presentation of the condition and its tendency to chronicity encouraged innovations, both in combinations of remedies and new chemicals.[33] There were many complaints of overtreatment.[34] Proprietary medical companies, which already had a significance market with topical antiseptic remedies, seized on the new epidemic, producing new products and rebranding older ones as having antifungal as well as antibacterial properties.[35] The most prominently advertised remedy in newspapers and magazines was a derivative of a veterinary liniment – 'Absorbine Jr.', marketed by W. F. Young, Inc.[36] The company claimed to have coined the term athlete's foot and in the late 1930s, the advertisements for Absorbine Jr. echoed public posters against venereal disease and referred to earlier fears, from the time of Typhoid Mary, to unrecognised carriers (see Figure 2.1).

Older products for 'skin disorders of the feet', such as Dr Scholl's 'Solvex', were rebranded to target the new consumers, thus, its advertisement claimed it was effective against 'gym or athlete's foot', 'foot itch' and 'golfer's itch'.[37] While doctors promoted the possibilities of prevention and commercial drug companies sold 'sure-cure remedies', there was also a sense that the high prevalence of tinea pedis meant

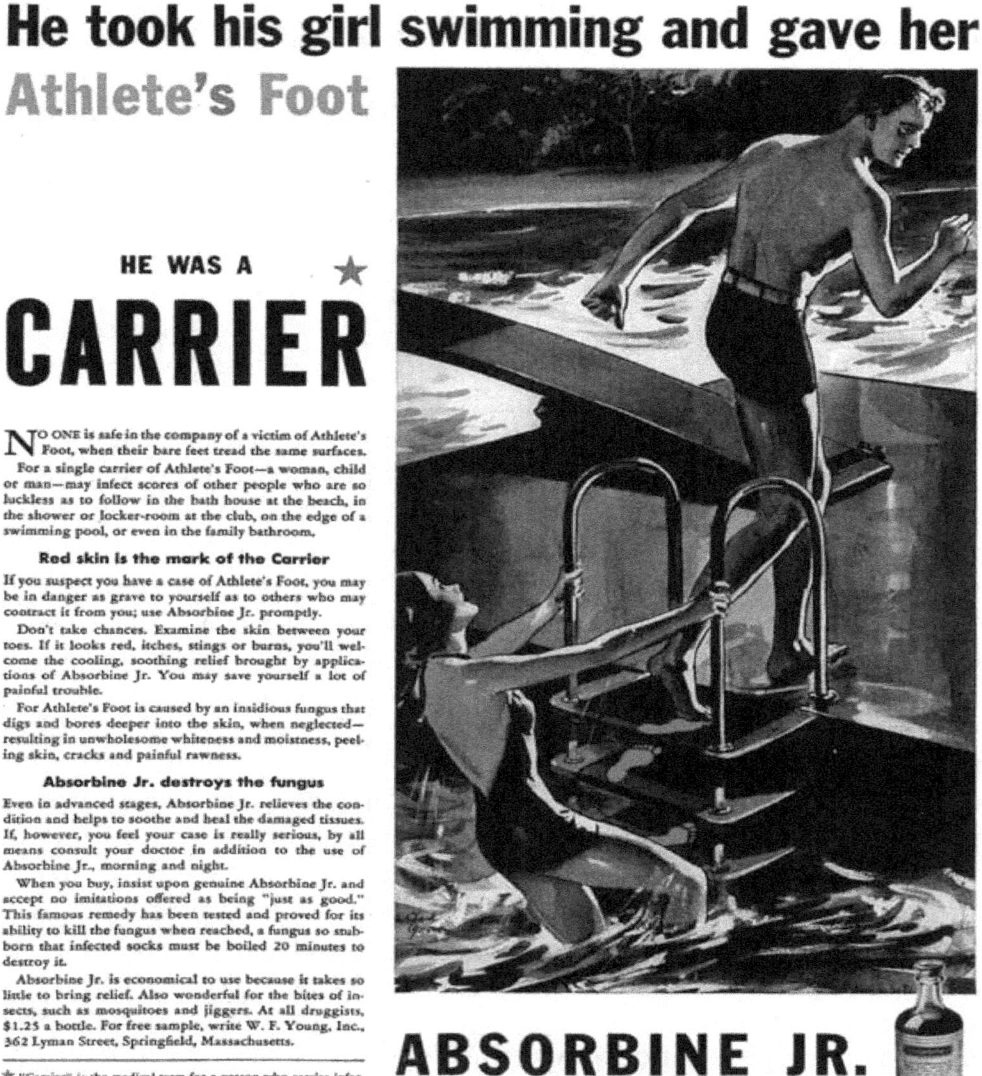

Figure 2.1 'ABSORBINE JR.' Athlete's foot advertisement, *Life*, 3(7)16 August 1937, 81. The advertisement is ©2013 DSE Healthcare Solutions, used under Creative Commons Attribution – Non-commercial

that it was an inevitable consequence of wearing socks and shoes; or, as it was later put, 'a penalty of civilization'.[38]

In Britain there was less medical and public awareness of tinea pedis and the term athlete's foot was not widely adopted until the late 1930s.

Medical writings concentrated on diagnosis and treatment in individual patients rather than any social group. However, doctors noted that it was a disease with 'something of the nature of a social qualification, being commonly met among the upper and middle classes' and, being mostly spread through bathing; it was, then 'paradoxically... a penalty of cleanliness'.[39] This changed in the 1940s, when Britain found its equivalent of American athletes – coal miners. Tinea pedis was identified as the commonest cause of miner's dermatitis, a new condition resulting, again paradoxically, from the provision of pithead baths for communal bathing at the end of underground shifts. The Sankey Commission, which had reported on the future of the coal industry in 1919 had recommended measures to improve the health and welfare facilities for miners and the largest proportion of its expenditure (35%) went on pithead baths.[40] Baths were introduced only slowly and the prevalence of tinea pedis only gained a national profile during the Second World War, when absenteeism due to illness and injuries was a threat to production in a pivotal industry.

Soldiers and miners

Concern about the incidence of tinea pedis amongst military personnel had been expressed between the wars. A study for the United States Navy published as early as 1924, showed 13% of all ranks were affected, but levels were as high as 91% amongst officers recruited from college. The same scenario was reported in the late 1930s in the Royal Navy, with the condition being prevalent amongst all ranks in tropical stations. Surgeon-Commander J. C. Souter expressed the opinion that tinea pedis was a submerged problem, where itching and discomfort was tolerated by men, 'yet every sufferer is a potential casualty' should the condition worsen, as it might on active duty when changes of clothing were difficult, or in the tropics.[41]

During the Second World War, skin diseases were a major cause of invalidism due to poor skin hygiene in combat locations, communal washing facilities and exposure to new pathogens.[42] In tropical theatres there were reports that skin conditions were responsible for three quarters of sick bay attendances in the Pacific.[43] One response at home was that in 1943, the Walter Reed Army Medical Centre in Washington established a mycology laboratory headed by Norman Conant who had started his career in Botany at Harvard, training with Raymond Sabouraud in Paris before taking a post in the Department of Microbiology at Duke University, specialising in mycology. He had worked on allergies and tinea, but gained international recognition in 1944 with the publication of a *Manual of Clinical Mycology*, co-authored with D. S. Martin, D. T. Smith, R. D. Baker and J. L. Callaway, all from Duke's Medical faculty. There were also problems at home amongst soldiers being exposed to geographically specific fungi at training bases in Western and Midwestern states, which we discuss in the Chapter 4.

However, the highest profile incident with tinea pedis during the war concerned a treatment on the home front. A mixture of phenol and camphor was very popular, but there were reports of overtreatment and high levels of exposure, leading to deaths.[44] The remedy was championed by Paul de Kruif in an article, entitled 'A Working Cure for Athlete's Foot' in *The Reader's Digest* in May 1942.[45] De Kruif is best known today for his book *Microbes Hunters* and for assisting Sinclair Lewis in the writing of *Arrowsmith*, but in the 1920s and 1930s he was a significant figure in American medicine.[46] He had worked for the Rockefeller Institute and become as publicist for medical science, serving as secretary to the President's Commission for Infantile Paralysis in 1934. However, by the 1940s he had become a controversial personality, mainly through publicising various medical innovations, of which his athlete's foot cure was seen as another questionable example.[47] Indeed, such was de Kruif's reputation that the FDA issued a public warning against the use of phenol camphor mixture later in 1942.[48]

Amongst British forces in South East Asia, the prevalence of all forms of ringworm was so serious that the Royal Army Medical Corps set up a research unit there on soldier's dermatitis. Surveys by unit staff revealed that amongst soldiers in Malaya and Hong Kong, 79.5% had tinea pedis and 33.5% had tinea corporis, tinea cruris or all three.[49] However, ringworm received most attention in Britain, not because of its military toll, but due to its incidence in workers at home, along with the investment in fungus research prompted by the discovery of the antibiotic properties of penicillin and emerging problem of systemic mycoses. In Britain, the Medical Research Council (MRC) appointed a Medical Mycology Committee in 1943.[50] One goal was to rationalise taxonomies and tinea pedis was a particular problem. At the time the following terms were used by doctors across the Empire: 'athlete's foot'; 'Hong Kong', 'Shanghai' and 'Singapore foot'; 'gym', 'golfers' and 'swimmers' itch; 'toe-rot'; 'ringworm of the feet'; 'Cantlie's foot tetter', 'eczematoid ringworm of the extremities'; 'dermatomycosis'; 'epidermomycosis'; and 'epidermophytosis'.[51] Perhaps this variety was further evidence of the novelty of the infection, or even the diversity of specific pathogens producing different types of lesion, but most likely it reflected the multiplicity of practitioners, locations and presentations.

The Committee's work during the war focused on coal miners. The first detailed study was made in 1943 by R. B. Knowles in the coalfields of the north Midlands and South Yorkshire. He confirmed the widely held view that the introduction of pithead baths in the 1920s and 1930s had created the problem.[52] After the nationalisation of the industry in 1946 and the creation of the National Coal Board (NCB), surveys and reporting on the welfare of miners increased.[53] One study of miners in Warwickshire in 1946 found that 52% of the men had 'intra-digital disease', 15% had 'foot lesions other than fungus infection', and only 33% had 'healthy feet'.[54] It was against this background that in November 1951, a Committee on Industrial Epidermophytosis (CIE) was established within the MRC's Industrial Health Research Board (IHRB). The Committee's membership indicates how tinea pedis had become a multi-specialist problem. The CIE was chaired by John T. Ingram, a dermatologist from Leeds, who had considerable experience in the army and was joined by two other dermatologists, George H. Percival (Edinburgh) and H. Renwick Vickers (Sheffield).[55] Geoffrey C. Ainsworth provided mycological expertise, D. D. Reid from the London School of Hygiene and Tropical Medicine dealt with medical statistics, while R. E. Lane from the University of Manchester provided wider occupational health expertise.[56] Another member was Archibald L. Cochrane, who was then at the MRC's Pneumoconiosis Research Unit in Penarth, and later became a champion of randomised clinical trials, where his legacy has been institutionalised in the network of Cochrane collaborations.[57] Also on the Committee were T. E. Howell, the Principal Medical Inspector of Mines at the Ministry of Fuel and Power, and J. M. Rogan, Principal Medical Officer at NCB.[58]

The initial brief was quite wide, but Ingram argued that the CIE should 'deal in the first place especially with epidermophytosis of the feet in coal miners and to leave all side issues . . . until later'.[59] Rogan stressed the NCB's economic objectives of reducing absenteeism and other costs, wanting the CIE to focus on practical measures, such as prevention and methods for mass treatment.[60] However, Ingram had other ideas and fostered work across specialisms in epidemiology, the natural history of the disease, clinical and mycological diagnosis, research on fungal growth, the chemistry of the skin and the histopathology of the condition.[61]

Finding out the nature and scale of the problem in miners was the priority. Epidemiological studies were commissioned from J. G. Holmes, a dermatologist in Cardiff, and Jimmy Gentles, a mycologist who, during his term of appointment, moved to the University of Glasgow. Early results came from a pilot that Rogan arranged for Holmes to conduct at a colliery in Allerton Bywater, near Leeds.[62] There were issues with compliance and Holmes complained that miners showed a 'lack of foot-consciousness, thoughtlessness and in a few cases, selfishness'.[63] A larger study of 2,101 men working in mines across the country was published in 1956.[64] Clinical examinations found that 1,900 men (90%) had some abnormality of the skin of the foot, yet in only 438 cases (21%) was there laboratory-confirmed fungal infection. However, rates varied, from 50% in one East Midlands pit to 3.5% in the Yorkshire coalfield overall. The problems of reconciling clinical and laboratory diagnoses were shown by the fact that 75 patients 'showed so-called "diagnostic" lesions without any evidence of fungus being found', while 4% of those with 'clinically normal feet' tested positive in the laboratory.[65]

The Medical Mycology Committee's post-war survey on the incidence of mycoses in Britain, published in 1948, confirmed a view widely held within the medical profession, that the incidence of tinea capitis, the new term for ringworm of the scalp, in children had risen during the war. The rise was attributed to the suspension of X-ray treatment, the relaxation in school hygiene, and to the evacuation of children, with a consequent decline in hygiene and greater exposure to cats, dogs and cattle.[66] An increase in tinea pedis in adults was explained by continuing improvements in hygiene, the exposure of men to infection in military settings, and the circulation of ringworm species around the world with troop movements.[67] A particular concern was the importation of *T. rubrum* to Europe from the Far East, as it was one of the most difficult ringworm species to treat. However, the reported incidence of tinea pedis in Britain was nowhere near that in the United States. In 1950, Jacqueline Walker reported on a survey of 1,010 army recruits, 857 of whom were free of infection and of the 123 suspected cases, only 39 (4%) were confirmed in the laboratory.[68] One reason for the low incidence was the relative paucity of sports and college facilities, and there were certainly fewer homes with bathrooms where infection could spread within families. The place where the spread of tinea pedis was most common was in elite public schools, which had the best sports facilities.[69]

One problem in surveys was the discrepancy between clinical and laboratory diagnoses. Doctors accepted that microscopy and culturing were more reliable than clinical methods; however, there were few laboratories available to provide the tests and a reluctance amongst dermatologists to use them.[70] For some, the reliability of laboratory results was a moot point. They depended on many factors: from the quality of the skin sample taken, through to the competence of staff in particular laboratories. Accuracy mattered more in epidemiological studies than it did in clinical practice. False positives in a low incidence population would skew the result significantly, whereas dermatologists and general practitioners were prescribing broad spectrum, topical fungicides for all presentations of 'inter-digital dermatitis' without laboratory confirmation. Better-targeted treatment would have prevented what one doctor later termed 'a chemical assault' on the feet of the nation in the post-war era.[71]

The uncertainties over diagnosis, especially when fungi were found without clinical disease in 'symptomless carriers', reopened the question: were the fungi causing tinea pedis external contagious agents caught from other people, or were they saprophytic parasites of the skin that only caused disease in certain conditions?[72] While patterns of infection in particular groups and the identification of infective fungi on floors in baths and showers pointed to the overriding importance of contagion, some doctors argued that infection was more complicated. The seed and soil analogy was used to suggest both that prior physico-chemical changes had to make the skin open to infection, as in pre-pubescent children, or that a 'factor X' was involved.[73] Such views were important because doctors were only too aware of the limitations of topical remedies and, hence, were keen to promote specific and general preventative measures.

Chemical abuse of the nation's feet

In the late 1940s, the American market was flooded with topical treatments for athlete's foot. Writing in *JAMA* in 1946, G. B. Underwood and colleagues wrote on the 'unbelievable chemical abuse' of the feet of Americans.[74] In their practice they reported:

> Feet are seen daily, painted all the colors of the rainbow or daubed so thick with salves that removal with a tongue blade is necessary to view the underlying dermatitis. The shoes smell of solution of formaldehyde and are caked on the inside with fungicidal powders. The patients, when questioned about the number of remedies used, shrug their shoulders and exclaim 'I couldn't begin to recall. I've used everything. You are the sixth or seventh doctor I have seen. I've had this stuff between my toes for years. Just when I think it is well, it's back again. Each time it comes back I try something else. I've spent a small fortune for remedies, and look at my poor feet.' These patients are sure of the cause of their dermatitis. It is the 'athlete's foot' or the 'fungus.'[75]

They reproduced examples of the ways that companies selling topical remedies portrayed athlete's foot as dire threats to individual and public health. Potions were said to 'Kill Athlete's Foot Germs on Contact', to cure 'Factory Feet' and warned 'YOU PROBABLY HAVE ATHLETE'S FOOT or will get it'. Brands had names like 'Soretone', 'Korium', 'Octofen' and 'Desitin'. Some remedies were cure-alls, such as '3X^{B}', which also helped with 'minor wounds, blisters resulting from ivy poisoning, or similar conditions, corns, calluses, tired feet, chafing, prickly heat or similar skin conditions'. Underwood and his colleagues reported analyses of 106 popular remedies, finding the most common ingredients were phenol, ethyl aminobenzoate and, most worryingly, mercurial compounds. The Mennem Company's leading brand 'Quinsana', whose advertising regularly featured the threat of catching athlete's foot on the beach, contained Hydroxy-Quinolene, Magnesium stearate and boric acid. Underwood and his colleagues ended with a plea to dermatologists to 'take steps to prevent the commercial commandeering of scientific reports and formulas', and called for the regulation of popular skin treatments.

Whether the rash of new products was due to a real increase in the incidence of fungal skin infections is unclear, but the post-war increase in tinea capitis in American schools suggests that there was more ringworm in communities.[76] Infected children were treated with X-rays, as well as topical remedies and there were calls for public health agencies to take up the matter.[77] Laboratory reports showed that the main cause was no longer *Microsporon canis* caught from pet and farm animals, but *Microsporon audouini*, the main European ringworm species.[78] State and county authorities started campaigns, which were claimed to be effective. The reported incidence of tinea capitis fell in the 1950s, even though X-rays, the former treatment of choice, was dropped because of concern about the long term health effects of exposure to radiation.[79]

The most notorious example of the enthusiasm for developing and trialling treatments for athlete's foot were the investigations on prisoners undertaken by Arthur Kligman in Pennsylvania and discussed in Arthur M. Hornblum's book *Acres of Skin*.[80] Kligman worked in the Department of Dermatology at the University of Pennsylvania Medical School, then headed by David Pillsbury. Prior to his work with prisoners, Kligman had made experimental studies of children in mental defective homes to test the effects of X-rays used to treat tinea capitis.[81] He wrote in 1952 that,

> The work was carried out at a state institution for congenital mental defectives...The experimental circumstances were ideal in that a large number of individuals living under confined circumstances

> could be inoculated at will and the course of the disease minutely studied from its very onset. Biopsy material was freely available. By contrast, Sabouraud's researches were largely limited to the clinical opportunities presented by ringworm patients appearing at the Paris clinic.[82]

This work was part of wider studies of treatments for ringworm, especially the new topical creams versus depilation, either mechanically or by X-rays.[83]

In 1957, Kligman published an article with John Strauss that opened with the following statement.

> So much has been written about the subject of athlete's foot that one can hardly add still another paper to an already mountainous pile without some justification. We thought we could gain some fresh appreciation of this disease by studying it experimentally in a prison population. With this group it was possible to do a number of things which would otherwise have been rather difficult. Rigid control over the subjects, adult males in the age range of 20–50 years, offered many experimental advantages.[84]

Kligman's research at the prison, which ran from 1951 to 1974, grew from initial studies of athlete's foot treatments, to medications for a wide range of other skin conditions and cosmetics. He worked closely with pharmaceutical companies and prisoners were paid to be human guinea pigs. Kligman became infamous because of the ethical status of his trials, however, in American dermatology he remained a hero, with his death marked by an article with the by-line 'Albert the Magnificent' and no mention of the criticisms of his work.[85] Controversy was fed by the fact that Kligman was unapologetic; he considered retrospective judgements of the ethics of his work unfair and that he defended it, arguing that medicine had benefited and 'no prisoner suffered long-term harm, as far as he knew'.[86] Nonetheless, the furore caused by criticisms of his work in the 1970s, including the development of the anti-wrinkle cream Retin-A, prompted stricter Federal regulations on medical experiments with prisoners and human subjects more widely.[87]

In both the United States and Britain, the reported prevalence of tinea capitis waxed and waned in the 1960s. One clear trend in the United States was the growing importance of infection with *T. tonsurans*, seemingly imported from Central America and the Caribbean, with *M. audouinii* seemingly in decline across the northern hemisphere.[88] Some dermatologists speculated that the fall in incidence in the late

1960s was due to the fashion for long hair in both men and women, and for 'Afros' amongst African-Americans, both being protective against hair root infection.[89]

Griseofulvin: 'Epoch making' antifungal treatment

From the early 1940s, state and pharmaceutical company laboratories sought novel approaches to fungal infections following the model of antibiotics with bacteria; that is, chemicals that could be injected or taken orally, that would act as 'magic bullets', affecting the pathogenic microorganism and not the host's cells. There had been hopes in the early 1940s that penicillin, or similar fungally derived products, would be antagonist to pathogenic fungi, but these were unfulfilled. Nonetheless, the treatment of fungal infections did benefit from the increase in the scale and intensity of biomedical and pharmaceutical research.[90] Nystatin, which we discuss in Chapter 3, introduced in the early 1950s, was the only success in the search for antifungal antibiotics for a decade; but it was ineffective against ringworm and could not be taken orally. Researchers turned to other approaches. One was to build upon the observation that vulnerability to tinea capitis seemed to end at puberty, which pointed to changes to the chemistry of hair follicles and the identification of heavy fatty acids that seemed to have antifungal properties. The most important was undecylenic acid and its salts.[91] The effectiveness of this fatty acid was similar to compounds already in use, but it had the advantage, allegedly, of being less irritant because it was 'natural'. In Britain, the following proprietary preparations that were widely used from the late 1940s, all contained zinc undecylenate: 'Tineax' from Burroughs Wellcome and Co.; 'Mycota' from Boots and 'Desenex' from Wallace and Tierman. The salts of two other fatty acids, proprionic and caprylic, were also used in the same way. The market leader in Britain was 'Mycil', produced by British Drug Houses (BDH). Its active substance was *p*-chlorophenyl-*a*-glycerol ether, marketed as 'chlorphenesin' and discovered in 1947 by Frank Hartley, then Research Director at BDH, in 1947.[92] In the United States, 'Desenex' ointment and foot powder, produced by Wallace and Tiernan, led the way, and were used in the Korean War and later enjoyed endorsement from celebrities from the National Football League, such as Johnny Unitas.

An editorial in the *Lancet* in July 1946 had wryly observed that most doctors 'take a personal interest in tinea pedis, for – like piles, toothache, and sore throats – if we manage to escape it ourselves, it will not be long before some member of our family is clamouring for attention'.[93] The editorial bemoaned the fact that, despite the flood of new remedies, most treatments had limited effectiveness, particularly in the longer term. Over a decade later, reviewing treatments for general practitioners in May 1958, Grant Peterkin, head of the Skin Department at the Edinburgh Royal Infirmary, reflected that old favourites, such as Whitfield's ointment and Lassar's paste, were still second to none.[94] He noted the recent impact of nystatin on the treatment of *Candida* infections, both in topical applications and when taken orally for intestinal infection, and regretted that there had been no similar advance with tinea pedis. However, he was hopeful: 'Yet it seems possible that in the future fungus infections of the skin may be eradicated by some antibiotic given parenterally [orally].'[95] By the end of the year his hope had been fulfilled with the announcement of the oral antifungal drug – griseofulvin.[96]

Griseofulvin had been first isolated from the fungus *Penicillium griseofulvum* by Harold Raistrick at the London School of Hygiene and Tropical Medicine (LSHTM) in 1939.[97] Raistrick was Britain's leading figure in the biochemistry of fungi, having worked on industrial fermentation for the government in the First World War and then for Imperial Chemical Industries (ICI), before his appointment to the LSHTM in 1929. He had worked on penicillin in the early 1930s, following up Alexander Fleming's early publications, and his laboratory had continued to use *Penicillium* spp. as experimental models.[98] Surprisingly perhaps, griseofulvin was not screened for antibiotic properties in the early 1940s and its antifungal potential was only recognised at the end of the decade, and then in an agricultural rather than medical context.

Researchers at the Butterwick Research Laboratories of ICI found that it produced 'curling' in the hyphae of certain fungal species, inhibiting cell wall formation and cell division.[99] Further work showed it to be an effective, broad spectrum fungicide, though it had no great advantage over existing and cheaper commercial compounds. Mycologists remained interested in the compound, as did researchers at Glaxo's Sefton Park and ICI's Alderley Park Laboratories. Parallel, but separate, investigations showed that griseofulvin had a low toxicity when high doses were given to experimental animals. It also proved to be valuable as a laboratory agent for inhibiting the growth of hyphae-forming fungi, even at quite low concentrations.[100] However, its potential as an oral antifungal seemed limited because it was largely insoluble in water and, hence, could not be made available for absorption through the gut.[101]

Griseofulvin's promise as a fungicide in agriculture led Glaxo researchers to test its toxicity to humans to determine safe exposures for farm workers.[102] These trials showed few, if any, toxic effects. However, commercial development was not fast-tracked because griseofulvin was expensive to produce. In the mid-1950s, Glaxo researchers learnt that two other groups were interested in griseofulvin: Gentles through his work for the NCB, and workers at ICI who were exploring veterinary and human uses. Both Glaxo and ICI had taken out provisional patents on different aspects of the production and use of griseofulvin, and in an unusual move, signed a joint agreement in the spring of 1957 on their respective rights in all areas, from patents through to licensing. Glaxo continued to work with Gentles on animal studies, which led to a publication in *Nature* in August 1958.[103] However, work at ICI showed that griseofulvin could affect mammalian cell division and this prompted further collaboration between researchers in both companies.[104] In comparing data, it seemed that the different results were due to the particle size and that the coarser Glaxo compound was safer. Three dermatologists approached Glaxo for samples to test in patients with ringworm: Gustav Riehl in Vienna, Harvey Blank in Miami and David Williams at King's College London. The first results from these clinics were presented in late 1958.[105]

David Williams and colleagues published a report of nine patients with *T. rubrum* infection who had been successfully treated with orally administered griseofulvin, supplied by Glaxo.[106] There was great excitement about the work. Williams concluded his article with the claim that griseofulvin 'represents a fundamentally new therapeutic approach'.[107] One Cambridge dermatologist, hearing of the development, had written to the MRC claiming that the work was 'epoch making'.[108] The London trial had followed on from a report in August 1958, by Gentles, of successful oral treatment of ringworm in experimentally infected guinea pigs.[109] Gentles had rushed to publish and was similarly excited; though he went for understatement, ending with the remark that this work 'may be of some important for future progress in this hitherto unrewarding field of investigation'.[110]

Gentles and Williams spoke on griseofulvin at the annual meeting of the British Dermatological Society in July 1959.[111] Gentles reviewed the clinical literature and the growing consensus that it was effective for two reasons: first, through its deposition in keratin (the structural protein of hair and nails), and second in being fungistatic, that is, inhibiting the growth of the fungus. This meant that it was likely to be effective in deep-rooted infections of the hair follicles and in toenails. David Williams began his talk by reflecting on the reputation of dermatology within the medical profession and how this might have to change.

> Once upon a time – and thus all good stories begin – there was an old retired general practitioner who said that he could treat all skin diseases although he could diagnose none. Those were the slap happy days when local treatment was a magnificent pseudo-science – not even now do we have much understanding of how local applications work – and internal treatment was a desperate matter of letting justice seem to be done, not too critically.... But in the last fifteen years there have been remarkable advances in the chemical and antibiotic field. Treatment is becoming so specific that there is much to be said for a proper diagnosis before starting it. Penicillin has made syphilis so rare that it is easy to forget its existence. Anti-tuberculous drugs have ruined for us a fascinating, a lovely group of dermatological conditions. And now griseofulvin.[112]

Williams stated that in his clinic the 'experience so far has been so gratifying that it is difficult to be restrained about what seems to be happening'. He gave the drug a ringing endorsement, stating 'griseofulvin is a remarkable drug with minimal toxic effects and that it has come to stay, we have no doubt'.[113] Questions remained about dosage, resistance, re-infection and toxicity, yet in a call-to-arms, he concluded, 'As Montgomery must have said, the break-through has been achieved and our forces can now pour through the gap to consolidate our gains.'[114]

Harvey Blank, who worked at the University of Miami School of Medicine, had also been prompted by Gentles's article to obtain griseofulvin from Glaxo.[115] He first tried it on 'a desperate and unique case' of *T. rubrum* infection, with some success, before a more organised trial on 31 patients with various forms of ringworm. The results were 'uniformly favorable', though he cautioned that toxicity still needed to be tested with prolonged use, and that it was too early to say anything about the likelihood of relapses. Nonetheless, the drug was cleared for use in the United States in July 1959, less than a year after Gentles's paper had been published.[116] Blank organised a symposium on griseofulvin in Miami in October 1959, funded by McNeil Laboratories, a subsidiary of Johnson and Johnson, at which 37 papers were given by speakers from 11 countries, including Gentles and Williams. The rapid spread and trialling of the drug indicates the intense medical interest, across so many countries, that there was in finding oral antifungal drugs. Introducing the proceedings in *Archives of Dermatology* in May 1960, Blank reflected that the development of griseofulvin 'appears to be assuming the proportions of an historical nature'.[117] A key factor in the enthusiastic response in the United States was to explore the potential of the drug to treat persistent infection, such as fungal nail infection – onychomycosis.[118]

The St John's Hospital Dermatological Society organised a British meeting on griseofulvin in May 1960, attended by 189 doctors and scientists, with 24 papers published in a special issue of the Society's *Transactions*.[119] It was already clear that the drug was being widely used in general practice, as well as in dermatological clinics, and this despite the fact that it was expensive.[120] The introduction to the volume drew parallels between the ten-year lag in recognising the therapeutic potential of penicillin, with the 20 years taken from Raistrick's isolation of griseofulvin to its first clinical use.[121] The meeting heard a report of the first controlled clinical trial, led by Brian Russell at St John's Hospital, which was about to be published in the *Lancet*.[122] The trial showed griseofulvin was 'a striking effective remedy' and that 'In retrospect, it is questionable whether a double-blind trial was necessary.' There were 64 patients in the study: just one person of the 31 receiving the drug showed no clinical improvement, whereas 30 out 34 patients given the placebo were 'unimproved'. However, the study showed that the drug was no cure-all. There was considerable variation in the responses of individuals and even the toes of the same person! In addition, when laboratory rather than clinical assessments of cures were used, things were less positive still. Thus, after many weeks and months of treatment, over half of patients continued to harbour the fungus in the skin between their toes, and 26 of 32 patients had some abnormality in their nails. The redeeming feature was that no side-effects were reported; hence, the very long-term treatments that seemed to be necessary were felt to be safe.

Summing up at the St John's Symposium, Brian Russell stated that griseofulvin should be the treatment of choice for all forms of tinea capitis, except that due to *M. canis*, and, disappointingly, tinea pedis due to *T. rubrum*.[123] The drug was also recommended for other types of ringworm and favus, but was said to be only moderately effective against animal ringworm species. Interestingly, its value was 'doubtful or occasional' against the species that had been the main cause tinea pedis in earlier decades: *T. interdigitale*, *T. mentagophytes* and *E. floccosum*. Russell emphasised again that griseofulvin was fungistatic and not fungicidal, hence, 'clinical clearance is not synonymous with cure', while 'mycological clearance', if it could be achieved at all, took much longer. He also pointed to issues with re-infection, carriers, immunological effects, and its impact on the ecology of the body, responding to some reports that griseofulvin opened the body to *Candida* infections.

Griseofulvin became available as a prescription drug in Britain in April 1959; marketed as 'Grisovin' by Glaxo and 'Fulcin' by ICI.[124] There was no expectation within Glaxo that griseofulvin would be another penicillin in terms of sales and profit. Hector Walker, the head of research and development, observed, 'Dermatologists – at least some of them – seem a little bit disturbed that a specific treatment is now available that represents a not unsizeable part of their total practice, and there are reactionary dermatologists just as there are physicians when new treatments appear.'[125] The expectation was that topical treatments for ringworm would continue to be preferred, with griseofulvin used for persistent infection and onychomycosis. Soon, even these qualified hopes were being moderated. An editorial in *Lancet* mocked the recent meetings on the drug.

> Massed choirs met at international symposia in Miami last October and in London under the wing of the St. John's Hospital Dermatological Society on May 13 and 14 to add their paeans of praise. They sang, for doctors, in surprisingly close harmony. The main theme has been the remarkable success of griseofulvin, with pitch according to skill and experience. More recent variations have wandered a little into the more pensive, minor keys as certain problems and failures have become evident.[126]

Two years later, there was another sceptical editorial, this time responding to an epidemiological study of tinea pedis by Mary English that showed that only a small proportion of lesions of the toe-webs were fungal in origin and that there very few healthy carriers.[127]

> Griseofulvin has not lived up to expectations, and often does not eliminate fungus from the feet. In acute cases, topical fungicides often do more harm than good... For chronic cases, Whitfield's ointment is still the most usual remedy, and some difficult cases are kept symptom free by wearing sandals.[128]

However, Glaxo had been working on the drug with its American licensees and in 1962 developed fine particle form – GRISOVIN FP – for clinical trials. This was better absorbed through the gut, giving more even blood levels of the drug, even at half of the previously recommended dose. Nonetheless, results were still mixed and worries about toxicity remained.[129]

Despite the problems, in the 1960s griseofulvin became a standard treatment for susceptible forms of ringworm and joined nystatin in the new armoury of antifungal antibiotics.[130] Research on this class of drugs burgeoned in the decade, as mycological researchers in universities, government laboratories and pharmaceutical companies joined the search for natural and synthesised compounds with similar properties.[131] In the wake of the thalidomide scandal and the introduction of stricter safety regulations, much of the further work on griseofulvin was on its toxicity.[132] However, while many side effects were identified, they were all either relatively minor (headaches, gastro-intestinal, photosensitivity, liver function, allergic reaction), or cleared up after treatment ended. Griseofulvin was given prophylactically to American troops in Vietnam, though this did not stop ringworm being a major cause of disability.[133] Only reduced exposure, in shorter combat rotations, affected the overall incidence of ringworm and relapses were blamed on poor compliance in prolonged treatment.[134]

Griseofulvin, as a treatment for most forms of ringworm, united athlete's foot with other sites of infection, such that tinea pedis became distanced from hygiene and fitness. This shift exemplified a trend in medicine from the late nineteenth century of moving definitions of infections based on symptoms to specific causes. Ringworm was not unified by a specific cause, because there were many fungal pathogens, but rather by a treatment – griseofulvin. The drug was a major contributor to athlete's foot and other forms of ringworm, becoming defined as types of 'dermatophytosis', a term which grew in popularity from the 1960s. It was in fact a quite general, hybrid causal-symptomatic definition, literally, skin infection with fungi.

Azoles: 'A major advance in medical mycology'[135]

The success of griseofulvin, more than the earlier nystatin for candidiasis, changed the prospects of antifungal therapy and further new drugs were anticipated.[136] In the event, a widely adopted, oral antifungal alternative to griseofulvin for dermatophytosis did not emerge for nearly 20 years, until in 1977 the Belgian company Janssen announced ketoconazole.[137] Branded as 'Nizoral', it was one of the group of synthetic compounds called 'imidazoles', or more generally 'azoles', that the company had been screening since the late 1960s. The first two widely used drugs from this work were announced in 1969: clotrimazole from Bayer and miconazole, also from Bayer, which were targeted at *Candida* infection and deep seated systemic mycoses. Ketoconazole was different. It was promoted as a broad spectrum antifungal that could be used to treat dermatophytosis as well as candidiasis, histoplasmosis and cryptococcosis.[138]

Following the precedent of griseofulvin, Janssen sponsored a meeting to review progress and spread the word. The first international symposium on ketoconazole was held in Medellin in Columbia in November 1979, linked to the Ninth Ibero-Latin American Dermatology Congress.[139] The participants concluded that they were at 'the threshold of an important new advance' and that ketoconazole was the orally administered drug that was effective for a range of conditions, from acute systemic mycosis through to the growing problem of onychomycosis, that clinicians had been looking for.[140] The drug had been developed by researchers at Janssen Laboratories from the modification of miconazole, which they made less toxic and more suitable for oral administration.[141] The new drug was effective against many of the regionally specific fungal infections discussed in the next chapter and with immunocompromised patients. The concluding address was given by William Dismukes, who worked at the University of Alabama School of Medicine in Birmingham and was a founding member of the newly formed, NIH funded, Mycoses Study Group. He hoped that ketoconazole would be 'the first "total" antifungal agent with a broad spectrum of activity' and that very promising results *in vitro* and early clinical trials now needed to followed by longer term studies.[142]

The question with ringworm was this, was ketoconazole more effective than griseofulvin? Two reports by clinicians were presented at Medellin, one from Oregon in the United States and other Mexico. The group from Oregon reflected that,

> During more than 20 years of clinical experience with griseofulvin, the subject of failure of therapy has received scant notice. Only rarely do patients fail to respond to this drug because of either resistance of the organism or inadequate tissue levels of griseofulvin. Much more commonly, dermatophytoses respond to the drug but then either fail to clear or recur soon after discontinuance of therapy.[143]

The conclusion of the Oregon study was that ketoconazole was effective in cases that did not respond to griseofulvin, but whether it should be the first choice was left open. The second report was similarly positive. Ketoconazole was approved for clinical use and became available in 1982. The results of comparative trials with griseofulvin were published in 1985, which found they were equally effective for hair, skin and nail infection.[144] On balance, griseofulvin remained the first choice therapy because of concerns about liver toxicity of ketoconazole, which was recommended for patients who were griseofulvin-intolerant.[145] In the 1990s, two new, broad spectrum remedies that could be used topically and given orally became available for ringworm: itraconazole, another triazole developed by Janssen and marketed as Sporanox; and terbinafine developed by Novartis and marketed as Lamisil. Thus, the options available to doctors for treatment at all sites, and with all types of infection increased. However, there was some evidence of the development of drug resistance and tinea pedis increasingly presented along with the more difficult to treat, onychomycosis. Many of the azole compounds, when patent protection lapsed, became available for topical use in over-the-counter creams, competing with every other post-war antifungal back to nystatin. The development of azole drugs consolidated the remaking of athlete's foot as another type of dermatophytosis.

In this chapter, we have charted the rise and fall of athlete's foot as a disease of fitness and hygiene. It is not clear if the reported rise in incidence in the 1920s was due to the greater awareness, or presence of new pathogens in Western populations, or new conditions for ringworm fungi to spread and flourish. At the time, the majority of doctors maintained the latter and, specifically, that ringworm of the feet was a 'penalty of civilisation'. In all contexts, medical and public concern was linked to new lifestyles, new clothing, new military conditions or new working environments, the latter especially so in Britain, where coal miners rather than athletes put the condition on the map. While medical advice initially stressed prevention over treatment, proprietary medicine manufacturers turned the full weight of product development and promotion on the condition, typically selling their wares as products of medical progress. Athlete's foot was also at the forefront of the antibiotic revolution with fungal infections, through the development of griseofulvin, coincidentally a compound derived from a species of the *Penicillia*. The arrival of griseofulvin and then in the 1970s of the azoles, accelerated the redesignation of athlete's foot and other ringworm infections as dermatophytoses. They were no longer framed as 'diseases of modernity', but as fungal infections that were conquerable, if not yet fully conquered, by medical progress.

3

An Integrated Study of Antibiotics and Candida

Initial reporting of penicillin as a wonder drug emphasised the fact that it was derived from a fungus, and a common one at that. Fungi of the genus *Penicillia* are ubiquitous in the soil and rotting matter across the world. They are most commonly seen in the bluish mould growing on old fruits and bread, and there are specific species associated with types of cheese: *P. camemberti* and *P. roqueforti*. Indeed, the species that Alexander Fleming derived his pioneering antibacterial from agent was the common *P. chrysogenum* (formerly *P. notatum*), that was common enough in London to blow in through the window of his laboratory.[1] The main antibiotics that followed penicillin were also derived from fungi: streptomycin from *Streptomyces griseus*, tetracycline from *Streptomyces rimosus*, cephalosporin from *Cephalosporium acremonium* and, as discussed in the previous chapter, griseofulvin from *Penicillium griseofulvum*. These discoveries changed the profile of fungi in popular culture, from agents of contamination and decay to those of medical progress and human improvement, and there was renewed recognition of their role in food and drink production.[2] Antibiotics affected fungal infections in medicine in two main ways: first, they prompted a search for antifungal as well as antibacterial agents and second, antibiotics seemed to open the body to new types of invasive fungal infection, the most serious of which was with *Candida albicans (C. albicans)*, which was well known as the cause of thrush or yeast infections.[3] Thrush was commonly seen as an oral infection, especially in babies, and a genital infection in adults, particularly women.

In medicine, the success of antibiotics in treating bacterial infections defined what many historians have termed the 'Therapeutic Revolution' of the mid-twentieth century.[4] The better control of bacterial infections allowed more ambitious surgical procedures and the pharmaceutical industry produced drugs for the cure or better management of a seemingly ever growing range of diseases. However, assessments of the impact of antibiotics nowadays balance the optimism of effective cures for bacterial infections, with the increase in the number and seriousness of antibiotic resistant bacteria.[5] In fact, antibiotic resistance was recognised in the early 1940s and by the early 1950s, streptomycin, which had radically altered the prospects of tuberculosis sufferers, had to be taken with two other drugs, isoniazid and para-aminosalicylic acid (PAS), in part, to overcome antibiotic resistance.[6] Less well recognised, and an important theme of this chapter, is of how antibiotics opened the body to new types opportunistic infections, with systemic mycoses amongst the most difficult to manage. Writing in 1955, Ernest Jawetz, a microbiologist at the University of California Medical Center, San Francisco, wrote that that the '"rise of the yeasts" during antibiotic administration has been noted quite generally' and that the 'pathogenic potential of these fungi has caused concern'.[7] At this time the causal organism was known as *Monilia albicans* (*M. albicans*) and the infection moniliasis, but this changed to candidiasis or candidosis with the renaming of the pathogen.[8] In this chapter we keep to the terms used by doctors and others in context; but be warned there were no sudden changes, thus, old and new terms coexisted for many years.

We begin the chapter with a discussion of thrush in the nineteenth and early twentieth centuries and its transition from an oral infection of weak children to a genital infection of women. In both cases, doctors framed the disease in terms of the metaphor of 'seed and soil'; namely, that to spread and develop pathogenic fungi required vulnerable human tissue, weakened by poor nutrition or other diseases. We then discuss the 'Antibiotic Era' and the inter-connected development of fungi as sources of antibiotics, including antifungals, and the claims that the use of antibiotics precipitated a general increase in fungal infections and new types of systemic fungal disease. The iatrogenic consequences of antibiotics have been discussed by doctors and historians in relation to the development of bacterial resistance, but hardly at all with regard to fungal infections.[9] The most prevalent of the new infections was systemic or invasive candidiasis, which was present in new patient groups; firstly, patients with leukaemia and those being treated for other cancers with steroids; later, transplant patients, and finally in the 1980s, people with HIV/AIDS. The common factor was that all were immunocompromised or -suppressed, showing once again the importance of the relationship between bodily 'soil' and fungal 'seeds'. We end the chapter with a discussion of one of the great popular health crazes of the last quarter of the twentieth century – 'The Yeast Connection' – whose advocates argued that many of the new chronic and debilitating ailments of modernity were due to *C. albicans* overgrowth in the body.

Thrush: Weak children

In the mid-nineteenth century, oral thrush was regarded by doctors as a form of stomatitis, the symptomatic name for inflammation of the mouth, which also included ulcers, bleeding gums and, most seriously, cranum oris or noma, a gangrenous infection of gums or cheek with tissue destruction. Typically, a thin white membrane covered the palate, with white spots on the tongue, but in serious cases the tongue, cheeks and lips were covered, with possible spread to the throat and oesophagus. The condition was most prevalent amongst premature babies and then at weaning, when food matter stuck to gums and the mouth lining, acting as both an irritant and medium for infection.[10] Local epidemics were reported in lying-in hospitals, mostly alleged to be spread by poor hygiene amongst breast feeding mothers. While the disease was typically short-lived, disappearing as the baby gained weight, in a minority of cases it spread to the gut or lungs, and death usually followed. Mothers would say that thrush had 'gone through' their children.[11]

With children, it was an important skill for doctors to be able to diagnose differentially thrush from diphtheria; indeed, before the notion of specific infections was accepted, doctors believed that the white growth of thrush often transformed into the membrane of diphtheria as the child's health deteriorated.[12] The only treatment was to clean the mouth after meals, irrigate the mouth with glycerine borax and improve the general diet. Public health doctors saw thrush as a marker of poverty; it was most common in children with poor dietary and digestive troubles, which had progressed to general debility and fatigue. Although said to be common, thrush was rarely discussed in the medical press because it was either readily treated or self-limiting. However, it was occasionally reported in adult patients in the terminal stages of consumption and cancer, which resonated with the common observation that fungi flourished on dying or dead matter.

Thrush: Women and the 'Whites'

With hindsight, medical mycologists have identified the first publication on vaginal thrush as being that of Stuart Wilkinson in the *Lancet* in 1849.[13] This article appeared in the context of the contemporary interest in fungal theories of disease and was published in the same issue as a discussion of the alleged cholera fungus.[14] Wilkinson wrote that he had observed filamentous fungi in discharges from a woman that he traced to her uterus, but noted the 'healthiness of the vaginal wall'. Interestingly, today the vaginal wall understood to be the main site of infection, so it is debatable if this was really the first ever case.[15] The report stands alone in nineteenth-century medical literature and there was little or no direct discussion of fungal infection of the vagina again until the twentieth century. So, what happened to Wilkinson's thrush? This is, of course, the wrong question. What Wilkinson described was not vaginal thrush in the modern sense of specific infection, but an instance of 'leucorrhoea' or 'the whites', discharges that doctors defined against 'red' menstrual conditions.

Leucorrhoea was difficult terrain for many doctors because it involved intimate examination of women and was associated with venereal diseases, which might mean difficult questions for patients.[16] Speaking in 1862, Grailly Hewitt, one of London's leading gynaecologists, observed,

> [L]et it be remembered that it is impossible for the practitioner to exercise too great caution in pronouncing an opinion for or against the specific nature of a discharge from the female generative organs. In the words of the late Dr Ashwell, 'it is always his duty to cure the disease, but rarely to venture upon an exposition of its nature. If he can positively affirm that it is of simple origin, let him do so, if suspicion has been aroused; if not, it is better to avoid any distinct allusion to the matter.'[17]

Nineteenth-century medical books on the 'diseases of women' discussed leucorrhoea as a symptom rather than a disease condition in its own right. White discharges pointed either to constitutional disease, anything from tuberculosis to hysteria, or to local problems with the ovaries, fallopian tubes, uterus, cervix or vagina, any of which might be related to gonorrhoea, syphilis or venereal disease. The doctor's prime task was differential diagnosis, prognosis and treatment. If local treatment was recommended, it tended to be the use of anti-inflammatories or 'milder' antiseptics, such as mercury, boric acid, permanganate of potash or silver nitrate.

The direct association of leucorrhoea and specific fungal infection was first made in 1931 by Everett Plass, Henry Hesseltine and Irving Borts, obstetricians and gynaecologists from Iowa, who identified a condition they termed 'Monilial vulvovaginitis'.[18] Their finding emerged from a study of vaginal discharge in two pregnant women, where gonorrhoea was first suspected as the cause, but all tests had proved negative.[19] The broader context for this work was the venereal disease services that were developed after the First World War, through which venereologists became more interested in conditions other than syphilis and gonorrhoea, especially non-gonococcal urethritis (NGU).[20] NGU was an interesting condition, its diagnosis combined clinical and laboratory methods and it was essentially defined by what it was not: persistent genital discharge from which gonococci were absent.[21] NGU was almost exclusively reported in men, with very few women acknowledged suffering similar symptoms due to inflammation of the urethra, vagina or cervix.[22] However, in women the principal infective agent found in cases of leucorrhoea and vaginitis was *Trichmonas vaginalis*, a protozoan that seemed to be more prevalent in the United States than Europe, and *C. albicans*.[23]

The other important context was Rhoda Benham's work on *Monilia* fungi and disease.[24] Benham worked at the Columbia-Presbyterian Medical Center, where she and her colleagues became leaders in the field of medical mycology in the United States.[25] In a paper in the *Journal of Infectious Diseases* in September 1931, she argued that *M. albicans* was a 'well defined species which can be recognized and differentiated from related forms by its morphologic and cultural characteristics' and that many other organisms, previously regarded as distinct, were in fact the same species.[26] She stated the case directly:

> The evidence brought out by the different methods of study of this group of organisms gave remarkably concordant results. The strains isolated from thrush, whether called *Monilia* or *Endomyces*, the strains called *M. psilosis*, isolated from sprue, and the strains from erosion inter-digitalis, mycotic paronychia, mycotic intertrigo, perleche and superficial glossitis all showed essentially the same morphology, the same fermentations, essentially the same antigenic properties, both on direct agglutination and on absorption of agglutinins, and the same pathogenicity for rabbits. If one were ignorant of the source of these cultures, one would be unable to distinguish, for example, *M. albicans* isolated from thrush from *M. psilosis* isolated from sprue, and it would seem necessary for the present to regard such forms as merely strains of one species.[27]

In the following year, she published a short paper in the *American Journal of Public Health*, again emphasising that *M. albicans* was the main pathogenic 'yeast' found in humans.[28] She showed that the *Monilia* infecting plants and animals were distinct, and suggested keeping the term *Monilia* that for the plant pathogens and adopting Berkhout's term, *Candida* spp., for human pathogens.[29] Many mycologists thought the term *Candida albicans* unsatisfactory because it literally meant 'whitening, white'. Writing in 1940 from Duke University School of Medicine, Donald Martin and Claudius Jones quoted a French study that had identified 102 synonyms for *C. albicans*, while an Italian review had listed 121, with only 51 overlapping![30] In 1935, Benham wrote what turned out to be a forward-looking chapter on 'Monilia and moniliasis' in Frederick Gay's encyclopaedic *Agents of Disease and Host Resistance*.[31] She stressed the role of the *Monilia* spp. in the following: occasional epidemics of oral thrush and in association with gingivitis; some skin lesions and allergic reactions; infections of the vaginal mucous membrane and of the penis; infection of the eyes of the newborn; some bronchial and pulmonary infections; and generalised disease, often affecting the brain.

Thrush: Mothers and babies

Gynaecologists and obstetricians also took more interest in fungal infections in the 1930s, especially in pregnant women, in whom hormonal changes were reported to increase susceptibility.[32] In 1937 Brooke Bland and Abraham Rakoff of Jefferson Medical College, Philadelphia described a study in which 12 pregnant women and 12 non-pregnant women were infected with *C. albicans*. As we might expect for the time, there is no evidence that informed consent was sought or given; though as a minor, mostly self-limiting infection, doctors would have judged any danger to patients as negligible and justifiable for the progress of medicine. They found that ten out of 12 pregnant women acquired the infection, against four who were not pregnant.[33] This experiment was followed up by infecting a further 38 pregnant women, 25 of whom developed disease. Thrush was also reported to be common in diabetics, who had the new status of being maintained with insulin injections.[34] One idea was that high glucose levels in the blood could precipitate infection, another was that poor peripheral circulation and changes in pH predisposed diabetics.[35] Thrush was one of the many infections that made the new diabetes 'a disease of complications'.[36]

In the late 1930s, doctors noted that thrush in newborn babies (neonates) was likely caught from mothers during parturition, and there was cross-infection across sites in the body.[37] In 1940 Glen Liston and

Lewis Cruickshank published two studies of leucorrhoea in 200 pregnant women in Edinburgh that showed 49 (25%) had *C. albicans* infection, as against 75 with *Trichomonas* and four with gonorrhoea.[38] Their work was discussed in the *Lancet*, in an editorial on 'Vaginal Discharge' in September 1940 that pointed to personal and social issues for the patient.[39]

> One of the most distressing complaints that the gynaecologist and general practitioner are called on to treat is vaginal discharge. To the patient it is demoralising, because of its intractability, and in a sensitive woman it may cause considerable mental trauma. To the layman, moreover, a vaginal discharge carries a sinister innuendo – many an innocent woman has suffered unmerited blame from husband or family for a non-venereal infection, and a discharge has even been the starting point of an action for divorce.[40]

The importance of differential diagnosis, of what was also termed 'vaginal mycosis', was emphasised, along with the new possibilities for treatment.

The *Lancet* editorial was followed up by three letters. Dr Mary Michael-Shaw of the Royal Free Hospital and Salvation Army Mothers' Hospital in London recommended using specialist laboratories for diagnosis. Along with the other correspondents, she discussed treatment and recommended Stovarsol (branded as Spirocid and Arsetosone), an arsenical originally produced in the Ehrlich's series that gave the world Salvarsan. Stovarsol was No. 594 and sometimes recommended for syphilis.[41] In his letter, Lewis Cruickshank recommended 'bi-weekly painting of the whole vagina, external genitalia, thighs and pubic region with 2% aqueous gentian violet', while other doctors described their successful treatments with antibacterial douches, using products such as Eli Lilly's Negatan (also called Negatol) and Monsol.[42] Drug companies, increasingly aware of the new market created by thrush infections, developed new formulations and carriers for topical antiseptics, such as gentian violet, marketed as 'gentia-jel'.

The accepted 'reference' study of neonatal oral thrush in Britain as an emerging problem was published in 1942 by two bacteriologists from Edinburgh, G. B. Ludlam and J. L. Henderson.[43] It was based on a survey of babies born at the Royal Infirmary in the city in 1940. The incidence of the condition diagnosed clinically was 6.4% (163 cases) in that year, down from 7.2% (168 cases) in the previous year, but the figure was believed to be higher, as many babies only showed symptoms after discharge. A group of '60 unselected infants' was tested by swabbing and laboratory testing, which revealed the fungus in 18.3% (11 cases), almost three times that diagnosed symptomatically. The authors suggested that the difference pointed to a significant level of latent disease, or benign presence of the fungus. Amongst babies with symptoms, the incidence was highest in premature babies, then in those partly or wholly bottle-fed, and lowest in those breast-fed. There was seemingly no discussion over whether thrush was increasing because of the rise in the number of hospital births, or the switch from breast to bottle feeding that was being reported in the 1940s.[44]

Paediatricians showed more interest in *Candida* infection as a potentially serious condition and warned that it could rapidly change from trivial to life threatening. If it spread to the oesophagus, stomach and intestines, symptoms were diffuse and often missed, with *Candida* infection often only recognised at post mortem.[45] Such concerns added to the uncertainties about the nature and management of thrush. On the one hand, it appeared to be very common and in the great majority of cases cleared up quickly, but on the other hand it might be a sign of poor general health or a warning of very serious underlying disease.[46] In succeeding years the clinical picture worsened further with claims that *Candida* infection could also spread to the lungs and even develop as systemic disease, similar to septicaemia.[47]

In 1952, Ian Donald, later a pioneer of ultrasound in obstetrics, then a Reader in obstetrics at the University of London, published on the infections seen at the Institute of Obstetrics and Gynaecology's 'D' Clinic in London over the previous five years.[48] The breakdown of the cause of infections in women, after gonorrhoea had been excluded, was *Trichomonas* vaginitis (TV) – 37.4%; *Monilia* – 16.2%, TV and *Monilia* – 7.7%; – miscellaneous 33.5%, and – 'insufficient information' 5.1%. The following year, in a series of 'Refresher Courses for General Practitioners', Scott Russell, Professor of Obstetrics and Gynaecology at the University of Sheffield, recommended rigorous cleansing and disinfection of the vagina before childbirth to flush out *Candida* and other pathogens.[49] There were critics who maintained that such measures made infection more likely, causing irritation and inflammation. They also argued that it was better to encourage the normal micro-flora of the body, which helped make the bodily soil less vulnerable to infection. Doctors also speculated that new clothing fashions and materials, such as tight-fitting nylon underwear that kept the skin warm and moist, had contributed to the increase in the incidence of thrush in women.[50] It was not without irony then that the most talked about underwear of the 1950s, though only seen in newspaper photographs and not by movie theatregoers, were the panties worn by Marilyn Monroe when she stepped into the updraft from the subway grate in the movie 'The Seven Year Itch'.[51]

Yeasts and 'the antibiotic era'

In June 1951, the Council on Pharmacy and Chemistry of the American Medical Association (AMA) agreed that a statement should be printed on bottles of three leading antibiotics (aureomycin, chloramphenicol and terramycin) to warn 'that patients receiving these drugs may be more susceptible to 'Monilial or other yeast-like organisms'.[52] This initiative was made in the context of patients showing all manner of adverse reactions to the new antibiotics. From the first use of penicillin, there had been many, many celebratory assessments of lives saved and improved by the new 'wonder drugs', but by the early 1950s these celebrations had been tempered. Concerns were expressed by doctors and the public about antibiotic use on several fronts: resistance in certain bacteria; allergic reactions in patients, including anaphylactic shock; and a growing incidence of superficial and invasive fungal infections.[53] In 1951, a collection of essays was published entitled *Penicillin Decade 1941–1951: Sensitizations and toxicities*.[54] Some of the most prominent side effects were noticed on the skin, in the form of rashes, and in the mouth, with inflammation and infection of various types, including *C. albicans* growth.[55] What attracted most attention was the development of so-called 'superinfections', as when *Staphylococcus aureus* colonised tissues from which other bacteria had been cleared by broad-spectrum antibiotics. Previously, doctors had used the term to refer to a secondary infection of the same pathogen, especially in cases of syphilis and tuberculosis, but in the 1950s the 'super' came largely to refer to secondary infections of a different pathogen and, in the case of secondary mycotic infections, the term 'fungal overgrowth' was coined.[56]

It is often forgotten that until the mid-1950s penicillin and other antibiotics were largely administered by injection or used topically, because the formulations available were poorly absorbed by the gut.[57] For external infections, penicillin was administered in creams and other carriers, including mouthwashes and pessaries, while aerosols were developed for throat and bronchial infections.[58] For most serious infections, penicillin was given by injection into muscles or via saline drip, which meant that it was most readily given to hospital patients. General practitioners were required to make three or four home visits each day to give injections to keep up the levels of the antibiotic in the system.

The awareness of the adverse effects of antibiotics grew with the arrival in the late 1940s of tetracycline, which was both broad spectrum and taken orally, and could cause the yellowing of teeth in infants and photosensitivity. Initially, fungal overgrowth was well down the list of concerns, top of which were allergic and toxic reactions, vitamin deficiency, the development of resistance and bacterial overgrowth.[59] Indeed, many reviewers implied that the extent and seriousness of fungal overgrowth had been overstated by medical mycologists talking up the importance of their specialism. The first clinical discussion of fungal overgrowth was in June 1949, when Harold Harris spoke at the New York Academy of Medicine on treating patients suffering from brucellosis with aureomycin and chloramphenicol.[60] He suggested that overgrowth was due to a combination of *C. albicans* gaining virulence in the absence of bacterial competition, the destruction of intestinal bacterial flora, and the lowering of the vitality of gut tissues. He worried too about the permanence of the changes and the development of more virulent strains of the fungus. In June 1951, James Woods and colleagues, from the Watts and McPherson Hospitals in Durham, North Carolina, published a study of 25 patients who had developed *C. albicans* infection after treatment with various antibiotics.[61] The study found no evidence that antibiotics had a stimulating effect of the fungus, but confirmed the view that the removal of competing bacteria cleared the gut for fungal colonisation. The report also suggested that treatment with vitamin B complex offered some amelioration, but could give no reason why, other than perhaps it improved the general nutritional status of the body. However, the immediate reason for the intervention of the Council on Pharmacy and Chemistry in June 1951 was because of reports that aureomycin, chloramphenicol and terramycin could precipitate fungal infection of the lungs, whereas the bowel infections noted previously had been 'of little consequence'.

Cases of broncho-pulmonary moniliasis had been reported in medical journals for decades.[62] The increased attention given to tuberculosis after the Second World War, because of mass X-ray screening and effective antibiotic treatment, revealed a greater prevalence of broncho and pulmonary mycotic disease.[63] A study by Robert Oblath and colleagues in California, published in July 1951, argued that *C. albicans* should be added to the list of mycotic pulmonary organisms alongside *Coccidioides immitis* and *Histoplasma capsulatum*, which we discuss in the next Chapter.[64] There were also reports of *C. albicans* infection of the heart (endocarditis) and kidneys. This gave wider recognition to the possibility that moniliasis was changing from an irritating, though relatively mild disease of mucous membranes in the mouth and genitalia, to a serious, often fatal disease of major internal organs. An editorial in the *British Medical Journal* in June 1951 noted the decision of the Council of Pharmacy and Chemistry, but was sceptical of the need for a similar warning about tetracycline in Britain. [65] The writer suggested that 'there was much more extensive use of these drugs generally in America' and that it had brought to light complications which were unfamiliar to doctors in Britain.

A year after the call for warnings on tetracycline packaging, an editorial in *JAMA* reaffirmed the action and concluded that 'The occurrence of moniliasis as a complication of antibiotic therapy has been definitely established.'[66] This claim was contested by Albert Kligman, whose work was discussed in Chapter 2.[67] Kligman argued that, with respect to the impact of wide-spectrum antibiotics, the 'incrimination of moniliasis as the cause of numerous side-reactions requires critical reappraisal'. He advanced four points. Firstly, much of the evidence for the enhancement of fungal growth came only from *in vitro* experiments.[68] Secondly, he suggested that 'reported instances of localized moniliasis are not actually cases of this disease', but rather instances of inflammation due to many causes, where *C. albicans*, a common non-pathogenic presence in many part of the body, might be expected to be found.[69] Thirdly, he argued that diagnoses had been made on insufficient evidence and, fourthly, that mycotic diseases had complex aetiologies, where a single factor, such as the presence of an antibiotic, was unlikely to be sufficient to produce disease. Kligman ended by warning that the development of antibiotic resistance in staphylococcal and streptococcal bacteria 'is likely to be of far greater significance than the problem of superinfections with fungi'.[70] Ernest Jawetz complained that Kligman was minimising the dangers of moniliasis, saying that 'the overgrowth of yeasts was mainly a saprophytic surface phenomenon'.[71]

However, Kligman's views were supported by clinical assessments in the mid-1950s. Louis Weinstein and Lois Finland, writing in the *New England Journal of Medicine* in February 1953 on 'Complications induced by antimicrobial agents', mentioned fungal infection very briefly and focused on hypersensitivity and superinfections from antibiotic-resistant bacteria.[72] In a paper the following year, Weinstein announced his findings on 3015 patients treated with antibiotics, where 52 or 1.74% developed superinfections, of which only seven were due to *C. albicans*.[73] In a study published in the *Lancet* in 1954, Jessie Sharp reported that the incidence of *C. albicans* in the throat, sputum and rectum of patients had doubled during oxytetracycline therapy. However, presence of the fungi was not necessarily associated with disease and the only concern expressed was that these patients would spread *C. albicans* at home when discharged.[74]

Despite the relatively low case incidence, antibiotic induced moniliasis (or as it was increasing referred to candidosis or candidiasis) attracted interest, not least because doctors linked it to the new phenomenon of systemic *Candida* infection in patients who were severely debilitated or immunocompromised from other diseases, or receiving toxic treatments for leukaemia, such as nitrogen mustard therapy.[75] The general point made by medical mycologists was that recent innovations were changing the internal milieu of the body to achieve radical therapeutic advances, but that this led to *C. albicans* emerging as a serious pathogen because it was already present in the healthy body, usually harmless or perhaps even in a symbiotic relationship.[76]

Nystatin – The first antifungal antibiotic

The narrative of the antifungal drugs in the antibiotic era is dominated by the discovery of nystatin by Elizabeth L. Hazen and Rachel F. Brown at the Albany Laboratory of the New York State Department of Health. Their story has been told in Richard Baldwin's book *The Fungus Fighters: Two Women Scientists and Their Discovery*.[77] Hazen had worked as a bacteriologist since 1931 and took the special course in medical mycology at the College of Physicians and Surgeons of New York, befriending Rhoda Benham. Brown was an organic chemist who had joined the Albany Laboratory in 1926 and worked on serum diagnoses, including the Wassermann Reaction for syphilis. They began to work together to try to find antifungal agents against *Coccidioides* and *Candida*, and in the fashion of the time turned to the soil and the chemicals produced by fungi.[78] Within two years, in a soil sample from a friend's garden, they found that the fungus *Streptomyces noursei* had yielded an antifungal compound, which they called fungicidin. It was both fungistatic – preventing the multiplication of organisms – and fungicidal – actually killing organisms.[79] The discovery was announced at a regional meeting of the National Academy of Science in October 1950.[80]

Two years later, Selman Waksman, who was then Professor of Microbiology at Rutgers University, New York and soon to accept the 1952 Nobel Prize in Physiology and Medicine for the development of streptomycin, bemoaned the fact that screening of new chemotherapeutic agents had been mostly for antibacterial, rather than antifungal activity.[81] He argued that there was no *a priori* reason why fungi had not developed antagonistic reactions to other fungi as well as bacteria. Indeed, both penicillin and tetracycline had proved effective in the treatment of actinomycosis, then classified as a fungal disease.[82] Waksman suggested that, as there were many effective topical antifungals, the research 'prize' would go to anyone finding an antifungal that could be injected, or taken orally to attack topical infections from within and combat the emerging problem of systemic infections. He pointed out that such chemicals would also be very useful in veterinary medicine, where fungal diseases were found to be endemic and often epidemic. Waksman identified the actinomycetes as the most promising group for antifungals and particularly *Streptomyces* spp., the potential of which had been demonstrated by Hazen and Brown. However, he was only able to report promisingly fungistatic and fungicidal results in laboratory studies.

Nystatin was introduced as 'Mycostatin' in 1954. Finance for its development came from a private foundation, the Research Corporation for Scientific Advancement (RCSA). This organisation, which had been created in 1912, received and distributed funds for what would now be termed near-market research and with nystatin the RCSA dealt with patents, licences and development. The drug was produced under an agreement, between E. R. Squibb and Sons, the RCSA, and Hazen and Brown, which saw part of the income from sales and royalties reinvested in research by the RCSA and in the newly created Brown-Hazen Fund. An indication of the success of nystatin was that by 1960, income to the fund had risen to $200,000, which was used mainly to support training programmes in medical mycology.[83]

Squibb issued Mycostatin in powder form, which doctors and pharmacists made up into ointments, lotions, pessaries and sprays with appropriate carriers.[84] However, it was soon available in tablets for oral administration to treat intestinal moniliasis where non-absorption was a boon as the compound remained at high levels in the gut.[85] It was marketed for the treatment of three conditions: oral thrush, vaginal thrush and 'monilial overgrowth' in the intestines. Doctors reported good results, and in topical applications patients welcomed not having to suffer the indignity of having their mouths and other parts painted with gentian violet.[86] There were no reported side effects from the topical application of nystatin, but when doctors tried injecting the drug there were problems: pain at the site of injection; then shaking, chills, fever and general malaise, and some long-term effects, such as sclerosing of the veins. Nystatin prompted the first international symposium on fungal therapy in Los Angeles in June 1955, where one question, perhaps surprisingly given the profile of nystatin, was: Why is topical therapy for the superficial mycoses so ineffective?[87] In all, there were 56 papers on every possible aspect of the topic, as the contents page revealed: 'therapy, epidemiology, biology, ecology, reservoir pathogenicity, and immunization in fungus diseases, a number of factors bearing indirectly on therapy, such as laboratory controls and hormonal influences'.[88] Nystatin was more effective than previously available compounds, but it was not a cure-all in the clinic.

The first British clinical report of the use of nystatin for vaginal thrush was in March 1955. Two women who had suffered for many months and endured the irritation, inconvenience and often the embarrassment of using gentian violet, enjoyed rapid symptomatic relief with nystatin pessaries.[89] The following March, two general articles on nystatin were published in the *British Medical Journal*, which prompted letters on local experience in Oxford and London.[90] In September 1956, details of larger clinical trials began to appear. Harry Pace and Samuel Schantz, from Brooklyn, presented details of 59 patients with laboratory confirmed *C. albicans* vaginitis that were treated simply by the insertion of nystatin tablets into the vagina. The average success rate was 98.3%: 100% amongst the 31 women who were pregnant and 96.3% in the non-pregnant.[91] A similar study by Warren Lang and colleagues at the Jefferson Hospital, Philadelphia, with 70 patients, again showed prompt symptomatic relief and near total success.[92] However, other reports were more mixed; for example, one study from Los Angeles published in 1957 showed 'excellent' results in 43% of patients, 'good' results in 53% and fair results in 4%.[93]

Trials in Britain were similar. In January 1957, Roy Jennison and J. D. Llywelyn-Jones at St Mary's Maternity Hospital, Manchester, reported 88% success with nystatin in cases of thrush, compared to 47% with gentian violet. Later that year, William Barr, at the Western Infirmary in Glasgow, published his trials with 64 women: 55 (86%) were 'completely cured' (mycologically clear); 62 (97%) were cured symptomatically; and only 10 (16%) relapsed.[94] He also gave the outcomes of 12 diabetic women with infection, where results were less positive: nine (75%) were cured symptomatically, but two of these had relapsed. Barr linked this to raised levels of sugar in the urine that provided a substrate for the fungi to develop.

In the 1950s, the most controversial use of nystatin was for intestinal *Candida* overgrowth in patients taking tetracyclines. In fact, the initial promotion of 'Mycostatin' had suggested its use in the 'prevention and treatment of intestinal moniliasis, or candidiasis, especially for patients taking oral antibacterial antibiotics for prolonged periods'.[95] Many studies had shown that after taking oral antibiotics, particularly for long periods, the number of patients with *C. albicans* in their faeces rose dramatically.[96] There were contrary views about what this meant. Some doctors argued that it caused diarrhoea and intestinal conditions; others suggested that most patients with positive rectal swabs had 'no complaints of diarrhoea, burning sensation on defecation, or soreness of the anus and surrounding skin'.[97]

One solution to the alleged problem of *Candida* overgrowth in the gut was to give patients on antibiotic regimes nystatin as a prophylactic. Andrew Childs at Ruchill Hospital, Glasgow, trialled this protocol in 1954 and in 1955 Squibb introduced 'Mysteclin', a combination of tetracycline and nystatin.[98] Squibb's advertising claimed that 'Mysteclin' was valuable for 'many common infections', including bronchitis, meningitis, pneumonia and tonsillitis, and by halting the overgrowth of *C. albicans*, it would also protect against 'gastrointestinal distress, anal pruritis, vaginitis, and thrush', any of which on occasion 'may have serious and even fatal consequences'. Such drug combinations worried those doctors concerned about the development of bacterial resistance and other complications of antibiotic therapy, and they were unhappy that the drug tacitly accepted the theory of antibiotic-induced fungal overgrowth.[99]

In the 1960s 'Mysteclin' became controversial in the new context of drug regulation. It was one of the antibiotic combinations that prompted an investigation, sponsored by the National Academy of Sciences and National Research Council, into fixed drug combinations in 1969.[100] Such drugs were seen by many physicians as 'irrational' and typical of the 'avaricious marketing' of pharmaceutical companies, but others worried at the impact of regulations.[101] In the event, 'Mysteclin' was banned by the FDA.[102] Squibb started a counter offensive. This gained notoriety when it emerged that the company had facilitated the writing of letters from physicians asking for the ban to be lifted and enrolled the heads of Harvard and Yale Medical Schools, who were also paid consultants to the company, to give evidence.[103] Squibb came up with a new combination, 'Mysteclin-F', in which nystatin was replaced by amphotericin B; the original formulation became 'Mysteclin-V'.[104]

By this time amphotericin B was a well known and widely used for systemic fungal infections. It had been isolated, like nystatin from a *Streptomyces* species (*S. nodosus*), in an antibiotic screening programme at the Squibb Institute for Medical Research in 1953.[105] Purification produced two compounds: amphotericin A and amphotericin B, and the latter was shown to counter systemic mycoses in experimentally infected mice and rats, and to do so through oral administration. Amphotericin B was licensed in 1955.[106] For a while, amphotericin B promised to be the penicillin of internal fungal infections, but its clinical use proved problematic. The compound was not readily absorbed by the gut, though Squibb overcame this setback by producing a suspension that could be given intravenously. It was tried with some success against localised and systemic cryptococcosis, blastomycosis, histoplasmosis and coccidioidomycosis, but the side effects were many, severe and potentially fatal.[107] Reactions included fever, and nausea and vomiting, and serious kidney damage. However, the drug was used in patients with life-threatening systemic fungal infections in what was sometimes called salvage therapy, with doctors and families calculating that the chance of a cure was worth the risks.

By the 1960s the two most common types of *Candida* infection, oral and vaginal thrush, were well understood by doctors, not least because the availability and success of nystatin had prompted greater medical interest. Oral thrush was readily diagnosed by the characteristic white patches and, if necessary, samples for microscopy and culturing were easily obtained. In neonates doctors found that infection was mostly caught from nurses and mothers; in Britain the incidence of *Candida* infection in pregnant women was around 15%.[108] However, diagnoses were a problem because of the problematic position of medical mycology. Rosalinde Hurley, who then held a joint clinical and microbiology post at Queen Charlotte's Maternity Hospital, London, pointed to a tension between laboratory-based, 'botany types' and clinic-based, 'medical types' in the specialism.

> A ridiculous situation had in the past been reached in clinical microbiology in which the microbiologist believed Candidal vaginitis to be a clinical diagnosis and the clinician believed it to be a mycological diagnosis. The two groups rarely seemed to have discussed the problem. The situation had now improved, if only to the point of admitting that a problem existed.[109]

It seems that the arrival of nystatin, with its broad-spectrum activity, meant that medical interest in the actual fungi producing infection, which had never been high, remained cursory.

The success of nystatin also led pharmaceutical and disinfectant companies to introduce products with, allegedly, similar properties, such as

'Sporotacin', candidicin, pimaracine and hamycin.[110] There is no doubt that self-treatment with the new topicals was widely practised. New prescription antifungals continued to be launched by pharmaceutical companies, including topical amphotericin B, with claims of 85–95% cure rates, though often several courses of treatment were necessary.[111]

The market leader from the 1970s was Bayer's 'Canesten', the active principle in which was clotrimazole, developed in its laboratories by Prof Karl Heinz Büchel and marketed in cream, spray and tablet forms. It was mainly used for vaginal infection, where it offered excellent symptomatic relief, but it was no cure-all, as the recurrence of infection was common.[112] Initially, 'Canesten' was a prescription product, but in the 1990s it became available over the counter. In pessary form, it remained the market leader for vaginal infection in 2000 and sold well in cream form for topical infections, including tinea pedis.[113]

Systemic candidiasis: 'A disease of the diseased'

The first book devoted solely to *Candida albicans* was published in 1964.[114] Its authors were Howard Winner and Rosalinde Hurley, both of whom worked in clinical pathology at the Charing Cross Hospital, London.[115] Hurley, who qualified in both medicine and law, went on to a distinguished career in medical microbiology, always championing mycology, and eventually working in medical regulation. The authors saw their book as a response to the increased incidence of the disease and the burgeoning literature on the topic, yet they were puzzled by the lack of agreement on many issues.[116] One key point of contention was, had there been a 'real' increase in the incidence of *C. albicans* infection, or was the increase only apparent and due to greater awareness and improved diagnostic methods? Winner and Hurley suggested it was the latter. A key piece of evidence was that reported mortality from systemic candidiasis (moniliasis had gone out of fashion) showed no increase at all in recent decades.[117] If there had been more infections in the general population, they argued, there should have been more deaths in special groups, as there would have been a greater likelihood of the development of systemic disease. They thought it unlikely that the availability of nystatin and amphotericin B had changed therapeutic outcomes in terminal cases. The only change in mortality from fungal disease since 1940 was the decline in deaths from actinomycosis, which was susceptible to penicillin.[118]

A second question was, to what extent was systemic candidiasis a primary rather than secondary disease? Winner and Hurley went with the latter, endorsing the old adage that *Candida* infection was primarily the 'local expression of a very bad state of the whole system', or was 'a disease of the diseased'. External infections were associated with predisposing conditions, so it seemed logical that the same applied to internal disease. Winner and Hurley were quite sceptical of the near orthodoxy that antibacterial antibiotics were an important predisposing factor to candidiasis and concluded, 'One is left unable to advance a precise explanation of the nature of the imbalance between host and parasite which changes a harmless symbiotic relationship into a disease which may have lethal consequences.'[119] The mortality rate with systemic candidiasis was nearly 90%, which was perhaps unsurprising as most sufferers had prior serious illnesses.[120]

The first international symposium on *Candida* infection was held in London in 1966, supported by the pharmaceutical company E. R. Squibb & Sons. The proceedings were edited by Winner and Hurley, and covered all aspects of the infection, but most attention was given to systemic disease, for which Squibb's amphotericin B remained the treatment of choice.[121] In the same year, Mildred Seelig, of New York Medical College, published on 'The role of antibiotics in *Candida* infection.' She noted that a review of mycotic disease in 1945 by Downing and Conant had observed that systemic or disseminated infections with *C. albicans* were rare.[122] Two decades later it was clear things had changed, for over half of Seelig's paper was devoted to systemic disease. The increased incidence was said to be hard to quantify, but Seelig was in no doubt that there had been a major change. She argued that this was due firstly to normally saprophytic organisms becoming pathogenic; and secondly, to the creation of new groups of vulnerable patients with altered internal bacterial flora and depressed immune systems. The former related to the increased use of antibiotics, especially combined and broad-spectrum formulations, while the latter was due to more invasive surgery and new therapeutics, such as with cortisone.[123] One example of the change was candidal endocarditis, which was rare in the 1940s, yet by 1961 it was 'an emerging peril in cardiovascular surgery'.[124] The predisposing factors were: the use of multiple antibiotics and adrenal corticosteroids; catheterisation and intravenous fluids; and general poor health of patients.[125] The number of cases associated with cortisone and adrenocorticotropic hormone (ACTH) was small, but they pointed to a new situation where deep-seated fungal infections developed as the result of the body's immunological and physiological functions deliberately altered by therapeutic regimes.[126] The novelty of such complications in the 1950s meant that many were written up for publication as rare or atypical cases, giving systemic fungal infections a profile that was greater than their clinical incidence.

The most controversial site for medical debates about the pathogenicity of *C. albicans* was the lungs, and this went back to tea taster's cough in Sri Lanka in the 1920s. Doctors had debated whether *C. albicans* was a harmless saprophyte as it was found widely in the sputum of children and adults, which acted as a reservoir for lung and tracheal infection.[127] Bronchopulmonary candidiasis was investigated in the laboratory and the clinic, with some studies suggesting that fungal infection worsened asthma and tubercular infection by altering lung tissue and function.[128] The number of cases was small, but they were challenging to diagnose and treat, with suspicions that broncho-mycotic disease was greatly underreported. Despite there being very few cases, chest physicians invested some effort in devising criteria to determine whether primary infection was due to *C. albicans*. These standards were very tight, requiring the fulfilment of Koch's postulates to confirm *C. albicans* and exclusion of other infections, such as tuberculosis.[129]

Winner and Hurley's view of bronchopulmonary candidiasis in 1964 was that nothing had been resolved 'due to the chronic nature of the disease, to the fact that histopathological studies are made later in the course of the illness . . . and that there is no clear-cut association of a particular clinical and a particular pathological feature at all stages of the disease'.[130] One question was, did it matter whether *C. albicans* was the primary or secondary infection? A second was, does this matter as the treatment would be the same? For many doctors it did matter and not only to help resolve aetiological uncertainties. They complained again that there had in fact been an 'overgrowth' of laboratory-based medical mycologists, which had led to fungal infections being over diagnosed and their clinical significance overstated.

Systemic candidiasis gained a higher medical profile in the 1960s and 1970s from its association with immunocompromised patients, either amongst those with diseases affecting the immune system, principally leukaemia in the 1960s, and in the growing number of patients on immunosuppressant therapies, principally anti-inflammatory drugs or anti-rejection drugs in transplant patients in the 1970s. In fact, the most important anti-rejection drug cyclosporine had been isolated from a fungus (*Tolypocladium inflatum*) by researchers at the Sandoz Company in Basel, Switzerland and initially viewed as an antifungal antibiotic.[131] However, in the 1980s the numbers of immunocompromised patients expanded greatly in profile and number with the arrival of HIV/AIDS. Very early in the epidemic, oral and oesophageal candidiasis were reported as opportunistic infections in AIDS sufferers; indeed, it was considered, along with Kaposi's sarcoma and pneumocystis pneumonia, as a marker of the disease.[132] By the mid-1980s, some estimates were that 75% of AIDS patients had oral candidiasis and doctors were recommending that any patient presenting with oral *Candida* infection in a high risk group should be screened for the infection.[133] From the early 1990s, when doctors differentiated between those who had AIDS related complex (ARC), – an early phase of the infection, and those with AIDS, the respective figures for *Candida* infection were 33% and 90%, respectively.[134]

From the early 1980s, doctors used nystatin and amphotericin B for oral thrush in AIDS patients, but the new azoles seemed to hold more promise.[135] They proved effective for the oral and oesophageal forms of candidiasis common in AIDS patients, though results for systemic disease were mixed.[136] However, another azole, fluconazole, came along in the mid-1980s. This drug, developed by Pfizer as 'UK-49,858' in their laboratories at Sandwich in Kent, was trialled as a superior alternative to ketoconazole, especially for all forms of candidiasis.[137] In 1989, de Wit and colleagues at the St Pierre University Hospital, Brussels, published the first trial comparing the new drug with ketoconazole in the treatment of oropharyngeal candidiasis in patients with AIDS and ARC.[138] They reported that fluconazole was not only more effective, but was less toxic and better tolerated.[139] However, it was unavailable in the United States and when the 'People with AIDS Health Group' heard of the potential of the drug, it acted as a buyer's club for patients. The Group announced that it would import the drug pending US approval, which was on an accelerated track, though not finally sanctioned by the FDA until January 1990.[140] Doctors added fluconazole to the range of drugs used, but treatment regimes varied greatly depending on the type of infection, likely patient compliance and cost. In addition, drugs were chosen in relation to the other fungal infections affecting AIDS patients, such as cryptococcosis, histoplasmosis and coccidioidomycosis.[141]

Candidiasis in AIDS patients, though common, was reasonably well controlled with azoles, along with better-tolerated forms of amphotericin B. Reported mortality from candidiasis peaked in HIV/AIDS sufferers in the mid-1990s, having done so in all patients in 1989.[142] What these trends meant was disputed. Frank Odds argued that the reported mortality for candidiasis was likely to be quite unreliable because it was not notifiable and diagnosis was variable. From close analysis of the available data for the United States, England and Wales, he concluded that while it was likely that there had been a 'real' increase in candidiasis mortality over the 1970s and 1980s, this had probably been 'exaggerated by a rise in enthusiasm for the study of candidosis [Odds preferred this term] and improved methods of diagnosis'.[143] However, he was in no doubt that the clinical incidence of the disease was higher because of the continuing rise in the numbers of immunocompromised patients and greater awareness of *Candida* infection.[144]

The fact that patients treated for systemic candidiasis were relatively small in number and typically had multiple disease problems meant that clinical trials with antifungals had not been of the same rigour as in other fields. In 1977, the NIH and National Institute of Allergy and Infectious Diseases (NIAID) had sought to develop better clinical trials with systemic fungal infections and convened a group to explore the matter. They met at Atlanta Airport and submitted a bid, led by William Dismukes, at University of Alabama School of Medicine in Birmingham for NIH funding.[145] The other members of the group were John Bennett (NIH), Gerald Medoff (St. Louis), Richard Duma (Virginia), Merle Sande (Virginia) and Harry Gallis (Charlotte) and they became known as the Mycoses Study Group (MSG). The MSG was awarded their first contract by NIAID in the following year and others followed for 27 years. This support allowed the establishment of 'a Central Administrative Core Unit based at the University of Alabama School of Medicine at Birmingham, a Central Biostatistics Unit, distinctly focused disease or population at-risk study groups with designated principal investigators, an annual meeting, and partial funding for various types of clinical trials or epidemiologic studies'.[146] The first trial, comparing amphotericin B alone and combined with flucytosine in the treatment of cryptococcal meningitis, was funded by NIAID and the John A. Hartford Foundation, and published in the *New England Journal of Medicine* in July 1979.[147] A year later they published guidelines for clinical trials with antifungal drugs and many other studies followed.[148]

A new problem in the final decades of the twentieth century was candidaemia – *C. albicans* infection of the blood that was mostly found as nosocomial infections, that is, those acquired in hospital. The 1979 edition of Frank Odds's *Candida and Candidosis* had no chapter on the condition, but the second edition in 1988 did, driven by the growing medical and public concern about hospital-acquired *Staphylococcus aureus* and in particular Methicillin-Resistant *Staphylococcus aureus* (MRSA).[149] Most nosocomial infection was bacterial, but up to 10% and rising was due to fungi, with *C. albicans* the most prevalent; indeed, mycoses were ranked third or fourth overall. Intensive care units were important places of infection because of the proliferation of sites where

C. albicans could either enter the body (e.g. catheters) or grow (monitoring sensors). In some cases, suspected septicaemia, the great dread of those managing high-dependency patients, was found to be candidaemia, which was soon placed amongst a number of systemic blood infections, termed 'fungaemia'. A review in 1995 claimed that over the 1980s the incidence of blood-stream infection due to *Candida* spp. increased by almost 500%, though again the question had to be asked, how much of this was due to greater awareness and better laboratory testing?[150]

The requirement for laboratory tests to confirm candidaemia and the new methods of identifying pathogens revealed that the dominance of *C. albicans* as the major cause of candidiasis was under threat from other species.[151] Whereas previously, *C. albicans* infection had been the default, the new molecular technologies of identification enabled faster and more accurate differentiation of species. These methods were used because clinicians needed to monitor the type and number of fungi due to the emergence of resistance to antifungal drugs. The development of resistance had been feared in the 1950s from the overuse of nystatin and amphotericin B, but this proved less of a problem in fungi than bacteria because resistance is not readily transmitted between strains. However, resistance did emerge in the late 1980s, following from the extensive and intensive use of fluconazole with AIDS patients. Initially, resistance was partial and overcome by increasing the dose, though in time other drugs became available, notably posaconazole and voriconazole. The pattern of drug use also affected the epidemiology of infective species; for example, use of fluconazole reduced the incidence of *C. albicans*, but facilitated the increase in *C. krusei,* which was resistant to the drug.[152] These epidemiological discoveries were made from case reviews and surveys of the usual suspects: patients with leukaemia; cancer sufferers and other patients on immunosuppressant therapies; those in intensive care or high-maintenance therapy, and those with HIV/AIDS. Moreover, it was of course around this group that the notion that candidiasis was 'the disease of the diseased' gained use and acceptance.

'The Yeast Connection'[153]

Writing in 1988 in the second edition of his book on *Candida*, Frank Odds was clear that there had been a 'public revolution in *Candida* consciousness' in the 1980s.[154] However, this was not due to greater awareness of systemic candidiasis, candidaemia, or infection in those with HIV/AIDS, but to two popular books: William Crook's *The Yeast Connection: A Medical Breakthrough* (1982) and Orian Truss's *The Missing Diagnosis* (1983).[155] Crook was a paediatrician, who had founded a Children's Clinic in the 1950s and served on the staff of the Jackson-Madison County General Hospital in West Tennessee. He developed an interest in chronic conditions in children, such as bedwetting, colic, migraine, fatigue and hyperactivity, coming to favour the idea that many of these were due to food allergies. He was a populariser, publishing in 1963 a general parenting advice book, *Answering parent's questions,* in the vein of Benjamin Spock, before three books on food allergies in the 1970s: *Your allergic child: a pediatrician's guide to normal living for allergic adults and children* (1973); *Can your child read? Is he hyperactive? A pediatrician's suggestions for helping the child with hyperactivity, behavior and learning problems* (1975); and *Are you allergic? A guide to normal living for allergic adults and children* (1978).[156] In 1979, Crook claimed that his life changed – he came across an article by Orian Truss on *Candida* infection and chronic diseases in adults in the *Journal of Orthomolecular Psychiatry*.[157]

Orian Truss had a private practice in Birmingham, Alabama and an interest in allergy and infection.[158] He was influenced by Linus Pauling's ideas on orthomolecular medicine.[159] Pauling had coined the term in 1968 to refer to 'the maintenance of health and cure of disease by regulating the concentration in the body of substances naturally found there'; this meant, literally, striving to have the 'right' chemicals at the 'right' levels in the body.[160] Pauling pursued this, most famously, in his support for megavitamin treatments, particularly vitamin C to manage the common cold, but initially his focus was on psychiatry. The subject was debated extensively in the early 1970s as dietary management was an attractive alternative to many of the new neuroleptic drugs and their side effects, but a report for the American Psychiatric Association in 1973 was highly critical.[161] However, orthomolecular medicine enjoyed popularity as an 'alternative' therapy, and, very unusually, one endorsed by a Nobel Prize winner for Physiology and Medicine.[162] Orthomolecular medicine was one of a number of alternative or fringe medical movements in the 1970s and 1980s that challenged orthodox medicine at every level and over the nature and treatment of most diseases.[163]

Orian Truss first aired his views on the health effects of yeast allergies and infections at the eighth Scientific Symposium of Academy of Orthomolecular Psychiatry in Toronto in May 1977. His talk was published in 1979. Truss argued that the persistence of a chronic infection in the body required 'the absence of an effective immunologic response to the pathogen' and that in chronic candidiasis, as in leprosy and tuberculosis, disseminated disease can be due to an 'antigenic load' overwhelming the immune defences.[164] In turn, a weakened immune system would predispose patients to local and general pathological conditions. He painted a picture of the patient with chronic candidiasis that would become very familiar in succeeding years; hence, it is worth quoting at length.

> A careful history that traces the illness from its onset suggests the diagnosis. It invariably includes a story of futile efforts by many competent specialists to establish an organic basis for the chronic illness, and of the almost irresistible recommendation of psychiatric therapy. Attention in the history should be directed to the influence of repeated pregnancies, birth-control pills, antibiotics, and cortisone and other immunosuppressants. The onset of local symptoms of yeast infection in relation to the use of these drugs is especially significant and usually precedes the systemic response. Repeated courses of antibiotics and birth-control pills, often punctuated with multiple pregnancies, lead to ever-increasing symptoms of mucosal infections in the vagina and gastrointestinal tract. Accompanying these are manifestations of tissue injury based on immunologic and possibly toxic responses to yeast products released into the systemic circulation. Many infections are secondary to allergic responses of the mucous membranes of the respiratory tract, urethra, and bladder, necessitating increasingly frequent antibiotic therapy that simultaneously aggravates and perpetuates the underlying cause of the allergic membrane that allowed the infection. Depression is common, often associated with difficulty in memory, reasoning and concentration. These symptoms are especially severe in women, who in addition have great difficulty with the explosive irritability, crying, and loss of self-confidence that are so characteristic of abnormal function of the ovarian hormones. Poor end-organ response to these sex hormones is confirmed by the common association of acne, impairment or total loss of libido, and the whole range of abnormalities of menstrual bleeding and cramps, as well as a very high incidence of endometriosis in those who have undergone hysterectomy. Many of these patients also start developing multiple intolerances to foods and chemicals, making it increasingly difficult for them to live in a normal environment. Many or all of these intolerances disappear as the yeast problem is brought under control.[165]

Table 3.1 Treatment of chronic candidiasis[166]

I.	**Non-immunologic measures that retard yeast proliferation**
A.	Passive: measures of avoidance
1.	Diet: low in carbohydrates and in foods with high yeast or meld content
2.	Antibiotics
3.	Contraceptive hormones
4.	Environments characterised by high meld-spore exposure
B.	Active: therapy with antifungal drugs: nystatin, amphotericin-B, flucytosine, ketoconazole
II.	**Measures to strengthen the immune response of the host**
A.	Passive (avoidance): immunosuppressant drugs
B.	Active
1.	Diet: adequate nutrients for proper immune response
2.	Correction of unrelated conditions that impair the immune response, for example, hypothyroidism
3.	Use of extracts of *C. albicans*
a.	Extracts
b.	Testing
c.	Treatment

Truss's treatments aimed to restore immunological 'competence' and, as seen below in Table 3.1, while his preventive and treatment regimens recommended avoiding antibiotics and immunosuppressants, they included the use of antifungal drugs. Therefore, while presenting himself to readers as a holistic, alternative practitioner, Truss was a quite pragmatic in his clinical work and used the full range of orthodox drugs, including nystatin and the new azoles.

Truss also drew inspiration from the work of Theron G. Randolph, the 'father of clinical ecology' and his idea that a key determinant for health in modern societies was to avoid exposure to chemical contaminants of air and water, including antibiotics.[167] Clinical ecologists were on the fringe of American medicine, as signalled in 1981, when the California Medical Association (CMA) adopted the position that clinical ecology does not constitute a valid medical discipline. The critique, widely endorsed by medical organisations, stated that scientific and clinical evidence does not support the diagnosis of 'environmental illness' and 'cerebral allergy', and that evidence is lacking for the concept of massive environmental allergy.[168]

In the preface of *The Yeast Connection*, William Crook wrote that he had read Truss's paper on *C. albicans* and chronic illness in the summer of 1979 and immediately tried the suggested treatment regime on one of his difficult patients, 'a 41-year old woman (I'll call her Nancy Jones) with severe chronic hives [urticaria], accompanied by mental confusion, fatigue and depression'.[169] He started her on nystatin and a yeast-free, low carbohydrate diet. Within six days her hives had improved, in weeks they disappeared and after almost a year all her symptoms had improved. Crook reported trying the regimen with another 20 patients.

> Nearly all were adults with complex health problems, including headache, fatigue, depression, recurrent vaginal infection, joint pain and sensitivity to chemical odours and additives. Almost without exception, they improved. And some improved dramatically.[170]

He continued ad hoc variations in his treatments, extending the range of conditions and ages, eventually to include his paediatric patients. In the meantime, Truss had been featured in the 'Dan Freeman Report' on CNN in September 1981, an appearance that allegedly brought more responses than any previous programme.

In was not long before Truss and Crook joined forces and they did so first at an 'informal' conference they called on '*C. albicans* and the relationship to human disease' in Dallas, Texas, in July 1982.[171] This was attended by 20 physicians and an equal number of patients. Crook made his television debut on the subject in Cincinnati in January 1983, in a broadcast that led to 7,300 requests for more information and his decision to write *The Yeast Connection*. In the meantime, Truss self-published *The Missing Diagnosis*; but it was Crook and his book that gained the public's attention, not least because he was accessible to the media and an effective communicator. The first print run of *The Yeast Connection* in 1983 quickly sold out. He claimed that 270,000 copies were purchased in the first two years. Crook wrote in the preface that, already, 'my recognition of "the yeast connection" has changed my life and my practice and had enabled me to help many, many patients conquer previously disabling illnesses'. The book was in its fourth edition in 1986.

Crook soon had wider ambitions, hoping to forge what he saw as 'The Coming Revolution in Medicine'.[172] He had written *The Yeast Connection* as a self-help manual, with checklists, diagrams, illustrations and clear preventive and therapeutic advice on necessary changes in lifestyle and diet, including recipes, and special measures for different patient groups. One of the most controversial features of the book was its 10-point self-diagnosis schedule, where three or four 'yes' answers suggested that 'yeasts played a role in your symptoms'.[173] The explanation of the causes of yeast overgrowth was presented in words and graphics. Crook's advice was threefold: first, 'avoid foods which promote yeast growth'; second, seek a prescription from your doctor for 'medication which helps rid your body of yeast germs' (nystatin or ketoconazole); and, third, make changes to your lifestyle and behaviour. In the early 1980s, taking prescription antifungal drugs was an integral part of the treatment and the merits of nystatin and ketoconazole were discussed in some detail.[174] However, later and in the hands of other advocates, the self-help and 'alternative' features took over, as the regime moved to a natural therapy, not least because many doctors refused patients antifungal drugs as they did not accept that 'fungal overgrowth' was a disease or syndrome at all.

The popular success of Truss and Crook brought imitators who linked *Candida* overgrowth directly to other, so-called, 'twentieth century diseases'.[175] In the hands of Truss and Crook, 'fungal overgrowth' had always been linked to allergies and infection, and to chemical sensitivities, hyperactivity and mental disorders.[176] Soon the illnesses they had identified were medicalised by other doctors, with such names as the *Candida* syndrome, *Candida* allergy syndrome, the yeast syndrome, polysystemic chronic candidiasis, chronic candidiasis syndrome and, most commonly, candidiasis hypersensitivity syndrome (CHS). In June 1984, Crook branched out from popular writing and appearances to advance 'The Yeast Connection' to the American medical profession. His chosen subject was depression and he wrote a letter to the *Journal of the American Medical Association* suggesting that the condition was 'commonly related to prolonged or repeated courses of broad-spectrum antibiotics or to birth control pills, which promote the overgrowth of *C. albicans* on mucous membranes'.[177] He acknowledged that the 'mechanisms involved still have not been clearly elucidated', but wrote that he had good evidence 'from clinical history, followed by a therapeutic response to oral nystatin and a yeast-free, low-carbohydrate diet'. His views were rounded upon by several correspondents, who dismissed his claims as lacking evidence and being based on multiple misconceptions.[178]

The following year, several medical organisations attacked Crook, Truss and their followers. The American Academy of Allergy and Immunology was worried by the attention being given to CHS and in August 1986 published a position statement in its journal.[179] The Practice Standards Committee found 'multiple problems with the candidiasis hypersensitivity syndrome'; principally that 'the concept is speculative and unproven' and that 'elements of the proposed treatment program are potentially dangerous'. The Committee stated that 'basic elements of the syndrome would apply to almost all sick patients at some time' and that 'the broad treatment program would produce remission in most illnesses regardless of cause.' Moreover, there was 'no published proof that *C. albicans* is responsible for the syndrome' or that 'treatment ... with specific antifungal agents ... benefits the syndrome.' The dangers in the treatment regimes were that the promiscuous use of drugs would produce resistant strains of *C. albicans* and of that there could be long-term effects with patients on systemic antifungals for many years. In November 1987, at a meeting on Controversies in Infectious Disease, John E. Edwards of (UCLA) attacked Crook and those on his bandwagon.[180] His description nicely captured the frustrations of regular medicine.

> Certain generalizations can be made regarding 'the yeast connection.' The symptoms described by the authors are generalized and affect nearly every organ system. As listed, some symptoms are widely diverse; for instance, both fatigue and hyperactivity are included. Nearly every normal individual has had certain of these symptoms during the course of a normal lifespan. Case reports are anecdotal. Possibly none of the authors have had formal training in the disciplines of allergy and immunology, infectious diseases, or mycology. After nearly a decade since the original description, no articles on this disease appear in peer reviewed journals included in the Index Medicus. There are no prospective controlled therapeutic studies, and there are no animal model data.[181]

A year later, the Canadian Paediatric Society warned that, 'Physicians must not be swayed by the attention that the syndrome has attracted in the lay press.'[182]

The Yeast Connection was published in Britain in the summer of 1988. Chronic candidiasis had been discussed in the popular press for a couple of years and linked to myalgic encephalomyelitis (ME) or post-viral fatigue syndrome (PVFS).[183] In *The Observer,* Sue Finlay wrote that ME was 'An illness doctors don't recognise', but which she had overcome by following the diet recommended in Leon Chaitow's *Candida albicans: Could Yeast Be Your Problem?*[184] Clinical ecologists also gained a hearing in Britain. One described *Candida* overgrowth as 'the quiet epidemic that is ruining modern lifestyles', due to the specific condition of 'dysbiosis [abnormal intestinal flora]' and to '[t]he burgeoning of complex viral infections such as AIDS and ME – and, to a lesser extent, Herpes'.[185] In these conditions, it was claimed, 'candidiasis was almost always present as an immune-sapping illness'.

Although there was a pathological theory behind *The Yeast Connection*, Crook relied on the claim that the real test of his ideas and recommendations was in the clinic. He once said, 'There's not a single test to prove it, but it works' and used emotive case histories to great effect; such as that of Darlene Lindbom of Paris, Tennessee, who 'went to two universities in a wheelchair. "You've got something like MS", they told her – she had spinal taps, biopsies, the lot. I put her on my special diet and nystatin. Now she's fit and runs a successful business.'[186] Crook visited London to promote his ideas in June 1988, which the *Guardian* styled the 'thrush theory'. He stressed the link to food allergies and found a forum with the British Society for Allergy and Environmental Medicine, which had links with the British Society for Nutritional Medicine.[187] Both meetings were regarded as 'alternative' by the mainstream British medical profession and studiously ignored.

In 1989 the first clinical trials with patients reporting the 'Yeast Connection' were published. Lisa Renfro and colleagues at the Department of Pediatrics and Family Medicine at Farmington, Connecticut, reported on 100 consecutive patients suffering from chronic fatigue, eight of whom believed their symptoms were due to chronic candidiasis.[188] The article concluded that the authors were 'unable to find physical or laboratory findings that were different from the 92 other patients with chronic fatigue'. However, they did find that 'patients with the yeast connection were more likely to be taking high doses of vitamins and were more likely to be getting help from non-medical caretakers. In fact, these caretakers might be the source of the diagnosis.'[189] They went on to conclude that all but one sufferer had depression or an anxiety disorder, and that, from the point of view of achieving a positive outcome, not dismissing chronic candidiasis might be beneficial in allowing a therapeutic relationship between doctor and patient to be maintained. The following year a similar study was published by doctors at the University of Alabama Medical School in Birmingham, Crook's local stomping ground.[190] This was a state-of-the-art randomised, double-blind trial of nystatin therapy in CHS, which concluded that, while patients on the trial improved, as was to be expected, the study had provided 'additional objective evidence that the syndrome is not a verifiable condition'.[191] An accompanying editorial in the *New England Journal of Medicine* anticipated that supporters of the yeast connection would not be impressed and, as expected, Crook and others wrote in pointing to successful treatment in with many patients.[192]

In Britain, the yeast connection only attracted sustained medical criticism in the early 1990s and then in the context of a complex debate that linked allergies, food intolerance and alternative medicine. These issues crystallised in a report by the Royal College of Physicians on *Allergy: Conventional and Alternative Concepts*, in 1992, which stated the '*Candida* theory is unsubstantiated'.[193] Responses quickly appeared in 'alternative' medical publications, particularly in the *Journal of Nutritional Medicine*; however, the specifics of the '*Candida* theory' were lost in a larger dispute on the status of 'alternative' medicine.[194] In July 1992, Keith Mumby, Britain's most high-profile clinical ecologist, appeared before the General Medical Council (GMC) and was found guilty of 'touting for charges' and failing to give a patient adequate medical attention.[195] This led the main author of the College's Report on *Allergy*, Barry Kay, to argue that the 'GMC should consider censoring all forms of diagnosis and treatment which, by reasonable standards, have consistently failed to show clinical efficacy'. Mumby was allowed to reply in an article entitled 'Science or flat earthers? The clinical ecologist replies'.[196] This was almost the last word, as the stridency and frequency of the medical establishment's assault of alternative practitioners waned, though patient demand in Britain and the United States continued to grow.[197] In medicine, CHS was gradually absorbed into a number of, what became known as, 'symptom-based conditions', which included chronic fatigue syndrome, fibromyalgia, multiple chemical sensitivities, sick building syndrome, Gulf War syndrome and irritable bowel syndrome.[198] Crook continued to publish, seeking niche markets with cook books and patient-specific audiences: women, children with, attention deficit disorder and autism, and people with chronic fatigue syndrome.[199] Many other authors expanded the genre, with titles such as *The Candida Control Cookbook* (1996), *Feast Without Yeast: 4 stages to better health* (1999), and *Complete Candida Yeast Guidebook: everything you need to know about prevention, treatment, & diet* (2000). However, the medical profession increasingly ignored CHS, except to dismiss it, especially because of the new emphasis on evidence-based medicine and the Gold Standard of double blind controlled clinical trials.[200]

Antibiotics were the icon of mid-twentieth-century medical progress and their development influenced *Candida* infection in complex ways. As thrush, the disease came to the fore in the post-war years when nystatin, the first antifungal antibiotic, was introduced and brought women with the vaginal infection to the clinic. Doctors believed that previously the condition had been self-treated or accepted, perhaps self-limiting, but had certainly been underreported. At the same time, the use of antibacterial antibiotics, especially broad-spectrum formulations, by clearing the body of its natural microbial fauna, seemed to open the body to topical infection. New clothing may have been a factor too, with stretch synthetic fabrics making underwear more close fitting and impermeable. Antibiotics were also implicated in systemic or invasive candidiasis, as the numbers of vulnerable patients multiplied. Amongst cancer patients, steroid and other treatments depressed the immune system, as did blood cancers like leukaemia. Some of the new systemic candidiasis patients suffered from iatrogenic conditions. The principal groups were transplant patients, those in intensive care, those maintained with serious chronic conditions and then people with HIV/AIDS. However, the rising tide of candidiasis was met with new antifungal antibiotics, especially azole drugs and, by the 1990s the management of systemic candidiasis was more successful. In the 1980s another new type of candidiasis emerged, CHS, which although dismissed by mainstream medicine as a fiction and a fad, became the archetypal 'disease of modernity'. Its alleged cause, overgrowth of *C. albicans* in the body, was linked to many features of modern life, including the overuse of antibiotics. It was not without irony, therefore, that, alongside lifestyle and dietary changes, taking the antifungal antibiotics produced by the modern pharmaceutical industry was also recommended.

4

Regionally Specific Fungal Infections

In 1950, the Biology Section of the New York Academy of Science (NYAS) held what it claimed to be the first conference on medical mycology in the United States.[1] What prompted the event was not the announcement of the discovery of nystatin by Hazen and Brown, as their publication was still in press, but the growing profile of fungi and fungal infections across the nation. Fungi, not least because of interest in penicillin, were attracting the interest of biologists and biomedical researchers who, alongside screens for antibiotic activity, were adopting them as experimental models in studies of nutrition, physiology and immunology.[2] All the leading names of the field from the 1930s attended the meeting: Carroll Dodge, Norman Conant, Rhoda Benham and Lucille Georg, and there were new faces who had developed expertise during the war and in particular localities. Speakers drew attention to the increased incidence of systemic candidiasis, signalling a switch in the medical mycological gaze from external (exogenous) to internal (endogenous) disease. Although the incidence of endogenous, systemic fungal infections was very low, they had very high mortality and presented unusual cases that fascinated physicians. In addition, there was a new awareness of the toll of morbidity from endemic, exogenous disease, as with athlete's foot and thrush, and with regionally specific, often sub-clinical infections, principally coccidioidomycosis, blastomycosis and histoplasmosis.

In this chapter, we tell the story of regionally specific fungal infections, and look at the rise of fungal-induced asthma, as one part of the twentieth-century story of the rise of allergies and asthma.[3] We begin by discussing the new epidemiology of endemic fungal infections that emerged in the late 1940s and the attempts by medical mycologists and other interested clinicians to attract more resources for research, prevention and control. We discussed the increased incidence of acute, invasive candidiasis associated with new medical treatments in the last Chapter; here we examine in turn the three principal chronic, though occasionally epidemic, regional mycoses prevalent in North America – coccidioidomycosis, blastomycosis and histoplasmosis. Our attention then switches to Britain and allergic fungal conditions, firstly, farmer's lung and then allergic bronchopulmonary aspergillosis (ABPA). This class of fungal allergens was 'discovered' in Britain and seemingly absent from North America, until expertise was transferred back across the Atlantic.

The new epidemiology of fungal diseases

In the early 1950s, medical mycologists, along with cancer physicians and chest surgeons, began to draw attention to a new problem posed by invasive fungal infections. Writing in 1953, David Smith, a colleague of Norman Conant at Duke Medical School described the new situation as follows.

> Unlike most bacterial and viral infectious diseases, the systemic mycotic infections are not transmitted directly from patient to patient; consequently, one would not expect to see epidemics caused by fungi. In most instances the mycotic infections are endemic and sporadic but true epidemics of sporotrichosis, coccidioidomycosis and histoplasmosis do occur when groups of non-immune individuals are exposed to an environment containing large amounts of the saprophytic form of the fungus. More than a thousand cases of sporotrichosis developed in the gold mines of South Africa when the timbers in the mine became infected with *Sporotrichum schenckii*. Epidemics of coccidioidomycosis occurred when companies of non-immune soldiers from the East marched in the dust of certain South-western deserts. Epidemics of histoplasmosis have occurred following the exposure of groups of nonimmune individuals to pigeon manure, chicken manure, bat manure in caves and to the dust of unused silos.[4]

Reviewing the epidemiology of fungal infections in the same year for the *New England Journal of Medicine*, Otis Jillson pointed to 'the recognition of the benign, common forms of histoplasmosis; the diagnosis and surgical treatment of coccidioidal pulmonary residua; the treatment of blastomycosis with stilbenes', and added the growing incidence of systemic mycoses.[5] Interestingly, he dealt with skin infections briefly and said very little about exogenous or endogenous candidiasis, at a time when nystatin was attracting attention.

At the 1950 NYAS meeting, Samuel B. Salvin, then at the Division of Infectious Diseases at NIH, placed the incidence of fungal diseases in context of other infectious diseases.

> Fungus infections in man, although less frequent than bacterial, are still numerically important. For example, of the 92,933 deaths due to infections and parasitic diseases in the United States in 1945, 284, or 0.3 per cent, were due to mycoses. This was approximately equal to the number of deaths reported as caused by scarlet fever, measles, or the typhus-like diseases (due to rickettsia), and was more than the total of all deaths recorded from rabies, smallpox, relapsing fever, leprosy, brucellosis, paratyphoid fever, plague, cholera, and anthrax. It should be realized, of course, that effective control measures are employed against some of the aforementioned diseases, whereas control methods against the mycoses not only are not practiced, but, generally, are not even known. It should also be borne in mind that the dermatophytoses, although characteristically nonfatal, are extremely common, probably equalling the most widespread of the bacterial or virus diseases in prevalence.[6]

In 1953, Walter Nickerson from the Department of Microbiology, Rutgers University, tried a creative presentation of mortality data to chart the rise of fungal infections.[7] He used graphs for the period 1945–1949 that showed starkly opposite mortality trends, where 'all infections' had dropped sharply, while that from mycoses had increased markedly. Nickerson had produced his graphic illustration by using very different scales for the two classes of infection. Deaths from mycoses were recorded as actual numbers, while those from all infections were recorded in thousands. The alarming increase of nearly 50% in fungal infection deaths was actually from 270 to 380, while the actual number of deaths from all infections had fallen 30%, from 93,000 to 66,000 deaths – still 170 times greater! In the event, the annual total deaths from mycoses in the next decade never reached 500.[8] More telling was Nickerson's point about morbidity; he stated that 'mycotic infections are probably the mostly widely distributed and most numerous types of infection, with dermatophyte infections, such as athlete's foot, alone as prevalent as the most widespread of the bacterial and virus diseases'.[9]

Medical mycologists had long argued for recognition of the distinctive pathogenicity of fungi. In 1940, Arthur Henrici, who worked in the Department of Bacteriology at the University of Minnesota, argued that most bacterial and viral infections developed rapidly, and then plateaued in severity, before falling away, because of either recovery or death. With fungal infections, however, a typical pattern was of the slow and incremental development of chronicity, and prolonged morbidity, often at sub-clinical levels.[10] The only bacterial diseases with similar patterns of pathogenicity were tuberculosis and leprosy. Henrici maintained that the slow increase in severity meant either that the infecting fungus progressively changed and developed pathogenic properties or that the resistance of the host was gradually worn down. There was no evidence of the former, so he focused on changes in the host and its 'soil', claiming that prolonged exposure to certain fungi and their toxins produced hypersensitivity in the host cells. Henrici referred back to the theories of Richard Pfeiffer and Clemens von Pirquet on overactive immune responses.[11] Pfeiffer's authority was drawn upon for the argument that fungal endotoxins inflamed and ultimately killed cells, creating a nidus for the fungus itself to grow. On the other hand, von Pirquet's work was used to suggest that host cells developed allergic-type sensitivity. Henrici favoured the latter, but stressed that because fungal infections were complex and variable, both mechanisms might operate, or be found with different species of pathogen.

The prevalence of sub-clinical, chronic disease was recognised by public health officials as characteristic of regionally specific mycoses in the United States. The new geography of endemic fungal infections was revealed by David Smith in 1953, on a map that showed the distribution of coccidioidomycosis, blastomycosis and histoplasmosis in the United States and northern Mexico[12] (Figure 4.1). The new epidemiological profile changed the position of medical mycology in the United States in the 1950s. This was evident first in the proliferation of new publications and courses.[13] Ana Espinel-Ingroff's analysis of the institutional development of medical mycology shows that new departments and new experts emerged in affected areas, for example, at Michigan State University (1951), Tulane University (1955), the University of California, Los Angeles (1956), the University of Oklahoma (1957) and Virginia Commonwealth University (1965).[14] Initiatives took place in varied settings, sometimes with public health departments, but mostly in university biology and microbiology departments. That said, leading figures and departments in the East remained important. Norman Conant, Chester Emmons and Libero Ajello continued to head key departments at Columbia, Duke and the National Microbiological Institute, which was reorganised from 1955 as the National Institute of Allergy and Infectious Diseases (NIAID) and, of course, the Centers for Disease Control and Prevention (CDC) in Atlanta remained influential.

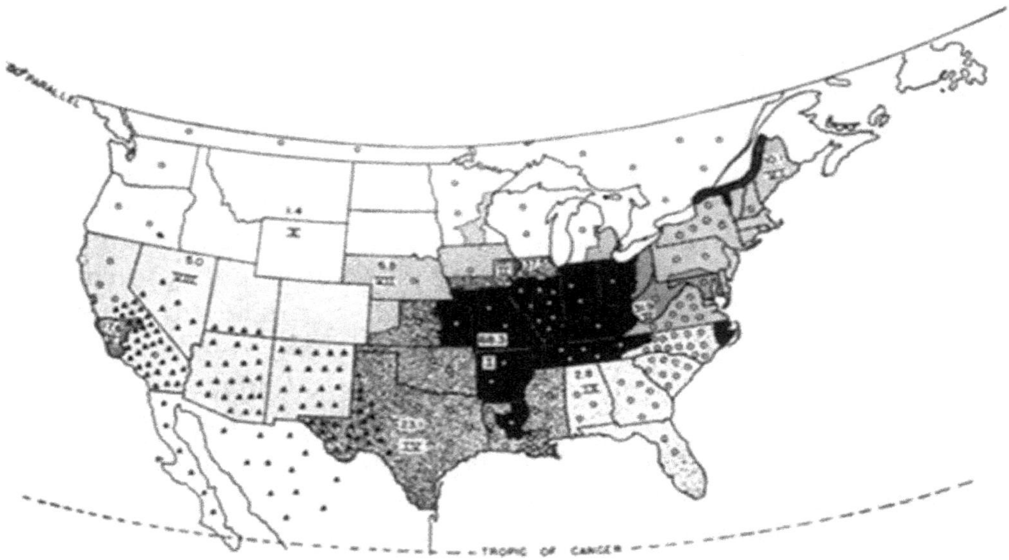

Figure 4.1 Distribution of histoplasmosis, blastomycosis and coccidioidomycosis in North America.[15] The histoplasmosis areas are shown in black, the blastomycosis as circles and the coccidioidomycosis areas as triangles. Smith, D. T., 'The diagnosis and therapy of mycotic infections', *Bull NY Acad Med*, 1953, 29(10): 778. This figure © 2013 New York Academy of Medicine used under Creative Commons Attribution – Non-commercial

Regional mycoses I: 'Valley fever' – coccidioidomycosis

The first regionally specific infection to attract attention was coccidioidomycosis through Emmons's work at NIH.[16] The very notion of the geographically specific infection had weakened in medicine in the second half of the nineteenth century with the move towards aetiological definitions of disease and the essential role of specific germs. However, there was new interest in the early twentieth century with vector-borne tropical diseases, where the range of insects was limited by biogeographical factors.[17] In the United States this was evident in the work on tick-borne Rocky Mountain Spotted Fever, which had its highest prevalence in certain states: North Carolina, Oklahoma, Arkansas, Tennessee, and Missouri.[18]

In the 1940s, coccidioidomycosis, also styled as 'San Joaquin' or 'Valley fever', was known to be caused by the fungus *Coccidioides immitis* (*C. immitis*).[19] Its mode of spread was seemingly simple: fungal spores, released from the soil, entered the body through the lungs, where an infection might develop. In fact, most people did not develop any symptoms and those that did experienced a cold or mild flu-like symptoms. In a tiny fraction of people, especially those with other diseases and with weakened immune systems, infection spread through the bloodstream to give disseminated coccidioidomycosis.

Research by Ernest C. Dickson and Charles Smith in the 1930s had revealed that infection with *C. immitis* was very common amongst those living in certain areas, and that it was best regarded as an endemic, chronic and benign infection.[20] It seemed that residents built up immunity from long-term, low-level exposure, hence most infection was sub-clinical and, as would be expected, clinical disease was most common amongst in-migrants who had not had the opportunity to build up immunity. Population movement and settlement westwards had been going on in the United States for many decades and it seemed likely that coccidioidomycosis emerged at this particularly moment because of the new speed and scale of migration, especially families fleeing dust blows in the prairies. Evidence to support this view came in the 1940s when coccidioidomycosis developed amongst the recruits brought to the region to train for the United States Air Force.[21] As the war effort grew, more troops arrived, which gave investigators the opportunity to make comparisons of incidence by sex, race and nationality. For instance, some 13,000 German prisoners of war were held at Florence, Arizona, where the incidence of coccidioidomycosis became so high that they were moved away, as United States government officials worried that such a high rate of infection would lead to them being charged with violation of the Geneva Convention on treatment of war prisoners.[22]

After the war, the military presence in the Southwest continued and expanded. So too did worries about coccidioidomycosis and this led in 1955 to the establishment of an annual meeting of the Veterans Administration-Armed Forces Coccidioidomycosis Cooperative Study Group (CCSG). This type of cooperative meeting had begun in the late 1940s as a way of developing and sharing expertise on the treatment of tuberculosis with streptomycin.[23] Initially, the main agencies were the Veterans Administration, the Army, the Navy, Public Health Services and the National Research Council. While the focus of the early annual conferences was squarely on tuberculosis, fungal infections were sometimes discussed, as in 1952 when trial coordinators noted that histoplasmosis lung infections had complicated their clinical trials by making differential diagnosis with X-rays more difficult.[24] The first coccidioidomycosis meeting in 1955 came from a direct concern with the growing incidence of the infection, especially at air bases, notably Williams AFB and Luke AFB in Arizona, Edwards AFB in California, and Lemoore NAS, also in California. The problem grew with the investments in military infrastructure that came with the Cold War. Williams and Luke became training centres, with a steady stream of non-immune recruits passing through, while Lemoore was further developed in the 1960s for strike aircraft, and Edwards became a centre for research, including rocketry, and eventually was a landing site for the Space Shuttle.

The construction of new runways and other facilities on these military sites disturbed the subsoil, which together with aircraft take-offs and landings circulated *C. immitus* spores to those living and working nearby.[25] Some civilian sufferers were treated by military doctors; however, they were mostly dealt with by local physicians, who also treated military personnel when they were referred to local hospitals for serological and radiological investigation. Thus, the leading authority on the disease in the military, from the 1940s to the 1960s, was Charles E. Smith, Dean of Public Health at the University of California Berkeley.[26] He had developed his expertise during the Second World War at Berkeley, where he established a research laboratory and diagnostic serological services.

In the 1950s *C. immitus* biology was found to be more complicated than previously recognised and the new understanding was set out in the first book entirely on the disease by Marshall J. Fiese in 1958.[27] Fiese was based at the Veterans Administration Hospital in Fresno and in his 'Foreword' to Fiese's volume, Charles Smith wrote that the work reflected the author's deep experience: '[Fiese] has seen and viewed.... countless roentgenograms[X rays], seen and studied the tragic autopsies, and perhaps most importantly of all, lived for years in the coccidioidal countryside.' An unusual feature of *C. immitis* was that, rather than being spread by spores, it was actually the cells of the hyphae, called conidia, that circulated in the air. Conidia were found to be tiny and readily carried in dust; hence, the popular representation of coccidioidomycosis as spread by 'flying conidia', or 'flying chlamydospores'.[28] When inhaled, the human body was shown to respond in one of three possible ways. First and most commonly, the conidia were destroyed by the immune system and a degree of immunity, albeit variable, to future infection was established. Alternatively, the conidia grew in the lungs in a spherical form, into bodies that released many more such 'spherules', producing inflammation and a chest infection. Lastly and least common, and only if the lung infection was severe, infection could spread in the blood and cause inflammation, especially in the skin and brain. The reported incidence of the severe form increased in the 1960s and was found principally amongst patients and former patients who were to some degree immuno-compromised.[29]

Local physicians in Arizona and California had mostly to deal with the second type of endemic infection, which was often self-limiting.[30] Particular occupational groups were at higher risk of developing the disease, notably, agricultural and construction workers. Archaeologists were another high-risk group, and often had severe infection because they were new to a region. The profile of coccidioidomycosis rose in sporadic epidemic outbreaks, as in California at the end of 1977. A large dust storm blew through Bakersfield on 20 December, depositing conidia to the north and west along familiar terrain in the San Joaquin Valley.[31] Cases were reported in two main areas: the known endemic area of Kern County around Bakersfield and a previously non-endemic area west of Sacramento. Within six months, 142 cases of clinical lung disease had been identified in Kern County and 379 at the University of California Davis (UCD), nearly 300 miles north, with sufferers from Los Angeles and Oakland, as well as Sacramento. Public health officials reported that rainfall immediately after the storm had probably reduced significantly the number of cases; however, they worried that conidia had drained into the subsoil and that new endemic areas might be created.[32] Demosthenes Pappagianis, a member of the Department of Medical Microbiology at UCD who had led the local response to the epidemic, became a leading researcher on the epidemiology of the disease in subsequent decades[33] (Figure 4.2).

In the early 1990s, there was another epidemic, later termed 'the great coccidioidomycosis outbreak'. Reported cases of the infection rose from a long-term average of 300–600, to 1,200 in 1991, to 4,541 in 1992 and 4,107 in 1993.[34] The foci were in the south of the San Joaquin Valley in Kern and Tulare counties. Pappagianis was brought in to investigate. He found no obvious precipitating reason for the outbreak, and instead looked to climatic factors, notably the long-term drought and high spring rainfall in 1991 and 1992, to soil disturbance from construction; and to possible new groups of susceptible in-migrants.[35] The outbreak brought national attention to coccidioidomycosis and a CDC-led investigation, whose interest was in both endemicity and the extent of acute and disseminated disease.[36] Their study concluded that with the aging of the US population and the increase in the number of immunosuppressed persons, severe pulmonary and disseminated coccidioidomycosis threaten to become important public health problems in areas of endemicity.[37] Pappagianis also contributed to an investigation of an outbreak following an earthquake in Northridge,

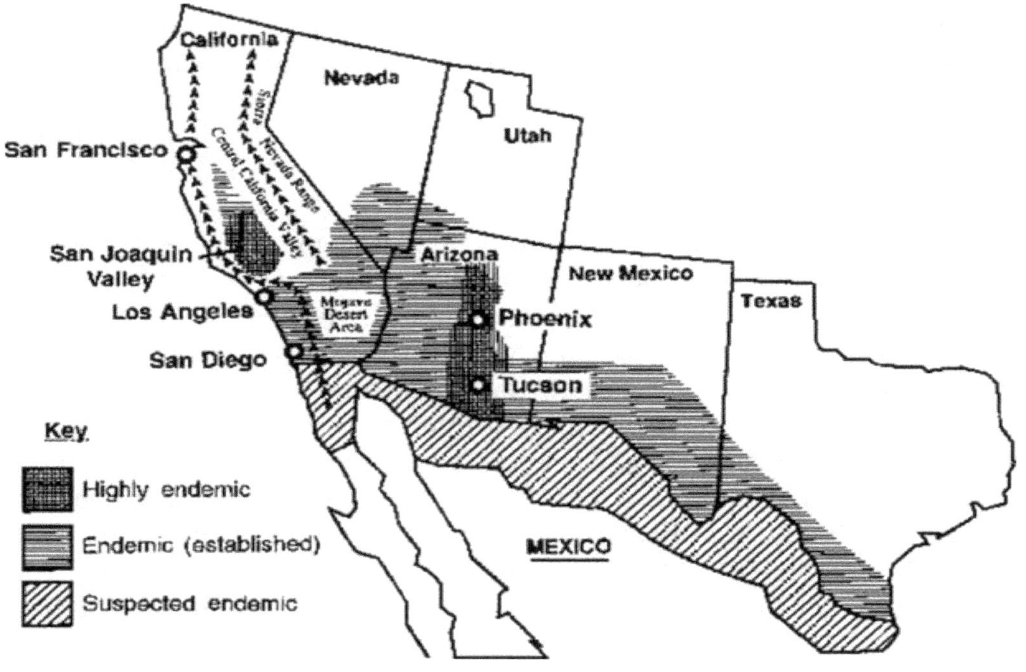

Figure 4.2 The geographic distribution of coccidioidomycosis. Cross-hatching indicates the heavily disease-endemic area, single hatching and the moderately disease-endemic area.[38] Kirkland, T. N. and Fierer, J., 'Coccidioidomycosis: A reemerging infectious disease', *Emerg Infect Dis* [serial on the Internet]. 1996, Sep.

California in January 1994, to which 203 cases were linked and three coccidioidomycosis deaths added to the overall toll of 57.[39]

In addition to Pappagianis, two other researchers stood out in the study of coccidioidomycosis during the period. One was John Galgiani, who worked at the Veterans Affairs Medical Center and University of Arizona, Tucson, and was the leading expert on coccidioidomycosis in that state. His specialism was immune responses and he was amongst the first to publish on coccidioidomycosis in AIDS sufferers.[40] Over many years he campaigned for recognition that coccidioidomycosis was becoming a disease of national importance, because of continuing high rates of in-migration to Southwestern states and the increase in the number of immunosuppressed patients. General population mobility was also a factor, with many cases presenting outside of endemic areas in out-migrants; indeed, he reported that 46% of coccidioidomycosis patients with AIDS were in non-endemic areas.[41] In 1996, coccidioidomycosis was being discussed as 'a re-emerging infectious disease'.[42]

Theo Kirkland and Joshua Fierer, respectively, from the San Diego School of Medicine and Department of Veterans Affairs Medical Center, San Diego, wrote that it warranted the label because 'the number of cases... has increased dramatically, and the clinical symptoms of this illness have changed in patients with acquired immunodeficiency syndrome (AIDS)'.[43]

The second key researcher was David A. Stevens, who was based in the Santa Clara Valley Medical Center, San José and the Stanford University School of Medicine. He became a leading authority on the clinical management of coccidioidomycosis, especially the use of chemotherapy. His expertise, developed along with that on the treatment of aspergillosis and other opportunistic mycoses, was recognised in leadership roles and honours in the Medical Mycological Society of the Americas (MMSA), International Society for Human and Animal Mycology (ISHAM) and the American Society for Microbiology (ASM). Stevens's early career work was on viruses, but he switched to fungi in 1974 with a study of immunity to *C. immitis* and then to its treatment.[44] With Hillel B. Levine, he pioneered the use of one of the new azoles, miconazole, for coccidioidomycosis.[45] In 1980, he edited a new textbook on the disease, contributing chapters on immunology, other syndromes, immuno-compromised hosts, chemotherapy immunotherapy, vaccination and a bibliography.[46] Stevens enrolled Pappagianis to write on epidemiology and serology, and Galgiani on ophthalmic disease.

By the 1970s, the Cooperative Study Group meetings, which began under military sponsorship, had moved to civilian control, with Stevens, Galgiani and Pappagianis taking leading roles. However, as early as 1957 a larger symposium had been called and that met every eight years or so, styling itself as 'international' for the first time when it met in Tucson in 1977.[47] This change reflected two developments: first, greater interest in the disease in Mexico and South America and second, the experience of physicians across borders with serological diagnosis and amphotericin B treatment of disseminated disease.[48] Furthermore, after the Californian coccidioidomycosis outbreak in 1977, a growing number of laboratories had begun to explore vaccine development, utilising the tools of the new molecular biology.[49] Indeed, a vaccine developed by Pappagianis and Levine went on trial in 1981, but this showed little or no benefit.[50] Attention was also directed to ethnic and social groups that were at greater risk from the disease, particularly black men, Native Americans, and pregnant women. With the former, researchers explored the contribution of racial susceptibility and environmental factors, with a consensus developing around the importance of the latter.

Researchers found that exposure, socio-economic position and access to health care were the most important determinants of vulnerability to infection and the development of disease.[51] Pregnant women were thought to be vulnerable because of changes in their immunity and hormonal levels, but close study showed them to have, at worst, only a tiny additional likelihood of developing disseminated disease.[52] In the 1980s, as would have been expected, more coccidioidomycosis was reported in immuno-compromised patients in Southwestern states, and also across the United States in people who had lived or travelled to the endemic areas. Thus, the work of regional coccidioidomycosis experts linked up with that of mycologically minded clinicians nationwide. Their research and clinical experience put them in a good position to assume national leadership roles in the field. For example, David Stevens led the NIH multicentre clinical trials group on antifungal drugs between 1990 and 2000 and chaired committees writing practice guidelines on aspergillosis as well as coccidioidomycosis.[53]

Regional mycoses II: Blastomycosis – North American and otherwise

Blastomycosis was a term invented at the end of the nineteenth century for eruptive skin lesions or granulomas, which were assumed to be caused by infective fungi. The prefix 'blasto-', from the Greek for 'budding' or 'sprouting', came from the clinical presentation of raised lesions that were disfiguring, especially so with facial lesions. In the 1900s in the United States, the name became associated with so-called Gilchrist's disease, first thought to be protozoan, but then linked to a dimorphic (two forms) fungus named *Blastomyces dermatitidis* (*B. dermatitidis*).[54] For a while the infection was termed 'North American blastomycosis' as researchers found that it was restricted to the geographical areas of the Ohio, Mississippi and Missouri River basins and the western shore of Lake Michigan. There followed, what contemporaries recognised as, 'an era of confusion during which the disease was confounded with other entities, particularly cryptococcosis and candidiasis' and 'Nineteen new names were suggested for the causative fungus.'[55] Consensus on the pathogenesis of the disease followed work by Norman Conant and colleagues at Duke Medical School in the late 1930s.[56] They endorsed the idea that there was a form of the disease specific to North America, though other forms of blastomycosis, due to other fungal species, were found on other continents. South American blastomycosis was a condition with similar symptoms, but produced by a different fungus – *Paracoccidioides brasiliensis*. Although blastomycosis typically first presented as skin lesions, there were many reports of disseminated disease, which suggested parallels with coccidioidomycosis. Doctors wondered if there was also self-limiting or sub-clinical pulmonary infection; however, there was no evidence of aerial transmission in the mode of *C. immitis*. There were few reports of blastomycosis fungus in the environment, and certainly none of concentrations likely to produce disease in humans. The mystery of the manner in which it spread led some doctors to call it the 'the enigmatic disease'.[57]

A study in the mid-1960s by Leo Furcolow, who was based in Kansas in the centre of an endemic area, showed that there had been only 685 confirmed cases of blastomycosis across five states between 1912 and 1964, a figure which he assumed grossly to under-estimate its actual incidence.[58] Furcolow found that infection rates were higher in males than females, and there was 'a slight excess of cases among Negroes'; both factors were linked to the view that blastomycosis was associated with outdoor work or sports. A similar geographical distribution of the incidence of *B. dermatitidis* was found in dogs, so perhaps they were hosts and further credence to this link was suggested by similarities with the epidemiology of histoplasmosis. Another difficulty in mapping the disease, certainly in comparison with coccidioidomycosis, was the absence of a reliable skin test, which meant that the epidemiological picture relied on symptomatic cases.

Disseminated blastomycosis attracted the attention of clinicians because of its high mortality rate, which was typically 80%, though treatment with amphotericin B brought this down to less than 20%.[59] A difference with other endemic fungal diseases was that immunosuppressed patients were seemingly less likely to become infected, though if they did, severe disease was common.[60] Epidemiological and clinical studies found no significant patterns in the incidence of blastomycosis, other than predisposing illness. However, it has been always been more common in men, seemingly because of outdoor exposure. Suspicions remained that its epidemiology was similar to coccidioidomycosis because the lungs were the primary site of infection, and its prevalence amongst in-migrants and construction workers.[61]

The low incidence of endemic blastomycosis, along with the limited systemic infection, meant that no critical mass of local specialist practitioners developed and the expertise of the few people with special knowledge was not in demand. However, scientists and clinicians in the regions affected were able to develop specialist practices by developing work on other low-level endemic mycoses, most notably histoplasmosis.

Regional mycoses III: Histoplasmosis[62]

Histoplasmosis is caused by infection with the fungus *Histoplasma capsulatum* (*H. capsulatum*), and is associated with specific localities; indeed, it was sometimes referred to as Ohio Valley Fever, though it soon became clear its prevalence was wider. Its endemic areas overlapped with those of other regional fungi and researchers' work straddled different mycoses. For example, Leo Furcolow became renowned for his work on blastomycosis and histoplasmosis, and Louis Ajello combined expertise on coccidioidomycosis and histoplasmosis.[63] However, unlike blastomycosis, whose low incidence meant less attention from the clinicians, histoplasmosis, similar to the medical history of coccidioidomycosis, gained prominence nationally as social changes led to an increase incidence and importance. Moreover, according to Thomas Daniel and Gerald L. Baum, a national research network emerged around the disease with work led by federal agencies.[64] For Daniel and Baum, one key figure in the United States was Jan Schwarz, a Jewish émigré based in Cincinnati, Ohio, who worked on tuberculosis, before taking Conant's course at Duke and converting to mycology. From his base in Cincinnati, at the centre of the *H. capsulatum* endemicity, he became a leading national expert alongside his friend Leo Furcolow, who became known as 'Mr Histoplasmosis'.

Retrospectively, the first case of histoplasmosis has been identified in the Panama Canal Zone in 1906, when Samuel Taylor Darling reported an acute lung infection, with fever and breathlessness, caused by a protozoan that he named *Histoplasma capsulatum*.[65] Sporadic cases were reported over succeeding decades and in 1934 its causal organism was shown to be a fungus rather than a protozoan.[66] However, the disease only attracted the attention of doctors in the 1940s in relation to pulmonary tuberculosis, first in the military and then after the war in sanatoria. Recruits for the military were screened for pulmonary tuberculosis, with both a chest X-ray, which revealed active or healed lesions in the lungs, and the tuberculin skin test, which through an immune response confirmed either active or previous infection. A significant number of recruits showed, perversely, lesions in the lungs with a negative skin test. One possibility was that immunity declined over time; another was that a second disease was causing the lung lesions, and it turned out that histoplasmosis was such a disease. Fortuitously, a means to investigate the matter became available with the development of a tuberculin-type skin test for the infection, using an antigen product called histoplasmin. One study showed that of 94 men with healed lung lesions, 24 cases were due to tuberculosis and 70 to histoplasmosis.[67] A later study by Furcolow, published in 1962, showed that histoplasmosis was responsible for lesions in 7.5% (3,366/44,882) of sanatorium patients from across the country, which indicated that nationally some 8,200 patients entered sanatoria with evidence of histoplasmosis, and that of these, 25% might have had active disease with tuberculosis.[68]

This work, facilitated by the Division of Mycotic Diseases at CDC and the US Veterans Administration, and orchestrated through a Cooperative Study Group from 1952, revealed three features of histoplasmosis. First, it showed that there were certain regions of the United States where infection with *H. capsulatum* was very common, but that the development of symptomatic disease was quite rare. It seemed that children living in endemic areas developed immunity from low-level exposure and that this gave long-term protection. Thus, those likely to develop illness were adult in-migrants without previous exposure.

Second, research on the aetiology of the infection was inconclusive for many years, but eventually yielded that the main source of infection was soil dust and that localities with accumulations of bird and bat droppings were particularly pathogenic. At times, histoplasmosis was known as 'cave disease'. Daniel and Baum describe the 'detective story' by which the aetiology was solved. Their narrative begins with a case at Camp Gruber in March 1944 when the soil as a source of the fungus was first indicated, but they show that it took several decades to determine a specific aetiology.[69] Nonetheless, greater medical awareness of histoplasmosis and improved serological diagnostic testing led to more cases being identified, especially of systemic infection where, as with similar invasive mycoses, amphotericin B was the treatment of choice.[70]

By the 1970s, the disease had gained a higher profile, as increased population mobility around the United States brought more non-immune people to endemic areas, while anyone with active infection who moved anywhere across the country and became immuno-compromised was vulnerable to severe infection. There were also a series of epidemic outbreaks, often with small numbers affected and typically quite localised, but they were unusual, even bizarre, and attracted press and medical attention. Daniel and Baum discuss three epidemics: Mason City, Iowa in 1962 (returning in 1964) which was traced to bird rookeries; Suwanee County, Florida in 1973, linked to bats; and, the biggest of all, Indianapolis in 1978, which returned two years later.[71] Final estimates for the Indianapolis outbreak were that 120,000 people were infected, with 448 persons developing clinical illness, 55 with severely disseminated disease and 19 deaths. Over the 1980s and early 1990s, histoplasmosis became associated in the public mind and amongst physicians with AIDS, being the commonest endemic mycosis affecting patients.[72] Surveys in the early 1990s showed that it was found in 2–5% of AIDS sufferers in endemic areas and was the first sign of infection in over half of these cases. Infection rates amongst AIDS patients as high as 25% were found in certain cities, notably Indianapolis, Kansas City, Memphis and Nashville. Patients had quite general symptoms and treatments with the new forms of amphotericin B were successful, though maintenance of antifungals, typically the new azoles, was essential to prevent relapse.

Farmer's lung and allergic bronchopulmonary aspergillosis (ABPA)

Unlike the United States, Britain had no regionally specific mycoses linked to environmental factors of soil and climate, however, there were geographically localised conditions linked to occupation, which emerged in the 1950s. The most important was farmer's lung, which was initially linked to the *Aspergilli* fungi and pulmonary aspergillosis.[73] Aspergillosis, the principal cause of which was *Aspergillus fumigatus* (*A. fumigatus*), was considered only at the very end of Henrici's encyclopaedic *Molds, Yeasts and Actinomycetes* in 1930, after coccidioidomycosis, dermatophytosis, American blastomycosis, histoplasmosis and sporotrichosis.[74] However, the 15th edition of *Taylor's Practice of Medicine* in 1936 presented aspergillosis as an occupational disease of handlers of birds and grain, along with those who sorted human and animal hair for various products, for example, wigs.[75] Also in 1936, Richard Fawcitt, a radiologist in Ulverston, Cumberland, discussed *Aspergilli* spp. as the main cause of broncho-mycosis in the local farming community.[76] The numbers affected were small, but this study and one by Fawcitt's colleague Munro Campbell, are seen in hindsight as the beginning of the recognition of 'farmer's lung' as an occupational disease.[77] Fawcitt had also found aspergillosis amongst housecleaners, which might have been linked to new domestic technologies, such as the vacuum cleaner, which spread spore-carrying dust from exhaust vents.[78]

By the end of the 1930s, fungal spores had been added to pollen and house dust as causes of asthma, the prevalence of which was rising and fascinating doctors because of its complex aetiology, variable presentation, and link between the physiological and the psychological. At this time the physical basis of asthma was discussed in terms of allergic, hypersensitivity states, where the body reacted abnormally to certain substances or 'allergens'.[79] The largest group of allergens was plant and animal matter in the environment, with pollen and aerial dust understood to be the main exciting causes of allergic symptoms. Doctors debated whether the increased prevalence was due to better recognition, or because modern lifestyles made the body more vulnerable and increased exposure to allergens, or because new allergens had been created by modern farming and industry. In 1936, Grafton Brown, a Washington physician who specialised in allergy, pointed out that fungal spores were ubiquitous, present throughout the atmosphere in huge numbers and much smaller than pollen grains.[80] He was surprised that researchers had not considered them as allergens in house dust, especially when scientists were familiar with fungi as contaminants of their culture plates and slides in microbiology laboratories. According to Charles Thom and Margaret Church, writing in 1926, 'the *Penicillia*, the *Aspergilli* and the *Mucors* are the weeds of the culture room' and, of course, one now celebrated incidence of fungal contamination led to the discovery of penicillin.[81] Surveys of aerial allergens increased in the 1930s, using aeroplanes to explore high altitudes and remote locations, including flights by Charles Lindberg to survey areas in northern latitudes.[82] While the spores of a large number of fungal species were found to be potential allergens, they ranked well below pollen and dust. levels of known fungal disease spores found in the atmosphere were well below those of *Alternaria*, an ascomycete species that caused disease in plants and which emerged as main fungal suspect in causing asthma attacks.[83] Next in importance were the *Aspergilli*.

In Britain, aspergillosis was discussed in detail in James Duncan's national survey of fungal disease in 1945, in relation to both pulmonary disease and farmer's lung.[84] With pulmonary disease, cases were few and far between, and difficult to diagnose because of confusion with tuberculosis. However, Duncan was clear that 'the fungus is an essential factor in the aetiology of farmer's lung', but doubted that it was a primary inflammatory agent.[85] In 1953, Thomas Studdert, an assistant physician at the Cumberland Hospital in Carlisle, contested earlier views,

> The currently quoted view that farmer's lung is an actual fungous (*sic*) infection of the lungs does not bear close examination. The explosive onset, spontaneous clearing, and radiological picture are totally unlike any true fungous disease, and no real evidence has been produced to support this theory.[86]

Studdert's alternative, still framed with the possibility of fungal involvement, was that farmer's lung was an allergic reaction 'to some material in the fungus-laden dust'.[87] By the mid-1950s, the number of fungi considered as allergens increased to include *Penicillia*, *Mucors* and other genera, yet their role was now seen as creating allergenic dust, or mechanical irritation of the bronchi and alveoli, rather than specific allergic reactions. A 1963 report by the British Industrial Injuries Advisory Council, that led to the scheduling of a variety of occupational lung conditions, linked farmer's lung to other 'dust diseases', such as thresher's lung, chaff cutter's lung and bagassosis (sugar cane handler's disease).[88] It maintained the association with mouldy hay and vegetables, but said nothing about the role of specific fungi.[89]

A key reason why *Aspergilli* spp. were dropped from discussions of asthma and occupational diseases in the 1960s was the creation of the new specific condition of ABPA.[90] In 1952, Kenneth Hinson, with colleagues at the London Chest Hospital, published a study of eight cases of pulmonary aspergillosis, three of which were said to be an allergic type previously unrecognised and 'caused by sensitization of the host to the fungus'.[91] The condition was characterised around several symptoms: a syndrome of recurrent fevers, a changing X-ray pattern showing progressive lung damage, peripheral blood eosinophilia, and purulent sputum containing the *A. fumigatus*. Hinson and his colleagues were seen to have described an unusual type of aspergillosis, itself still very rare, so their claim was neither challenged nor endorsed; but it remained on the record. ABPA, as it was later styled, was not characterised by the invasive growth into tissues, rather fungi simply grew in pulmonary fluids and on the surface of lung tissues, causing inflammation.

ABPA attracted increasing attention in Britain through the 1950s and 1960s as doctors dealt with more patients with chronic lung diseases. It is again a moot point whether the decline in the incidence of pulmonary tuberculosis revealed previously submerged diseases, or whether the spectrum of disease that now faced doctors was genuinely new. Over the 1960s, there was increased incidence of lung cancer, chronic bronchitis and emphysema, which were linked to the effects of cigarettes, smoke pollution and occupation diseases. The growing incidence of non-specific chronic lung disease was captured in 1962 in the creation of the new, condition of chronic obstructive pulmonary disease (COPD).[92]

In both the United States and Britain there was more research on occupational diseases, which led to a greater differentiation of causes, linked to improved prevention and new regulations.[93] However, ABPA was only reported in Britain and particularly in London, where the concentration of patients with chronic chest conditions allowed Jack Pepys, who was one of Britain's leading experts on allergies, to report new findings in 1959. He had investigated 145 patients who had *A. fumigatus* in their sputum, finding that 16 exhibited ABPA, according to Hinson's 1952 criteria.[94] Pepys published a second study in 1969, in which he reported on 111 patients.[95] He wrote that the primary indicators of ABPA were transitory pulmonary shadows, eosinophilia of blood and sputum, evidence of allergy to *A. fumigatus* and fungal mycelia in sputum. Corticosteroids were the recommended therapy, having been shown to be more effective than bronchodilators and other symptomatic treatments. The condition was typically debilitating, leading to progressive deterioration in lung function, though in some patients the condition 'burnt out' and they 'recovered'.

American allergists and pulmonary specialists were curious about why ABPA was not found across the Atlantic. In 1969, Raymond Slavin and colleagues at the St. Louis University School asked:

> Why is [allergic] aspergillosis such a rarity in the United States? It would seem that the climate and geography of England does not make a profound difference since *A. fumigatus* is commonly reported in air sampling surveys in this country. In addition, as stated previously, secondary aspergillosis is not uncommon. It appears then that a failure of recognition and errors of omission account for the rarity of allergic aspergillosis in the United States... With the proper appreciation of the characteristics of allergic aspergillosis, both laboratory and clinical, this disease may be more frequently recognized and take its place with such hypersensitivity pneumonitides as pigeon breeders' disease, bagassosis and farmers' lung.[96]

As late as 1977, APBA was being discussed as an 'emerging disease' in the United States, due 'to increased awareness by physicians, increased referral, better diagnostic modalities, and earlier bronchography'.[97] Studies in the 1970s comparing the incidence of APBA in London and Cleveland showed similar levels of sensitivity to *A. fumigatus* antigens in asthmatics in both cities (23% and 28%, respectively), with the differences in prevalence attributed to exposure.[98] However, the incidence of the condition was on the rise in both countries, contributing to the overall increase in asthma, which has been widely discussed and attributed to many factors, from greater awareness to modern lifestyles. ABPA was soon recognised in most countries as the most common form of fungal-induced allergic lung disease and, though a largely chronic condition, was known to produce acute episodes.[99]

By the early 1980s, ABPA was a disease defined by eight diagnostic criteria, which were: asthma, an immediate positive skin test to *Aspergillus* antigens; presence of antibodies for *A. fumigatus*; elevated total serum immunoglobulin E (IgE); bronchial damage revealed by X-ray; high levels of white blood cells; proximal dilatation of the bronchi and elevated serum immunoglobulin levels of IgE-Af and lgG-Af compared with mould-sensitive asthmatic patients.[100] This demanding series, which combined clinical, X-ray, laboratory and functional criteria, meant that differential diagnosis against other lung conditions, such as pneumonia, bronchiectasis and carcinoma, was difficult in practice. There were problems about standardisation between individual clinicians, let alone across clinics and countries. Treatment was largely symptomatic, mostly with prednisone, an anti-inflammatory corticosteroid; however, some doctors tried antifungal antibiotics, given by inhalation and as well as systemically.[101] The chronic character of ABPA led to investigations into the degree of the destruction of lung tissue in severe cases, recognition of which led eventually to the designation, by David Denning and his colleagues in Manchester, of a group of patients with the new condition of severe asthma associated with fungal sensitivity (SAFS).[102]

By the early 1990s, ABPA was mainly identified with two groups: chronic asthma sufferers and people with cystic fibrosis. In both groups, inflamed lung tissues, accumulated exudates, dilated bronchi, impaired breathing and other factors created the conditions for *Aspergilli* to grow and prompt an allergic response. Epidemiological studies suggested that 1–5% of asthma sufferers were affected by ABPA, which was, of course, a fast growing number of individuals. In 1991, the American Academy of Allergy, Asthma and Immunology (AAAAI) formed an ABPA Committee, which attempted to determine the incidence of the condition. Initial results suggested ABPA affected less than 1% of asthma patients, though without a standard diagnosis and poor reporting the figure was speculative.[103]

A higher incidence of ABPA was found amongst people with cystic fibrosis, which was a rapidly growing group due to the increase in life expectancy because of improved management of the condition.[104] Studies at the end of the 1970s showed that around 10% of children attending the cystic fibrosis clinics had the symptoms of ABPA.[105] However, fungal allergy was just one of a number of lung infections this group was vulnerable to and it was far less prevalent than those caused by bacteria and viruses.[106] A study published in 1990 reported that the main pathogens affecting people with cystic fibrosis were *Pseudomonas aeruginosa* (60%) and *Staphylococcus aureus* (27%), with ABPA in the range of 0.5–11%.[107] However, it was more common in older children and adults, at around 25%; hence, its importance was likely to grow.[108]

In 2001, a report by staff at the CDC in Atlanta presented an overview of mortality from invasive mycoses in the United States from 1980 to

1997.[109] The data they collected showed that 'deaths in which an infectious disease was the underlying cause, those due to mycoses increased from the tenth most common in 1980 to the seventh most common in 1997', with the annual number of deaths increasing from 1,557 to 6,534. They confirmed that there had been 'a marked upward trend in overall mortality due to the invasive mycoses', and highlighted the growing importance of immuno-compromising conditions, particularly HIV/AIDS.[110] What was interesting was that the regionally specific mycoses discussed in this chapter only registered in the summary when they affected patients with HIV/AIDS, indeed, the disease was 'a major determinant of the trend in overall mortality from histoplasmosis'.[111] However, the report supported the view that social changes were major factors in the fluctuating incidence of fungal disease, as with coccidioidomycosis in Arizona, where the increase was due to 'an influx into the state of older nonimmune individuals who were susceptible to acute infection and more likely to manifest symptomatic illness'.[112] In other places, it was not so much the arrival of virgin human soil, but the wider and more intense circulation of the 'seeds' of infection, literally thrown up by construction and extreme climate events.

In discussing overall mortality, the CDC report confirmed what doctors' experience had told them:

> The two major factors responsible for the emergence of fungal infections have been the HIV disease epidemic and the many advances of modern medicine (including solid organ and bone marrow transplantation) that enable or prolong the survival of critically ill and susceptible patients. In addition, the aging of the population has increased the number of susceptible persons.[113]

To which should be added greater medical awareness, plus new and more sensitive diagnostic technologies. However, the report showed that antifungal drugs had reduced mortality in certain groups and from certain infections; the main exception was aspergillosis, the mycosis most associated with 'advances in modern medicine', which we move on to in the next chapter.

5

Technology and Aspergillosis

Aspergillosis is the least well known of the diseases we discuss in this book, in part because there is no common presentation as with ringworm and thrush, and in part because it only emerged as a serious condition late in the twentieth century. We discussed *Aspergillus* spores as allergens in the last chapter and in this chapter we consider its other forms.[1] The first modern English language book on aspergillosis was a collection of essays published in 1985, some 20 years after that for candidiasis and 150 years after ringworm.[2] The first international meeting on aspergillosis was in 1971 and was linked to concern about farmer's lung.[3] Serious medical interest in aspergillosis only took off in the 1980s, with the emergence of invasive aspergillosis as an opportunistic, life-threatening infection of immuno-compromised patients. This condition had attracted some medical attention from the 1960s as a complication of leukaemia and its profile grew with the development of high tech surgical and medical interventions, such as transplant surgery, intensive care and immunosuppressant treatment regimes.[4] However, the public profile of *Aspergilli* fungi was much higher, not as infectious disease agents, but as producers of toxic chemicals that developed on rotting foodstuffs and introduced to the world a new class of poisons: mycotoxins. *Aspergilli* fungi produce compounds called aflatoxins and the detection of these prompted a debate about whether they were newly recognised, or newly produced. This ended with a consensus that they were genuinely novel and came from the unforeseen consequences of new technologies of transporting, storing and processing foodstuffs.

In this chapter, we first discuss what became known as the 'aflatoxin scare' of the 1960s, which led to the creation of a new research field of fungal toxins more widely, in large part prompted by fears that they were significant carcinogens. This episode eventually led to new standards of food storage and transportation across the world. Scientific and medical interest in the *Aspergilli* developed in the second half of the twentieth century for three reasons. Firstly, it came from the close relation of the *Aspergilli* to the *Penicillia* and technologies of antibiotic production. Secondly, the identification of various forms of aspergillosis through improved medical technologies, notably X-rays and antibiotics, which in patients with tuberculosis, literally and metaphorically opened their lungs to secondary aspergillosis infection. Finally, by the late twentieth century invasive pulmonary aspergillosis (IPA) was the most important and prevalent form of *Aspergillus* infection and a major problem in many medical fields. This infection can be regarded as an exemplary iatrogenic disease; it became the bane of human transplantation surgery, leukaemia treatment, and intensive care units and like candidiasis has been styled a 'disease of the diseased'.

Aspergillus flavus and aflatoxins[5]

In 1960, 100,000 turkeys died of a mysterious disease in southern England, mostly within 80–100 miles of London. Young birds simply collapsed in pens and fields, while adult birds showed a general malaise, with nervous symptoms, before dying. Post mortems revealed inflammation of the gut and liver damage, suggesting poisoning of some type rather than a feared contagion, such as Newcastle disease.[6] The outbreak spread to ducks and pheasants, which led to major investigations by the British government's veterinary agencies and agricultural feedstuff companies, notably British Oil and Cake Mills (BOCM). The problem was not followed in detail by the press, in part because it was localised and in part, because viral fowl pest was a much larger problem at that time.[7] Nonetheless, considerable efforts were made by government and corporate laboratories to find the cause of what veterinarians termed turkey 'X' disease.[8]

Following outbreaks in other parts of the country, suspicion fell upon feedstuffs and particularly Brazilian groundnut meal that had been given to poultry for the first time in 1960. Experiments at BOCM showed that the disease could be produced by feeding Brazilian groundnut meal, however, further work at the Home Office Forensic Laboratory failed to find any specific poison. Pathological investigations at Unilever Research Laboratories, the company that was the major importer and processor of groundnuts, first showed that turkey 'X' disease mainly affected the liver and, if rats were fed groundnuts for six months, some developed liver cancer.[9] In December 1961, the same group announced that they had identified a specific poison for turkey 'X' disease, a toxin produced by *A. flavus* that they called 'aflatoxin'.[10] In fact, four specific toxins were soon identified, which were subsequently labelled by their fluorescent profile with marker chemicals. Those that showed blue were designated B_1 and B_2 and those that were turquoise green G_1 and G_2. Aflatoxin B_1 was shown to be the most toxic form, causing acute hepatitis, immunosuppression, and hepatocellular carcinoma.[11] Research on *A. flavus* revealed further complexity as, rather than a single species, it turned out to be best characterised as a 'species complex'. Amongst the 11 species was *A. oryzae*, known in Japan as the '*kõji* fungus', which rather than being associated with toxins and poisoning, had been used for centuries in the production of sake, miso and soy sauce.[12] Indeed, it was termed the 'national fungus' by Professor Emeritus Eiji Ichishima of Tohoku University in the journal of the Brewing Society of Japan in 2006.[13]

The scare in Britain attracted considerable interest across the world and led to the development of a new field of research on mycotoxins. In the case of aflatoxins, investigators found the toxin in food imports sourced from East and West Africa and possibly India. A number of experimental studies showed that liver disease and liver cancer could be produced in a number of animal species, but the threat to human health remained unproven. An editorial in the *British Medical Journal* in February 1962 warned against any panic over foodstuffs imported from developing countries, but called for improved monitoring and more research on liver disease in countries where groundnuts and similar foods were dietary staples.[14] The following year, aflatoxin was found in peanuts in the United States, which when fed to ducklings produced the characteristic disease syndrome and cancers.[15] The NIAID began to fund screening programmes to find and identify mycotoxins.[16] While there remained no direct evidence of a threat to human health, in part because any exposure was likely to be sporadic and at low doses, reports of cancer from fungal metabolites grew. Amongst the most worrying were those from 'antibiotic species': for example, liver tumours in rats fed rice infected with *Penicillium islandicum* and, to the dismay of dermatologists, mice fed griseofulvin.[17] In 1965, the FDA introduced a standard for safe aflatoxin levels in foodstuffs of 30 parts per billion in peanut products, with levels above that requiring action. This policy set in chain new research projects on methods of monitoring and changes to regulatory responsibilities.[18]

The discovery of aflatoxin led to what was soon coined 'the mycotoxin Gold Rush', as researchers across the world investigated a whole new class of poisons and their health effects.[19] The American Society for Microbiology held a session on the subject at its annual meeting in July 1965 and other conferences followed. Why was so much effort and so many resources mobilised to meet 'a seemingly obscure toxicity syndrome in poultry flocks'?[20] First, doctors and food producers feared that aflatoxin was the tip of a toxin iceberg and that the long-term effects of fungal poisons had been overlooked. Reviews suggested that aflatoxins might have been the cause of previously unexplained outbreaks of disease in guinea pigs in 1954, dogs in 1955, and cats and rabbits in 1957.[21] There was also the possibility that other fungi might be contaminating different foodstuffs, with most concern about those imported from developing countries, where standards of husbandry and storage were suspect. In addition, the conditions and time taken in transporting products with the development of international markets meant there were more opportunities for deterioration and, hence, the production of toxins. Thus, there was impetus from state agencies and the public for scientists to develop a better understanding of the problem, and new methods to test and monitor for toxins. The globalisation of the food industry had created a completely new threat to human and animal health.

A second factor stoking interest was the fear that mycotoxins were possibly major causes of cancer; hence, new technologies of food production, storage and transportation might have been contributory factors to an increase in the incidence of the disease in the twentieth century.[22] The 1960s saw growing awareness of the long-term effects of chemicals in the environment, as the warnings of Rachel Carson's *Silent Spring* finally hit home, and as we discussed in Chapter 3, the 1960s and 1970s saw the development of clinical ecology and its warnings of direct and indirect environmental threats to human health. These concerns had focused on man-made chemicals, but now there was a further twist; new technologies were turning foodstuffs and natural products into sources of danger. Liver cancer was known to have a distinctive geographical distribution and had become a model for field studies of the causes of cancer.[23] The disease was most common in sub-Saharan Africa and Denis Burkitt, already famous for his identification of what became Burkitt's lymphoma, highlighted the possible impact of aflatoxin in his survey of cancers in East Africa in 1965.[24] In 1966, Richard Doll, well known for his work linking cigarette smoking and lung cancer, estimated that liver cancer rates in developed countries could be cut 10 to 15-fold, if people were able to reduce their exposure to carcinogens.[25]

At the end of the 1960s, John Higginson, a leading cancer epidemiologist, reviewed what might be possible in terms of prevention from all causes, in an analysis that divided aetiology into four categories: cultural, occupational, miscellaneous and unknown.[26] Unsurprisingly, lung cancer was 90% cultural. Colon and rectal cancers were 99% unknown. Liver cancer was 40% cultural and 60% unknown. With the latter, Higginson associated aflatoxin with DDT as possible triggers, but conceded that, though there was experimental evidence of carcinogenesis in animals, there was insufficient evidence of a danger to human health and he saw no case for tightening regulations.[27] While epidemiological studies remained inconclusive, the potency of aflatoxins as carcinogens made them useful agents for laboratory studies, particularly by inducing hepatomas in rats and rainbow trout.[28]

In 1979, one review of the burgeoning research on aflatoxins in the previous decade observed, 'Unfortunately the amount of factual information seems to be out of all proportion to the amount of light shed on the particular mechanisms by which aflatoxins damage susceptible cells.'[29] A similar conclusion with regard to safety policy was reached in a review by a committee constituted at the Institute of Medicine in Washington, and published in 1979 by the National Academy of Sciences (NAS).[30] The context was concern about whether saccharin, the most commonly used artificial sweetener, was a carcinogen and aflatoxins, along with mercury and nitrites, were included as comparators.[31] The review was very controversial. It recommended that food safety policy be made 'simpler, more flexible and more comprehensible', and that regulatory agencies be granted greater 'discretionary authority'. The suggestion was that the FDA could allow 'small amounts of carcinogenic additives in the food supply as it sees fit'. The review also suggested that an assessment of health risk *versus* economic benefit was necessary, plus an evaluation of the comparative risk of different foods.[32] But who would undertake the work and how risks were to be judged was left open.

The research trajectory with regard to the necessity for risk assessment with aflatoxins exemplified the problems of translating science into policy. Firstly, the link between the toxicity of aflatoxins in animals and humans was uncertain, and it had proved impossible to establish tolerance levels. Secondly, it seemed likely that there should be different safe levels for different foodstuffs, and that this would have to take into account secondary effects, for example, human exposure to milk from cows fed contaminated grains. Thirdly, the sporadic incidence of aflatoxin contamination, along with the potentially high price of prevention, meant that benefits seemed unlikely to be worth the cost. Finally, the number of stakeholders involved meant that it had proved very difficult and time consuming to have changes approved; for example, the five-year delay in reaching a decision on the 1974 FDA proposal to reduce the tolerance level of aflatoxin from 20 parts per billion (ppb) to 15 ppb.

The NAS review was framed within the overall context of the decline in deaths from infectious diseases, the rise in those from cardiovascular disease and cancer, and the changes to the human environment brought by technological development.[33] In the specific area of food, the authors pointed to technical advances having shifted hazards 'away from microbial contamination that produced acute disease soon after exposure', to 'chemicals in small quantities and other hazards introduced by environmental contamination as well as by food production and processing'.[34] The recommendation for regulatory flexibility came from the aim of allowing agencies to find a middle way between unrestrained use and a ban, as well as a desire to allow them to keep up with progress in research, production and monitoring.[35] In other words, the problem of aflatoxins was being defined largely in terms of the risks created by modern methods of food production, distribution and consumption; nonetheless, it was expected to be solved by those very same technologies.[36] One factor, echoing issues with regionally specific fungi, was that risks varied with place and individual lifestyles, particularly dietary, meaning that national, let alone international, standards were likely to be hard to agree and even harder to enforce.[37]

Aspergillosis: 'A Rare Disease', 1900–1960

Poultry were important in the story of *Aspergilli* fungi and human health at both ends of the twentieth century, as aspergillosis was recognised as a lung disease of fowl and cattle, and an occupational disease in humans around 1900.[38] Veterinarians reported the disease to be most common in birds, including chickens, turkeys and certain waterfowl, where it caused pneumonia and other lung diseases.[39] Mammals were said to be less susceptible, but it was reported in cattle and dogs. Veterinarians blamed contaminated grain, but argued that certain predisposing conditions were necessary, such as the animals being in poor general health or living in insanitary conditions. 'Brooder pneumonia', an American term for aspergillosis, came from its presence in intensively reared fowl. In humans, the disease was found mainly in those who worked with birds and cattle, those who handled grain or worked in dusty conditions. The primary presentation in humans was as bronchial or lung disease, though it was also reported sometimes to affect the cornea of the eye and the middle ear. The classic accounts of the disease came from Paris and its prevalence amongst 'les gaveurs de pigeons', the men who force-fed the birds being reared for food.[40] They did so by mixing grain and water in their mouths, chewing the mixture to a pulp and then spitting it forcibly down the gullet of the birds. This practice was undertaken on an industrial scale, with each man allegedly feeding 2,000 birds each day.

Pulmonary aspergillosis attracted the attention of doctors because of the similarities of its symptoms and pathology with pulmonary tuberculosis, and over whether it was a cause of a disease known as 'pseudo-tuberculosis'.[41] The great anti-tuberculosis campaigns, which began across Europe and North America at the end of the nineteenth century, brought more patients with lung diseases into the medical gaze, and doctors were required to differentiate those who would benefit from the new initiatives in treatment and care, such as those to be offered the sanatorium treatment.[42] There was also unhappiness that 'pseudo-' diseases still existed in an era when developments in pathology had led to greater specificity and aetiological constructions of disease. The Pathological Society of London formed a Committee on Pseudo-tuberculosis in 1899 and its report recommended that the name be dropped from the medical lexicon and that only lesions caused by the Koch's bacillus be termed tubercles. All other pulmonary lesions were to be referred to as 'nodules', one class of which was 'aspergillar nodules'.[43]

The first book on *Aspergillosis* was published in France in 1897 by Louis Rénon, who was Chef de Clinique a la Faculté de medècine de Paris.[44] Renon's work was one inspiration for an MD thesis on *Aspergillosis* submitted to the Victoria University of Manchester by Thomas Rothwell in 1899.[45] Rothwell's supervisor, Sheridan Delépine, Professor of Pathology, had published on *Aspergillus* skin infection 1894 and was active in tuberculosis research.[46] Rothwell reviewed the literature on the disease and experimental work on the fungus, before describing his own studies on the inoculations of spores into guinea pigs.[47] There had been work in Germany by Paul Grawitz, who was interested in immunity and the question of why a seemingly saprophytic organism became pathogenic; he asked: was this due to a change in the fungi, or the resistance of the host organism?[48] Louis Renon's 300-page book on, what he acknowledged was, 'a rare condition' discussed the disease in animals and in the laboratory, before considering 'Aspergillose de l'homme'.[49] With human disease, his main concern was whether infection was primary or secondary, and he concluded that it could be both, with *A. fumigatus* the most pathogenic species. Rothwell's thesis had similar conclusions, concentrating on the differences between *A. fumigatus* and the more benign *A. niger*.

Humphry Rolleston, a leading London physician who specialised in pulmonary tuberculosis, published an account of pulmonary aspergillosis in 1898.[50] He stated that it was almost exclusively a trade disease amongst millers, agricultural labourers, and others who worked with contaminated grains and with processes that created dust. He was clear that both *A. fumigatus* and *A. niger* could also infect the ear and skin, and wondered how many people diagnosed as suffering from pulmonary tuberculosis might really have aspergillosis, or have the fungus and bacillus acting synergistically.[51] The symptoms of pulmonary aspergillosis – a cough, purulent expectoration, coughing blood, bronchitis, consolidation at the top of the lung and raised temperature – were similar to those of pulmonary tuberculosis, which left the microscopic examination of sputum as the only means for differential diagnosis. As a primary infection, the prognosis with aspergillosis was 'less grave' than for pulmonary tuberculosis, but as a secondary complication it was said to be very serious and 'in fact a terminal complication'.[52]

In the inter-war period aspergillosis disappeared from the medical gaze; and when it was discussed it was to admit ignorance, especially of its relation to pulmonary tuberculosis.[53] Instead, the period witnessed great interest in the use of the *Aspergilli* in human food production, building on knowledge from Japan. The *Aspergilli* became a prime interest of industrial chemists, they were termed 'cell factories', because of their role in the production of citric, gluconic, itaconic and kojic acids, in what would now be termed biotechnology.[54] From 1917, *A. niger* was the mainstay of citric acid production, using technologies that were later adapted for the production of penicillin.[55] Scientists at Pfizer, then a fine chemicals business, with industrial as well as pharmaceutical products, had developed large-scale methods to meet the demands of the rapidly growing soft drinks and processed food industries.[56] In the 1930s, fermentation research was developed at the Industrial Farm Research Division (IFRD) of the United States Department of Agriculture. For example, in 1937 scientists from the Division published a paper setting out how to increase the efficiency of gluconic acid production with *A. niger* in submerged cultures.[57] This biotechnological application of the *Aspergilli* directly benefited the wartime initiatives with the new antibiotics, for example scientists from the IFRD moved to the Northern Research Laboratory at Peoria when it was established in December 1940 to work on 'deep culture' production of penicillin.[58] Thus, the link between *Aspergilli* and antibiotics was not, as with *Candida*, that new drugs opened the body to secondary fungal infections, rather it was the vital role the genus played in the production of antibiotics and hence the development of modern pharmaceutical industry.

As discussed in Chapter 3, the discovery of penicillin began a search for new fungal-derived antibacterials and the botanical similarities between *Penicillium* spp. and *Aspergillus* spp. meant that the latter became prime targets. Selman Waksman had first explored the antibacterial substances produced by *A. fumigatus* in the 1940s.[59] He identified a compound that he called 'fumigacin', which had an antibacterial spectrum similar to penicillin, but was weaker and never developed for clinical use. No doubt expecting similar products to penicillin, researchers coined the terms 'Aspergillins' to refer to the range of antibiotic substances derived from the *Aspergilli*. The most successful of the compounds was aspergillic acid, which had some effect against *Mycobacterium tuberculosis*.[60] Indeed, for many years *Aspergillus* spp. and *Streptomyces* spp. were regarded as most likely to produce anti-tuberculosis drugs, and, of course, the latter eventually yielded streptomycin.[61]

While mycologists and industrial biologists worked intensively on the fungus, aspergillosis continued to be largely ignored by doctors and the only publications were on 'rare' and 'unusual' cases of invasive disease. The Second World War gave no military, social or epidemiological stimulus to the incidence or profile of aspergillosis, as there had been with ringworm and troop invalidism, *Candida* and the spread of antibiotics, and migration and the geographically specific mycoses. In the United States, John Downing and Norman Conant in their 1945 review of mycotic infections for the *New England Journal of Medicine* did not mention aspergillosis.[62] Eight years later, in his review in the same journal, Otis Jillson was cursory on the topic, noting several recent reports where aspergillosis was usually caused by *A. fumigatus* and that there was no effective treatment.[63] However, he pointed to the difficulties with diagnosis, even at autopsy, because *A. fumigatus* was such a common contaminant in pathological and bacteriological laboratories, and hospital buildings.

In Britain, aspergillosis was discussed in detail in James Duncan's fungal disease survey in 1945, in relation to both pulmonary disease and farmer's lung.[64] With pulmonary disease, cases were few and far between, and difficult to diagnose because of confusion with tuberculosis. However, in the 1950s a new disease entity was recognised: *Aspergillus* fungus balls, or aspergilloma.[65] They were first reported by doctors in France, seen in chest X-rays from patients with cavities in their lungs left by healed tuberculosis lesions. This was a growing group due to the effectiveness of triple antibiotic therapy, with streptomycin, para-aminosalycilic acid (PAS) and isoniazid. However, the growths were not just found in former tubercular patients, they were also associated with other chronic lung conditions, of which there was growing awareness and investigation; for example, histoplasmosis and cavitating lung cancer.[66] A survey in 1968 by the Research Committee of the British Thoracic Association looked at 544 patients with persistent lung cavities larger than 2.5 cm in diameter.[67] Using X-rays, they found 11% of patients showed evidence of aspergilloma, with a further 4% probable cases. They also tested their blood serum for *Aspergillus* precipitins, which revealed 25% of the group were positive, though half these patients showed no X-ray evidence of infection. A follow-up study of the same group of patients, published in 1970, revealed that the presence of an aspergilloma did not increase mortality.[68] The important factor in mortality was that aspergilloma patients had worse coughs and were more liable to serious complications, such as haemoptysis. In around 10% of patients the aspergilloma had disappeared spontaneously, which led to the conclusion that treatment was, perhaps, unnecessary because they were benign, saprophytic growths. Where treatments were given, the procedures were similar to those developed for tubercular lesions. Thoracic surgeons, especially in the United States, removed the infected part of the lung (resection), while physicians used antifungal drugs. Only amphotericin B was effective and given by intra-cavity injection into the lung.[69] By the 1980s treatment had become more conservative, with surgery reserved for patients with severe haemoptysis.[70]

In the 1990s, aspergilloma was subsumed into the class of chronic pulmonary aspergillosis (CPA), which also included chronic cavitary pulmonary aspergillosis (CCPA), where patients had cavities without fungal balls, and chronic fibrosing pulmonary aspergillosis (CFPA), which developed when a primary infection remained untreated and scarred the lungs. In most cases, patients with CPA were found to have an underlying disease, typically tuberculosis, ABPA, lung cancer, COPD, emphysema, asthma or silicosis. As such, CPA typified the view that, like invasive candidiasis, aspergillosis was a 'disease of the diseased'.

Invasive aspergillosis

In the 1960s, the incidence of invasive candidiasis was much higher than that of invasive aspergillosis, but this changed in the next half century. Looking back from 1965, Samuel Asper and Andrew Heffernan reviewed the numbers of those diagnosed with aspergillosis in Johns Hopkins University Hospital from 1941 to 1963.[71] Their work was prompted by the aflatoxin scare and based on a re-examination of the autopsy reports of 26 cases, to determine if patients with aspergillosis had also suffered from liver disease.[72] They found no correlation, but determined to extract something useful from their data they turned their attention to aspergillosis in general, responding to reports that it was on the rise. At Johns Hopkins, its incidence had increased, but only slowly and it was still relatively rare. In the 23 years surveyed, there had been 26 cases, amongst 202 patients with fungal infections identified at autopsy. The total number of autopsies was 14,819, so the incidence of recognised fungal infection, which was no doubt an under-estimate, was quite low at 1.3%. However, there was a marked recent increase in aspergillosis, with 23 cases occurring in the ten years up to 1963 (Figure 5.1).

The authors regarded their most interesting finding as the association of aspergillosis with leukaemia, the incidence of which had nearly

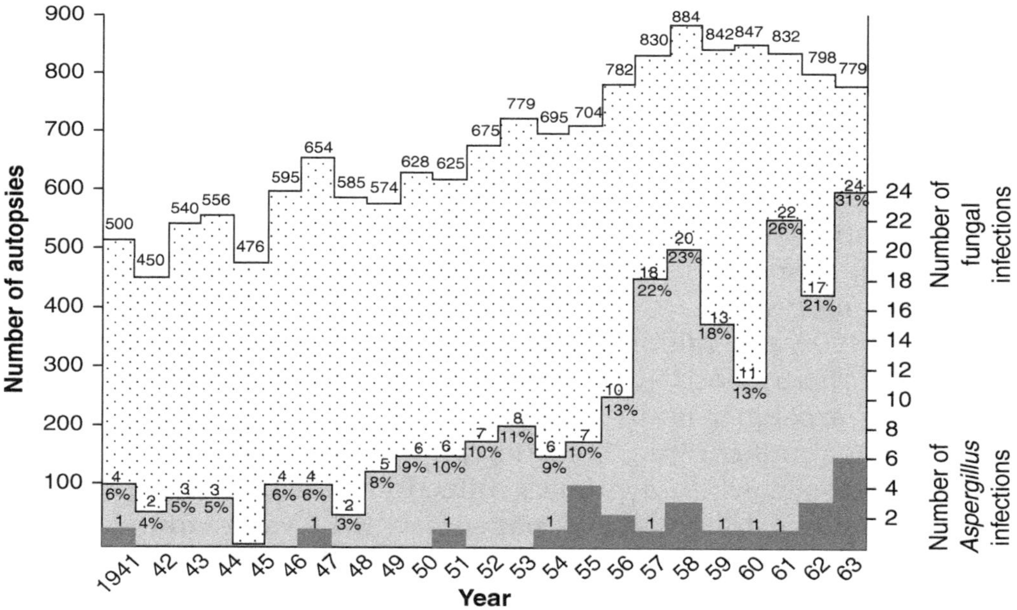

Figure 5.1 Incidence of fungal infections (including aspergillosis) found at autopsy at the Johns Hopkins Hospital, 1941–1963.[73] Asper, S. P. and Heffernan, A. G. A., 'Insidious fungal disease', *Trans Am Clin Climatol Assoc*, 1965, 76: 101. This figure © 2013 American Clinical and Climatological Association used under Creative Commons Attribution – Non-commercial

doubled since the 1940s, during a period when treatments had intensified.[74] Asper and Heffernan observed,

> It may well be, as others have suggested, that unique forms of therapy for leukemia, which alter host-parasite relationships, are the factors responsible for the increasing incidence of aspergillosis. In the weeks before death, all the leukemic patients had received antibiotics and steroids and all but one had received cytotoxic agents.[75]

They did not speculate on which of these treatments might be responsible for predisposing patients to aspergillosis, or the extent to which the leukaemia itself was a factor.

Other doctors had already speculated on the role of fungal infections in leukaemia deaths. Two years previously, in 1963, John Gruhn and John Sansom, of the Mount Sinai Hospital, Chicago, wrote that many studies suggested 'that the profound leukopenia [decrease in the number of white blood cells] induced by antileukemic drugs appeared to increase susceptibility to infections'.[76] A literature review found reports of mycoses in leukaemia patients at between 14% and 30%, while their own retrospective look at 25 autopsies found a 24% incidence in the period 1941–1961, increasing to 39% in the last five years. In total, candidiasis was found in 19 patients and aspergillosis in eight.[77] The authors concluded that leukopenia, antibiotics and steroids were all factors in fungal infections, though suggested that antibiotics were more important with candidiasis, and steroids with aspergillosis. [78] This conclusion chimed with earlier studies by Herschel Sidransky in New Orleans, who had explored the relative importance of steroids and antibiotics in experimental studies of aspergillosis with mice.[79]

The evidence mounted that the rise in aspergillosis cases was largely due to the rise in leukaemia cases.[80] In 1970, Robert C. Young and colleagues published on the pattern of aspergillosis found in the 98 patients autopsied at the Clinical Centre of the NIH between 1953 and 1970.[81] Leukaemia and lymph node cancers accounted for 86% of cases, with lung disease the main clinical manifestation. Aspergillosis had only rarely been diagnosed ante mortem. Three years after the NIH report, Richard Meyer and colleagues at the Memorial Sloan-Kettering Cancer Center, published a study that showed the prevalence of aspergillosis in leukaemia patients was rising quickly, such that in the first half of 1971, '41 per cent of the patients who died with acute leukemia had evidence of aspergillosis'.[82] A study published in 1972, also from the Mount Sinai Hospital, New York, reported that amongst

65 leukaemia patients: 16 had candidiasis, aspergillosis and four phycomycetes (common moulds).[83] Their finding chimed with those in other hospitals, where fungal complications ranged from 14–30%.[84]

The increase in the prevalence of fungal infections associated with leukaemias led doctors to seek better diagnostic methods and treatments, especially new ways to use amphotericin B, the only antifungal effective against *A. fumigatus* at this time.[85] In cases of IPA, looking for increased levels of the fungus in sputum was an obvious diagnostic test, however, as the infection was deep seated in cavities and even contained within an aspergilloma, it was possible that very few fungi would reach the throat or mouth. Indeed, sputum tests were regarded only as indicative, because of the ubiquity of the *Aspergilli* in the environment, in hospitals, and in the sputum of healthy individuals. The alternative test was for *A. fumigatus* antibodies in blood serum. The test used so-called 'precipitins', that is, proteins or other antigenic material from the fungus that would combine with antibodies to produce a cloudy precipitate when mixed with serum. This test had problems of specificity and sensitivity, again because of the presence of *A. fumigatus* in the environment and because of variable reactions to different antigens.[86]

From the early 1970s, aspergilloma was counted as a type of IPA, though it was identified and treated at outpatient chest clinics and framed, alongside pulmonary tuberculosis as a public health problem. In April 1970, the *British Medical Journal* published an article on the incidence of systemic mycoses in Britain, based on diagnoses made by the Public Health Laboratory Service in the week ending 3 April 1970, which was said to be typical.[87] Aspergilloma and aspergillosis were by far the largest reported infections: 225 cases of aspergilloma were due to *A. flavus*, 19 to other *Aspergilli*, and 15 to all other fungi. As discussed in Chapter 4, the *Aspergilli* loomed large amongst allergens, but the number of patients affected was below that with *C. albicans*. The report again emphasised that fungal diseases were neglected conditions, but the authors wanted to demonstrate that laboratory testing was available and that aspergillosis should be on clinicians' radar.

In the 1960s a new patient group emerged as potential sufferers of invasive aspergillosis – renal transplant recipients. The first modern kidney transplant, between identical twins, was performed by Joseph Murray in California in 1954.[88] As the donor and recipient were genetically and immunologically identical there was no problem of organ rejection. The number of operations between identical twins and close relatives increased, with Murray leading the field in the management of immunosuppression with local irradiation, specific cytotoxic drugs, initially Azathioprine, and corticosteroids (presnidone). The first renal transplant operation in Britain was also between identical twins, by Michael Woodruff in Edinburgh in 1960. By the mid-1960s, Murray and a growing cadre of transplant specialists had developed regimes to better match tissue types and to manage rejection and other complications, which enabled transplants between individual of similar tissue-type and this led the number of renal transplant operations to increase rapidly. Over the same period, the median survival time of recipients rose, with those receiving organs from live patients doing better than those receiving cadaver kidneys.

The major problem in the early years of renal transplantation was rejection, but as this was better managed and recipients lived longer, other complications came to the fore, principally cardiovascular disease, osteoporosis and infection. The most important infection was with cytomegalovirus, which affected the liver and lungs, and pneumocystis pneumonia. A significant minority of recipients developed mycoses due to a variety of opportunistic fungi: cryptococcosis, candidiasis and aspergillosis.[89] With aspergillosis, infection rates were relatively low, but mortality rates were high because of the difficulties with diagnosis and treatment. However, clinicians' awareness of the problem led to the introduction of prophylactic measures, for example, better surgical hygiene and patient care to prevent opportunistic infection and the pre- and post-operative use of antifungal drugs. A particular problem with renal transplant was that the most effective therapy for invasive aspergillosis was amphotericin B, where nephrotoxicity was the major side effect. Aspergillosis was also a problem in heart transplant patients; indeed, the condition reached the pages of the national press in 1969 when Britain's third heart transplant patient, Charles Hendrick, died four months after his operation from aspergillosis. The press described aspergillosis as a 'very rare' infection and one that Hendrick's doctors took a long time to diagnose, ultimately giving amphotericin B too late to save his life.[90]

Amphotericin B had the reputation amongst some doctors of being a treatment that was worse than the disease; it was often kept back for so-called 'salvage therapy' – a final attempt at therapy in the terminally ill or palliation.[91] However, in 1973, Bill St Clair Symmers, a pathologist at the Charing Cross Hospital and Medical School, complained of 'pharmacophobia' amongst physicians about amphotericin B.[92] He discussed five cases of invasive fungal infection, none was aspergillosis, where the drug was not used because of fears of nephrotoxicity and the patients died. He argued that the patients should have been given the chance of overcoming the infection and that dialysis might have been used 'to tide the patient over in the event of severe renal damage', or that 'the loss of both kidneys is not necessarily fatal or incompatible with a useful life nowadays'.[93] This view received support from Ross Forgan-Smith and J. H. Darrell of the Royal Postgraduate Medical School, who argued that, provided doses were kept low and blood urea monitored, the drug was safe and that kidney damage was often reversible.[94] One reason why physicians were reluctant to use amphotericin B was that diagnosis remained difficult. It seemed that many of those advocating its use were pathologists and medical mycologists, who had the benefit of post mortem evidence, which had not been available to clinicians. Despite its problems, amphotericin B remained the first choice therapy for invasive aspergillosis into the 1980s and was valued because it was also effective against other opportunistic fungal infections that might be present, such as candidiasis and cryptococcosis.

The primary site of aspergillosis remained the lung and inhalation the main route of infection, thus, chest physicians and infectious disease clinicians, who saw most patients of this type, became the experts on the disease. One issue that remained vexing was whether aspergillosis was always a secondary infection, with opinion shifting to the view that it could be primary in patients whose health was poor due to heart or lung problems. Better diagnosis revealed, or perhaps improved treatments produced, a new type of disease – chronic pulmonary aspergillosis (CPA). The term was first used in the late 1970s to differentiate patients with infection from those with chronic allergic reactions, but as noted above was adopted for all types of chronic infection, including aspergilloma.[95]

Azoles again

The story of invasive aspergillosis in the last quarter of the twentieth century was dominated by the development, trialling and clinical use of new antifungal drugs. The biggest change in preventive and therapeutic possibilities came in the 1980s with the introduction of triazole antifungal drugs. These compounds, of which the most promising were itraconazole and fluconazole, were produced from the series that began with clotrimazole.[96] Itraconazole was found in a programme of screening by Janssen Pharamceutica in Belgium.[97] The compound was first used in trials in 1982 and was given final approval in Britain in 1989 and the United States in 1992.[98] The momentum behind the search for new antifungals was evident in the fact that an international symposium on itraconazole was held in Oaxaca, Mexico, as early as October 1985, a full four years before its first regulatory approval.[99] Fluconazole enjoyed the same treatment, with Pfizer Pharmaceuticals sponsoring a symposium on early trials in Dorado Beach, Puerto Rico, in October 1988.[100] There were hopes that the drug would be valuable against oropharyngeal candidiasis in AIDS patients and this excited public and medical attention.[101] However, fluconazole's promise with aspergillosis was not realised.[102] Nonetheless, it was valued because of its broad-spectrum activity, with both superficial and systemic mycoses, and convenient oral administration.[103] In an article in the *Journal of Antimicrobial Chemotherapy* in January 1987, Roderick Hay had noted the great potential of triazole compounds because their targets were not well covered by existing antifungals.[104] However, he added that 'It will be a challenge to devise suitable methods of establishing their therapeutic roles in systemic fungal disease.'

Itraconazole was valuable with aspergillosis and prompted the first ever international symposium on '*Aspergillus* and aspergillosis'.[105] Held at the University of Antwerp in June 1987, and jointly sponsored by ISHAM and the Janssen Research Foundation, the event attracted 145 participants from 25 countries. The proceedings were co-edited by two Janssen Research Foundation scientists and Donald Mackenzie, who worked at the Mycological Reference Laboratory in London. All aspects of aspergillosis, allergic, toxigenic and pathogenic, were discussed, but the focus was on invasive disease and its treatment, with the majority of papers on treatment and prophylaxis with, unsurprisingly, itraconazole. The number of laboratories and clinicians that had been given the drug for trials was quite large. An underlying thread in the meeting was that amongst the general medical profession, aspergillosis and other fungal infections did not have the profile their prevalence and severity deserved. Indeed, delegates worried that the perception across medicine was that medical mycologists and clinicians were again exaggerating the importance of fungal infections to bring attention and resources to their area of specialist work.[106] One example was the problem of fungal infection in hospitals where building works were in progress. A lot of publicity had been given to how such works could be life threatening to immunosuppressed patient because of the liberation of fungal spores, yet infection control specialists had dismissed this as small beer in comparison to the dangers of hospital acquired bacterial infections, such as MRSA.

In his concluding comments at the Antwerp Symposium, Heinz Seeliger, Director of Institute for Hygiene and Microbiology at the University of Würzburg, suggested that itraconazole appeared to have started 'a new area of chemotherapy'.[107] Such hopes were soon to prove premature and several issues arose. First, it proved difficult to find sufficient cases for conclusive clinical trials, both to secure regulatory approval and to evaluate the new drug against amphotericin B.[108] When itraconazole finally passed all the trial stages and gained FDA approval in 1992, it was essentially as a 'salvage therapy'. Second, one of the alleged advantages of itraconazole was oral administration. However, Janssen found it hard to produce a formulation that was absorbed well enough to deliver a consistent effective dose.[109] Also, the active principle had to be protected from stomach acids, which meant patients had to swallow a large, coated capsule. Evidence also emerged in the early 1990s of a relatively large number of conflicts with other drugs, especially those likely to be taken by immuno-compromised patients. At the same time, new forms of amphotericin B were developed to mitigate its toxicity, mostly by binding the drug to lipids to avoid kidney damage, but these innovations were not taken up rapidly as they were not supported by randomised trials.[110] Trials with invasive aspergillosis were problematic because the number of patients were not only small, but were dispersed across the country, had different forms of the infection in different regions of the body, and they suffered from a wide range of underlying conditions.[111]

Nonetheless, by the mid-1990s, whilst still limited, treatment options for invasive aspergillosis had improved. Clinicians had gained better understandings of drug actions, more choices and protocols for different sites and types of infection. It was still the case, however, that many patients with the disease were diagnosed too late for effective therapy, though on this front there were promising new approaches from molecular biology for earlier and more accurate detection. One hope was that improved and standardised methods would make the recognition of infection easier for non-specialists. A lot of research was undertaken on antigen tests, but a breakthrough came with microassays to detect sugars released by growing *Aspergillus* hyphae.[112]

The profile of invasive aspergillosis grew because of its high mortality and the growing number of patients affected due to the greater use of immunosuppression with transplant, cancer and other patient groups.[113] Aspergillosis was an emerging infection in intensive care units, where monitoring and maintenance technologies, along with more aggressive therapies, opened the body to opportunistic infection. There was evidence in the mid-1990s from the United States and Germany that it had replaced candidiasis as the principal hospital-acquired fungal infection.[114]

A report on the changed picture and growing problem of invasive aspergillosis was presented in a European Science Foundation in 1998.[115] The summary gave range of incidence in different patient populations with health compromising underlying conditions at up to one in four for leukaemia patients and around one in eight for transplant recipients. (See Table 5.1): By comparison, the rate of infection amongst ordinary patients was less than 1%. A similar report by the *Aspergillus* Study Group in the United States, published in *Medicine* in 2000, based on data from 595 patients collected from 89 physicians, found a similar pattern.[116] At this time, the main treatments remained amphotericin B and itraconazole, separate or in combination, which still gave complete cures in only 27% of cases. The conclusion of reviews at this time was, as it had been for decades, that 'new approaches and new therapies are needed to improve the outcome of invasive aspergillosis in high risk patients'.[117]

There was, however, another new triazole in the pipeline – voriconazole.[118] This was another antifungal drug from the Pfizer research laboratories at Sandwich in Kent. It was produced from their programme to improve the effectiveness and range of triazoles.[119] The compound, first named UK-109,496, was subject to intensive *in vitro* testing in the 1990s, with new experimental methods and protocols used in comparative tests against amphotericin B and itraconazole.[120] Trials with mice and guinea pigs showed voriconazole to be an effective, broad spectrum antifungal, with high activity against *Aspergillus* spp.[121] Clinical trials showed that voriconazole had advantages over existing

Table 5.1 Incidence of invasive aspergillosis according to underlying condition.[122]

Condition	Range (%)
Lung transplantation	17–16
Allogeneic bone marrow transplantation	5–15
Acute leukaemia	5–24
Heart transplantation	2–13
Pancreas transplantation	1–4
Renal transplantation	0.5–10
AIDS	0–12
Multiple myeloma (stage III)	~4
Severe combined immunodeficiency	~4
Solid tumour and lymphoma	~1 – 3
Autologous bone marrow transplant	~1
Connective tissue diseases	~1

therapies in three areas: antifungal activity, administration and side effects. The drug was approved in the United States in May 2002 and in Europe the following year, primarily for the treatment of invasive aspergillosis. Its superiority over amphotericin B was celebrated in the *Lancet* in October 2002, though the advantages were relative: just over half of patients with invasive aspergillosis responded to voriconazole compared to just under a third on amphotericin.[123] Nonetheless, clinicians continued to be cautiously optimistic, not just about this drug, but because it pointed the way forward to more and better antifungals.[124]

Aspergillosis remains a rare disease, though in the first decade of the twenty-first century it became the largest cause of death from fungal infection in Britain and was second only to candidiasis in the United States.[125] Its impact in medicine was significant as it became associated with high profile settings: 'high tech' medical and surgical sites, particularly cancer and transplantation clinics, intensive care units and in the many clinical encounters that used immunosuppressant therapies. In one sense, aspergillosis was an exemplary iatrogenic condition – an unintended result of medical progress.[126] Indeed, the history of aspergillosis in the twentieth century can be mapped on key concerns and innovations. Pulmonary aspergillosis first attracted attention in the context of new interest in pulmonary tuberculosis around 1900 and re-emerged with mass X-ray and effective antibiotic treatment in the 1940s. *Aspergilli* spp. were also part of the rise of allergy and asthma, the development of antibiotics, and the discovery of mycotoxins. The profile of the infection was in step with larger epidemiological changes in mortality and especially morbidity: the decline in infections and the rise of cancers and other degenerative conditions, where chronicity and aggressive treatments opened the body to opportunistic infection. Serious disease was most common in a new type of patient – the post-transplant, immuno-compromised patient, who had been created and had to be maintained by modern medical technologies.

Summary and Reflections

Our aim in writing this book, apart from presenting the first history of fungal diseases, was also to contribute to the historiography of medicine. In this conclusion, rather than restate and revisit our histories of particular mycoses, we focus on crosscutting themes concerning the history of infectious diseases, the limits of the medical gaze, the history of medical specialisation and biographies of disease.

Our narrative has shown the value of approaching the history of infection in the twentieth century in terms of 'seed and soil'. Our reading of the medical record has been against the grain of the common focus on the 'seeds' – the specific causative organisms – of disease. It is no surprise that doctors' histories of infections are in this genre, after all the major trend in medicine in our period has been to define diseases in terms of their causes (aetiology), and from the middle of the century, to treat disease by targeting those specific causes with drugs, surgery or other technologies. The history of pulmonary tuberculosis exemplifies this trajectory. First, its medical name changed from phthisis (wasting) or consumption, a symptomatic definition, to TB.[1] The latter conflated pathology ('Tuberculosis') and aetiology (*Tubercle bacillus*), and approaching the disease in terms of its 'seeds' was reinforced after 1950, when antibiotics arrived as the long sought after 'magic bullets' that selectively killed the *T. bacillus* in the body. Doctors' histories of TB tended to write off pre-1950s treatments as 'unscientific' and ineffective, as they had focused on making the human 'soil' unsuitable for the *T. bacillus*, either by strengthening the body through the sanatorium regime, or removing the nidus of infection by surgery. Historians of medicine have been less judgmental and, in recovering the thinking and practices of the pre-antibiotic era, have shown the contingent nature of assessments of scientificity and efficacy, and suggested that for many patients, now abandoned treatments that aimed to improve bodily 'soil' did 'work'.[2]

The role of the 'soil' in the history of infectious diseases is implicit in Thomas McKeown's famous explanation of the decline in mortality from infectious diseases in Britain in the nineteenth century.[3] In his analysis, he discounted the influence of factors linked to the 'seeds' of infection, such the changing virulence of germs, along with medical and public health measures targeted at germs, and concluded that the principal cause of the decline was rising standards of living and improved nutrition, which had strengthened the body's soil and resistance to infection. The fact that many people whose body was infected with a specific germ did not develop disease was well known to doctors and especially with TB, as skin tests had long shown that while up to 90% of adults had been infected with the bacillus, only a fraction went on to develop the disease and fewer died.

In our discussion of fungal infections, we have also extended the metaphor of the 'soil' beyond its normal references to the individual body and its vulnerability to infection, to an ecological one that also embraces social and geographical settings, and to how these affected opportunities for the spread of infection as well as susceptibility. Our chapter sub-titles refer to particular types of 'soil' in this extended sense. Thus, for ringworm in children the 'soil' included an institution – schools, and for adults with foot infection, the 'soil' was a lifestyle – athleticism. With endemic mycoses, such as coccidioidomycosis, where the fungi were in fact literally in the soil, our larger notion of 'soil' included the social changes that brought in-migration and economic development. Warwick Anderson has recently highlighted the importance of the ecological tradition in work on infectious diseases in the twentieth century, but he shows that this expanded approach remained nevertheless predominantly 'biological', with any social and technological dimension implicit.[4] We have made the latter components explicit.

This book can be characterised as a history of diseases at the periphery of the medical gaze, or at the ends of the spectrum of infectious diseases. At one end, infections such as ringworm and thrush were ubiquitous, everyday and mostly either self-limited or self-treated, involving at most a single consultation with a doctor. This is not to deny that such infections can be chronic and hard to eliminate, even since the arrival of oral antifungal drugs. At the other end, infections such as candidaemia and invasive aspergillosis were rare and unusual, sometimes termed 'orphan diseases', and commonly fatal until recent decades.

But what can a study of these diseases at the margin contribute to our understanding of the middle, the majority and the mainstream? Above all, our analysis reminds historians that the minor, self-limiting and self-treated conditions are common across medicine and not just with infectious diseases. Illness 'ice bergs', the many episodes that do not reach the medical gaze, were and are present across all areas and most diseases. Yet, gaze of historians has always tended to be 'above the water'. For example, histories of the 'Great Influenza Pandemic' of 1918–1919 emphasise that between 20 and 40 million people died of the infection or complications such as pneumonia, yet the average mortality rate was around 2% (varying between 1% and 10%) amongst those who suffered.[5] This rate was very high compared to the normal experience of influenza, where case fatality rates was and remains typically less than 1%.[6] Both figures make our point that the majority patient experience of influenza was and is one of recovery; with an illness of variable severity, which was and is typically self-treated and not require medical attention, if indeed, the sufferer had access to, or could afford, professional consultation. Moreover, then, as now, those likely to die of pneumonia were and are people with underlying health problems; in other words, those with weakened 'soil'.

The investigation of rare and unusual diseases highlights the importance of the adaptation of mainstream ideas and practices to novel problems, and the opportunities to 'experiment' with new methods of diagnosis and treatment. In an era when standardisation and formal protocols dominate medical practice, our study of 'orphan mycoses' has shown the variability, complexity and individuality of clinical practice and the many resources, theoretical, practical and material, that doctors drew upon, and still draw upon, in all aspects of clinical work. The ways in which uses of amphotericin B, one the earliest antifungal antibiotic drugs, has been reinvented many times exemplifies this adaptability and shows the need to think about invention and innovation as processes rather than events. The very recognition of 'orphan diseases' in part derives from novel medical and social technologies of surveillance, which have provided new types of recognition of infection, such as X-rays and immune reactions, and new attitudes to risk associated with social, economic and technological changes, such as the negotiation of thresholds for intervention in public health and with specific populations.

Marginality has been studied by historians and sociologists of science as a 'context' that stimulates innovation.[7] These ideas have been critiqued empirically and for having loose definitions of marginality and innovation, but in this study we have discussed a group – medical mycologists – who were routinely designated marginal by their professional peers and saw themselves as such.[8] At the end of the twentieth century, medical mycology remained a small and marginal field; indeed, some in medicine argued that it was often oversold, with specialists exaggerating the importance of fungal diseases as causes of morbidity and mortality. We do not want to enter this debate, but instead reflect on the development of medical mycology as a specialism. As we noted in the Introduction, historical studies of specialisation in medicine are now less teleological and more nuanced, but there remains a focus on major specialisms and what might be termed 'mono-specialists'. As we have shown, most medical mycologists were 'multi-specialists', or had a number of 'specialist practices', even in the United States where the size of agencies, such as CDC and NIH, or the foci of regionally specific infections made mono-specialist careers possible. Indeed, a feature of our story is that the tension, expected in the 1930s and 1940s, between 'botany types' and 'medical types', which can also be seen as between laboratory and clinic, did not develop.[9] Cooperation and collaboration were characteristic as roles co-existed and were combined. In part, this was because of interdependence, especially as clinicians relied on laboratory-based experts to confirm and refine their diagnoses and, then after the 1950s, for the development of antifungal antibiotics. Solidarity was also prompted by size and marginality, which meant that creating and maintaining critical mass was a priority and specialist organisations, not least ISHAM which spanned the Americas and not just North America, were pivotal in this respect. In the United States, a presence at NIH and CDC was a boon. In contrast, medical mycologists in Britain had to be content with a single organisation, the BSMM, though this effectively lobbied national and, latterly, European agencies. Needless to say, the relatively small size of the field meant that individuals were very important, as too were personal connections and networks, which were facilitated by air travel from the 1950s, which made international meetings, both disciplinary and those sponsored by pharmaceutical companies on single drugs, more common and better attended. Our focus on diseases has meant that we have not dwelt on the careers of individual medical mycologists, though the repeated mention of names of key individuals, often with many infections and in multiple contexts, is testimony to their success in combining specialist practices.

The biographical mode is now fashionable in the history of medicine, not only for doctors, scientists and institutions, but diseases too.[10] We have not termed our narratives of fungal infections biographies, but have kept with 'histories'. Roger Cooter, while appreciating the richness of much of the new biographical genre, has criticised it for tending to be essentialist and singular, taking diseases as given, rather than looking at their construction and many identities.[11] Cooter was after all making these observations in the *Lancet*, the implication of his remarks being that historians of disease need to recognise that 'modern', singular narratives are no longer tenable in 'the face of contemporary impressions of fragmentation and the collapse of universal meanings'.[12] Our study supports this view. For example, consider the many views put forward on how to explain the rise in the incidence of fungal infections in the twentieth century. Some doctors maintain the increase was real and material, some said that it came from new conceptions of what constituted an infection, others said it was product of new medical technologies of surveillance and diagnosis, and others that it was iatrogenic. To these views can be added claims that the apparent rise came from changing public attitudes to infection and expectations of medical power. Our conclusion is that all the above forces were in play in the rise of mycoses, shaping, not just epidemiological patterns, but experiences and meanings; hence, despite the subtitle of this volume, over the twentieth century, mycoses can be seen as paradigmatic postmodern diseases.

Notes

Fungal Disease: An Overview

1. In the book, we use the terms 'fungal infections' and 'mycoses' (or singular fungal infection and mycosis) interchangeably, mostly following the usage of our historical actors in time and place.
2. The term 'ringworm' is very old and came from the circular patches of peeled, inflamed skin that characterised the infection. In medicine at least, no one understood it to be associated with worms of any description.
3. Porter, R., 'The patient's view: Doing medical history from below', *Theory and Society*, 1985, 14: 175–198; Condrau, F., 'The patient's view meets the clinical gaze', *Social History of Medicine*, 2007, 20: 525–540.
4. Burnham, J. C., 'American medicine's golden age: What happened to it?', *Science*, 1982, 215: 1474–1479; Brandt, A. M. and Gardner, M., 'The golden age of medicine', in Cooter, R. and Pickstone, J. V., eds, *Medicine in the Twentieth Century*, Amsterdam, Harwood, 2000, 21–38.
5. *The Oxford English Dictionary* states that the first use of 'side-effect' was in 1939, in H. N. G. Wright and M. L. Montag's textbook: *Materia Med Pharmacol & Therapeutics*, 112, when it referred to 'The effects which are not desired in any particular case are referred to as "side effects" or "side actions" and, in some instances, these may be so powerful as to limit seriously the therapeutic usefulness of the drug.'
6. Illich, I., *Medical Nemesis: The Expropriation of Health*, London, Calder & Boyars, 1975.
7. Beck, U., *Risk Society: Towards a New Society*, New Delhi, Sage, 1992, 56 and 63; Greene, J., *Prescribing by Numbers: Drugs and the Definition of Disease*, Baltimore, Johns Hopkins University Press, 2007; Timmermann, C., 'To treat or not to treat: Drug research and the changing nature of essential hypertension', Schlich, T. and Tröhler, U., eds, *The Risks of Medical Innovation: Risk Perception and Assessment in Historical Context*, London, Routledge, 2006, 144.
8. Rippon, J. W., 'Symposium on medical mycology', *Mycopathologia*, 1987, 99: 144. The *Fusaria* is a genus of soil-borne fungi, most of which are harmless, but some are well known to cause wilt in plants. Quorn, a meat-like product recommended for vegetarians, is produced from *Fusarium venenatum*.
9. Crook, W. G., *The Yeast Connection: A Medical Breakthrough*, Jackson, T., Professional Books, 1983.
10. Dubos, J., *Man Adapting*, chapters 7, 9 and 10; idem, *Mirage of Health: Utopias, Progress, and Biological Change*, New Brunswick, Rutgers University Press, 1959.
11. Dubos, J. and Dubos, R., *The White Plague: Tuberculosis, Man and Society*, London, Victor Gollancz, 1952.

12. Martin, G. W., 'Are fungi plants?', *Mycologia*, 1955, 47(6): 779–792; Whittaker, R. H., 'New concepts of Kingdoms of organisms', *Science*, 1969, 163: 150–161; Hagen, J. B., 'Five Kingdoms, more or less: Robert Whittaker and the broad classification of organisms', *Bioscience*, 2012, 62(1): 67–74.
13. Stringer, J. R. et al, 'A new name (*Pneumocystis jiroveci*) for pneumocystis from humans', *Emerg Infect Dis*, 2002, 8(9): 891–896.
14. Edman, J. C. et al, 'Ribosomal RNA sequence shows *Pneumocystis carinii* to be a member of the fungi', *Nature*, 1988, 334: 519–522; Armengol, C. E., 'A historical review of *Pneumocystis carinii*', *J Am Med Assoc*, 1995, 273(9): 747, 750–751.
15. Ainsworth, G. C., *Introduction to the History of Medical and Veterinary Mycology*, Cambridge, Cambridge University Press, 1987, 1–3.
16. Ainsworth, G. C., 'Agostino Bassi, 1773–1856', *Nature*, 1956, 177: 255–257; Arcieri, G. P., *Agostino Bassi in the History of Medical Thought*, Florence, L. S. Olschki, 1956.
17. Ainsworth, G. C., *Introduction to the History of Plant Pathology*, Cambridge, Cambridge University Press, 1981.
18. Bateman, T., *A Practical Synopsis of Cutaneous Diseases according to the Arrangement of Dr. Willan, Exhibiting a Concise View of the Diagnostic Symptoms and the Method of Treatment*, London: Longman, 1813; idem, *Delineations of Cutaneous Diseases: Exhibiting the Characteristic Appearances of the Principal Genera and Species Comprised in the Classification of the Late Dr. Willan*, London, Longman, Hurst, Rees, Orme, and Brown, 1817.
19. Jacyna, S., 'Pious pathology: J. L. Alibert's iconography of disease', Hannaway, C. and La Berge, A., eds, *Constructing Paris Medicine*, London, Clio Medica/The Wellcome Series in the History of Medicine, 185–219.
20. Lailler, C.-P., *Leçons cliniques sur les teignes, faites à l'hôpital Saint-Louis, par le Dr C. Lailler*, Paris, V.-A. Delahaye, 1878.
21. Worboys, M., *Spreading Germs: Disease Theories and Medical Practice in Britain, 1856–1900*, Cambridge, Cambridge University Press, 2000, 28–42.
22. Zakon, S. J. and Benedek, T., 'David Gruby and the centenary of medical mycology, 1841–1941', *Bull His Med*, 1944, 16: 155–168; Codell Carter, K., *The Rise of Causal Concepts of Disease*, Aldershot, Ashgate, 2003, 32–37 and 72–79.
23. Pelling, M., *Cholera, Fever and English Medicine, 1825–1865*, Oxford, Clarendon Press, 1978, 146–202.
24. Swayne, J. G. and Budd, W., 'An account of certain organic cells in the peculiar evacuations of cholera', *Lancet*, 1849, 54: 398–399.
25. Worboys, *Spreading Germs*, passim.
26. Sims Woodhead, G. and Hare, A., *Pathological Mycology: An Enquiry into the Etiology of Infectious Diseases*, Edinburgh, Young J. Pentland, 1885.
27. Muir, R. and Ritchie, J., *Manual of Bacteriology*, Edinburgh, Young J. Pentland, 1899, 133–138; de Bary, A., *Comparative Morphology and Biology of the Fungi, Mycetozoa and Bacteria*, Oxford, Clarendon Press, 1887.
28. Hawksworth, D. L., 'Geoffrey Clough Ainsworth (1905–1998): Mycological scholar, campaigner, and visionary', *Mycological Research*, 2000, 104(1), 110–116; Buczacki, S., 'Ainsworth, Geoffrey Clough (1905–1998)', *Oxford Dictionary of National Biography*, Oxford University Press, 2004 [http://www.oxforddnb.com/view/article/71235, accessed 3 May 2013].

29. Ainsworth, G. C., *Introduction to the History of Mycology*, Cambridge, Cambridge University Press, 1976; idem, *Introduction to the History of Plant Pathology*, Cambridge, Cambridge University Press, 1981.
30. Ainsworth, *Introduction to the History of Medical*, ix.
31. For an alternative approach to that adopted here, see: Wainwright, M., 'Some highlights in the history of fungi in medicine – A personal journey', *Fungal Biology Reviews*, 2008, 22: 97–102.
32. Espinel-Ingroff, A. V., *Medical Mycology in the United States: A Historical Analysis (1894–1996)*, Dordrecht, Kluwer Academic Publishers, 2003. The book was based on her 1994 PhD, Espinel-Ingroff, A., *Medical Mycology in the United States: 100 Years of Development as a Discipline*, PhD dissertation, Virginia Commonwealth University, Richmond, 1994. Also see, Espinel-Ingroff, A. V., 'History of medical mycology in the United States', *Clinical Microbiology Reviews*, 1996, 9(2): 235–272.
33. Daniel, T. M. and Baum, G. L., *Drama and Discovery: The Story of Histoplasmosis*, Westport, CT, Greenwood, Press, 2002. A version of the earlier chapters was published as Baum, G. L. and Schwarz, J., 'The history of histoplasmosis 1906–1956', *N Engl J Med*, 1957, 256: 253–258.
34. Fiese, M. J., *Coccidioidomycosis*, Springfield, IL, Charles C. Thomas, 1958; Odds, F. C., *Candida and Candidosis*, Leicester, Leicester University Press, 1979.
35. Hischmann, J., 'The early history of coccidioidomycosis: 1892–1945', *Clin Infect Dis*, 2007, 44(9): 1202–1207.
36. However, the 'The Aspergillus Website' has an excellent 'History' section, with an extensive collection of primary sources that we have used extensively in researching this book. 'The Aspergillus Website', Historical Papers Database and History Section. Accessed 25 March 2013, http://www.aspergillus.org.uk/indexhome.htm?secure/historical_papers/index.php~main.
37. Rosenthal, T., 'Perspectives in ringworm of the scalp: Treatment through the ages', *Arch Derm Syphilol*, 1960, 82(6): 851–856.
38. Seidelman, R. D. et al, '"Healing" the bodies and souls of immigrant children: The ringworm and Trachoma Institute, Sha'ar ha-Aliyah, 1952–1960', *Journal of Israeli History*, 2010, 29(2): 191–211.
39. For works that deal with the issue of specialisation of medicine, see, Rosen, G., *The Specialization of Medicine with Particular Reference to Ophthalmology*, New York, Froben Press, 1944; Stevens, R., *Medical Practice in Modern England: The Impact of Specialization and State Medicine*, New Haven, Yale University Press, 1966.
40. Weisz, G., *Divide and Conquer: A Comparative History of Medical Specialization*, New York, Oxford University Press, 2006, xxix–xxx.
41. This point is made by Stephen Caspar in his review of George Weisz's *Divide and Conquer in Medical History*, 2006, 50: 545–547.
42. Digby, A., *Making a Medical Living: Doctors and Patients in the English Market for Medicine, 1720–1911*, Cambridge, Cambridge University Press, 1994.
43. Macfarlane, J. T. and Worboys, M., 'The changing management of acute bronchitis in Britain, 1940–1970: The impact of antibiotics', *Medical History*, 2008, 52: 47–72.
44. Scambler, G. and Scambler, A., 'The illness iceberg and aspects of consulting behaviour', in Fitzpatrick, R., ed, *The Experience of Illness*, London, Tavistock, 1984, 35–37.

45. Porter, R., 'The patient's view: Doing medical history from below', *Theory and Society*, 1985, 14: 175–198; Condrau, F., 'The patient's view meets the clinical gaze', *Social History of Medicine*, 2007, 20: 525–540.
46. Galgiani, J. N., 'Coccidioidomycosis: Changing perceptions and creating opportunities for its control', *Ann N Y Acad Sci*, 2007, 1111: 1–18.
47. Editorial, 'Thrush', *JAMA*, 1927, 89: 1429–1430; Plass, E. D. et al, 'Monilia vulvovaginitis', *Am J Obstet Gynecol,* 1931, 21: 320.

1 School Settings and Ringworm

1. Sanderson, M., *Education, Economic Change and Society in England 1780–1870*, Cambridge, Cambridge University Press, 1995; Simon, B., *Studies in the History of Education*, London, Lawrence and Wishart, 1966; Digby, A. and Searby, P., eds, *Children, School and Society in Nineteenth-Century England*, London, Macmillan, 1981; Nasaw, D., *Schooled to Order: A Social History of Public Schooling in the United States*, New York, Oxford University Press, 1979.
2. Richardson, N., *Typhoid in Uppingham: Analysis of a Victorian Town and School in Crisis, 1875–7,* London: Pickering & Chatto, 2008.
3. Pusey, W. A., *The History of Dermatology*, Springfield, Ill., C. C. Thomas, 1933; Crissey, J. T. and Parish, L. C., *The Dermatology and Syphilology of the Nineteenth Century,* New York, Praeger, 1981. On Robert Willans see: Brunton, D., 'Willan, Robert (1757–1812)', *Oxford Dictionary of National Biography*, Oxford University Press, 2004. http://www.oxforddnb.com/view/article/29438. Accessed 8 February 2013.
4. On Plumbe see, Rosenthal, T., 'Samuel Plumbe', *Arch Derm Syphilol*, 1937, 36(2): 348–354.
5. Plumbe, S., 'History, Pathology and Treatment, of Ring-worm and Scald-head', *Lancet*, 1835, 926.
6. Ibid.
7. Brown, H., *Ringworm and Some Other Scalp Affections: Their Cause and Cure*, London, J. & A. Churchill, 1899.
8. Buchan, W., *Domestic Medicine: Or, A Treatise on the Prevention and Cure of Diseases*, London, 11th Edition, London, 1790, 555–556.
9. Beeton, I., *Beeton's Book of Household Management*, London, S. O. Beeton, 1861, No. 2667–2668.
10. Plumbe, S., 'Remarks on the Contagious Ring-worm of the Scalp', *Lancet*, 1835, 858.
11. There is an excellent history of ringworm in France, see: Tilles, G. and Tilles, G., *Teignes et Teigneux: Histoire Medicale et Sociale*, Paris, Springer, 2008.
12. Allan, G. A. T., *Christ's Hospital*, London, Town and County, 1984.
13. Plumbe, S., 'History, Pathology and Treatment of Ringworm and Scald-head', *Lancet*, 1835, i: 926–928 and ii: 50–51; Rosenthal, T., 'Samuel Plumbe', *Arch Dermatol*, 2008, 16: 36–43.
14. *Lancet*, 1835, 683–688.
15. Plumbe, 'History, Pathology', 928.
16. Plumbe, S., *An Address to the Governors of Christ's Hospital, on the Causes and Means of Prevention of Ring-Worm in That Establishment; To Which Is Attached,*

a Few Rules for the Domestic Management of the Scholars during Their Vacations, London, 1834.
17. Mayne, R. G., *An Expository Lexicon of the Terms, Ancient And Modern, in Medical and General Science*, Pt 2, London: J. Churchill, 1854, 265.
18. Lawrence, C., '"Incommunicable Knowledge": Science, Technology and the Clinical "Art" in Britain, 1850–1910', *Journal of Contemporary History*, 1985, 20: 503–520.
19. *Lancet*, 1875, i: 888.
20. Ibid.
21. *Lancet*, 1908, i: 822.
22. Lawrence, C., *Medical Theory, Surgical Practice: Studies in the History of Surgery*, London, Routledge, 1992.
23. Rook, A., 'Dermatology in Britain in the Late Nineteenth Century', *Br J Dermatol*, 1979, 100(1): 3–12.
24. Erichsen, J. E., *The Science and Art of Surgery*, London, J. Walton, 1869, 8.
25. Rook, A., 'James Stratin, Jonathan Hutchinson and the Blackfriars Skin Hospital', *Br J Dermatol*, 1978, 99: 215–219.
26. Ibid., 216.
27. Russell, B. F., ed, *St John's Hospital for Diseases of the Skin, 1863–1963*, Edinburgh, E. & S. Livingstone, 1963.
28. *Lancet*, 1864, ii: 538. The three supporters withdrew their support when they realised Milton's practice was mainly on the treatment of spermatorrhoea, the involuntary discharge of semen.
29. Hadley, R. M., 'The Life and Works of Sir William James Erasmus Wilson, 1809–84', *Medical History*, 1959, 3: 215–247; Power, D'A, 'Wilson, Sir (William James) Erasmus (1809–1884)', revised Geoffrey L. Aserton, *Oxford Dictionary of National Biography*, Oxford University Press, 2004. [http://www.oxforddnb.com/view/article/29702, accessed 15 August 2008].
30. Quoted in Hogg, J., *Parasitic or Germ Theory of Disease: The Skin, Eye, and Other Affections*, London, Baillière, Tindall and Cox, 1876, 33.
31. Asherson, G. L., 'Fox, William Tilbury (1836–1879)', *Oxford Dictionary of National Biography*, Oxford University Press, 2004. [http://www.oxforddnb.com/view/article/10048, accessed 15 August 2008]; English, M. P., 'William Tilbury Fox and Dermatological Mycology', *Br J Dermat*, 1977, 97: 100–112; Cooper, J., 'Anderson, Sir Thomas McCall (1836–1908)', revised, J O'D Alexander, *Oxford Dictionary of National Biography*, Oxford University Press, 2006, [http://www.oxforddnb.com/view/article/30414, accessed 6 October 2008; Anon, 'Thomas McCall Anderson, Obituary', *Lancet*, 1908, i: 468–471.
32. Tilbury Fox, G., *Skin Diseases of Parasitic Origin*, London, Robert Hardwicke, 1863; idem, 'The True Nature and Meaning of Parasitic Diseases of the Surface', *Lancet*, 1859, ii: 5–7, 31–32, 201, 260–261, 283–284 and 507–508; M'Call Anderson, T., *On the Parasitic Affections of the Skin,* London, Churchill, 1861.
33. Tilbury Fox, *Skin Diseases,* v–vi; Anderson, *On the Parasitic Affections*, 1–2.
34. Hogg, J., 'The Vegetable Parasites of the Human Skin', *BMJ*, 1859, i: 241; Hillier, T., 'On Ringworm and Vegetable Parasites', *BMJ,* 1861, ii: 552 and 577; Worboys, M., *Spreading Germs: Disease Theories and Medical Practice in Britain, 1865–1900*, Cambridge, Cambridge University Press, 2000, 73–107.
35. Wilks, S., 'Address in Medicine', *BMJ*, 1872, ii: 146–153.

36. Ibid., 149.
37. Colan, T., 'Parasitic Vegetable Fungi and the Diseases Induced by Them', *Lancet*, 1874, ii: 755–757 and 832–833.
38. Liveing, R., 'Lecture on the Peculiarities of Ringworm and its Treatment', *Lancet*, 1879, ii: 642–644, on 643–644.
39. Worboys, *Spreading Germs*, *Passim*; M'Call Anderson, T., 'Introductory Lectures to the Study of the Diseases of the Skin', *Lancet*, 1870, i: 149–151.
40. *Lancet*, 1861, ii: 449–450.
41. Pelling, M., *Cholera, Fever and English Medicine, 1830–1865*, Oxford, Clarendon Press, 1976, 146–202.
42. Tilbury Fox, W., 'On the Identity of Parasitic Fungi Affecting the Human Surface', *Lancet*, 1880, ii: 260–261; *Lancet*, 1867, ii: 266–267.
43. *Lancet*, 1889, ii: 1232.
44. Stark, J., *Industrial Illness in Cultural Context: 'La maladie de Bradford' in Local, National and Global Settings, 1878–1919*, Unpublished PhD Thesis, University of Leeds, 2011; Jamieson, A., *An Intolerable Affliction: A History of Lupus vulgaris in Late 19th and Early 20th Century Britain*, Unpublished PhD Thesis, University of Leeds, 2010.
45. British Association of Dermatologists, *A Biographical History of British Dermatology*, London, British Association of Dermatologists, 1995.
46. Tilbury Fox, W., 'Ringworm in Schools', *Lancet*, 1872, i: 5–6.
47. Hirst, J. D., 'Public Health and the Public Elementary Schools, 1870–1907', *History of Education*, 1991, 20: 107–118.
48. Harris, B., *The Health of the Schoolchild: A History of the School Medical Service in England and Wales*, Buckingham, Open University Press, 1995, 32–47.
49. 'Report of the Lancet Sanitary Commission on the Sanitary Condition of our Public Schools', *Lancet*, 1875, i: 795–796, 859–861 and ii: 111–112, 314–315, 422–423, 574–575, 682, and 785–787.
50. See the case of George Beavis who in November 1875 was fined for neglecting to send his daughter to school. Hansard, HC Deb 11 February 1876, 227: 227–229; *Times*, 3 February 1876, 5c; 9 March 1876, 6e.
51. Liveing, 'Lecture on the Peculiarities', 643–644.
52. Mansell, K., *Christ's Hospital in the Victorian Era*, Whitton, Ashwater Press, 2011.
53. Alder Smith, H., *Ringworm: Its Diagnosis and Treatment*, London, H. K. Lewis & Co. Ltd, 1880; 2nd Edition, 1882; 3rd Edition, 1885; Aldersmith, H., *Ringworm and Alopecia Areata*, 4th Edition, London, H. K. Lewis & Co. Ltd, 1897.
54. Tilbury Fox, W., 'On Ringworm of the Head and its Management', *Lancet*, 1877, ii: 643–644.
55. Alder Smith, *Ringworm*, 1882, vii.
56. Many general patent medicines included ringworm as one of the conditions they cured. Specifically, the most widely advertised topical remedies were Beatson's Ringworm Lotion, Bateson's Specific and Cuticura Soap. Holloway's Ointment was advised to be used in conjunction with Holloway's Pills, and those seeking a systemic cure could try was Orange's Universal Cerate and Vegetable Purifying Pills.
57. *Manchester Times*, 2 February 1889, 2 and 9 February 1889, 8.
58. *Morning Post*, 10 May 1889, 4; *Reynolds's Newspaper*, 26 May 1889, 1.

59. Worboys, *Spreading Germs*, 234–276.
60. Newson Kerr, M., *Fevered Metropolis: Epidemic Disease and Isolation in Victorian London*, Unpublished PhD Thesis, University of Southern California, 2007; Harris, *The Health of the Schoolchild,* passim.
61. On the Ringworm School see http://www.workhouses.org.uk/index.html?MAB/MAB.shtml, accessed 13 August 2010.
62. 'Dr Payne's Report on Ringworm', 1891, London Metropolitan Archives (LMA) MA, NSSD/79.
63. 'Dr Eddowes Report on Anerley School', 27 May 1893, LMA, NSSD 80.
64. Ibid., 30 December 1893. It was likely he used an ointment based on chrysophanic acid, ichthyol and salicylic acid. Eddowes, A., 'Treatment of Ringworm', *BMJ*, 1893, i: 785–786.
65. Abraham, P. S. and Eddowes, A., 'Contagious Skin Diseases in Schools', *Lancet*, 1894, ii: 275.
66. Morris, M., 'Ringworm in Elementary Schools', *Lancet*, 1891, ii: 348.
67. Anon, 'Enlargement of Functions of the Metropolitan Asylums Board', *Lancet*, 1897, i: 1483.
68. Baxter Forman, E., 'A Lecture on Medical London', *Lancet*, 1899, i: 213.
69. Downs School Sub Committee Minutes, 1903, LMA, MAB-5–17, MAB/0509, Sub-Committee Minute Book, pp. 43–44 and 61.
70. Anon, 'Ringworm and the Metropolitan Asylums Board', *Lancet*, 1904, i: 318–319. Also see: Admission and Discharge Registers, 1903–1906, LMA, MAB-22–8, MAB/2326, p. 1, 54, 64, 93 and 133. The first four children admitted on26 February 1903 were typical, staying respectively 26, 17, 13 and 8 months.
71. Abraham and Eddowes, 'Contagious', 275.
72. Ibid.
73. Morris, *Ringworm*, 1898, 69.
74. Brown, *Ringworm and Other Scalp Affections,* 1–3.
75. Tilles and Tilles, *Teignes et Teigneux*, 85–99.
76. Sabouraud, R., *Les Trichophyties humaines,* Paris, Rueff and Cie, 1894.
77. Civatte, A., 'Obituary: Raymond Sabouraud', *Br J Dermatol*, 50, 1938: 206–210.
78. Sabouraud, R., 'La Question des Teignes (Au Congress de Londres)' *Annales de dermatologie et syphiligraph,* 1896, 7: 1333–1357. Also see: Morris, M., *Ringworm in the Light of Recent Research,* London, Cassell and Co., 1898, v; Editorial, 'The Parasites of Ringworm', *Lancet*, 1893, i: 1204.
79. Aldersmith, *Ringworm,* 1897, 6.
80. Colcott Fox, T. and Blaxall, F. R., 'An Enquiry into the Plurality of Fungi Causing Ringworm in Human Beings, as Met with in London', *Br J Dermatol*, 1896, 8: 241; Roberts, L., 'The Present Position of the Question of Vegetable Hair Parasites', *BMJ*, ii: 1894, 685–688.
81. Sabouraud, R., 'X-ray Treatment of Tinea tonsurans', *International Clinics*, 1904, 2, 41–49; Sabouraud, R. et al, 'La Radiotherapie die teignes a l'ecole Lallier en 1904', *Bulletin de la Société française de dermatologie et de syphiligraphie*, 1905, 16: 10. Also see: Sabouraud, R., *Maladies Cryptogamiques, Les Teigne*, Paris, Masson & Cie, 1910; Tilles and Tilles, *Teignes et Teigneux*, 100–106.
82. *Lancet*, 1903, ii: 1102.

83. However, see: Shoemaker, J. V., 'Ringworm in Public Institutions', *Trans Am Med Assoc*, 1878, 29: 139–147.
84. Pulliam, J. D. and van Patten, J. J., *History of Education in America*, New York, Pearson, 2006.
85. Turner, J. P., *Ringworm and Its Successful Treatment*, Philadelphia, F. A. Davis, 1921; Burnett, J. C., *Ringworm: Its Constitutional Nature and Cure*, Philadelphia, Boericke & Tafel, 1892.
86. Kraut, A. M., *Silent Travelers: Germs, Genes, and the Immigrant Menace*, New York, Basic Books, 1994, 58–67; Allen, S. K. and Semba, R. D., 'The Trachoma "Menace" in the United States, 1897–1960', *Surv Ophthalmol*, 2002, 47(5): 500–599.
87. Markel, H., '"The Eyes Have It": Trachoma, the Perception of Disease, the United States Public Health Service, and the American Jewish Immigration Experience, 1897–1924', *Bulletin of the History of Medicine*, 2000, 74: 525–560.
88. Buckley, A. M., 'The X-ray Treatment of Ringworm of the Scalp', *JAMA*, 1913, 56: 1766.
89. Bunch, J. L., 'Sabouraud's Method of Ringworm Treatment', *Lancet*, 1905, i: 414–416.
90. Natale, S., 'The Invisible Made Visible: X-rays as Attraction and Visual Medium at the End of the Nineteenth Century', *Media History*, 2011, 17(4): 345–358; Pamboukian, S., '"Looking Radiant": Science, Photography and the X-ray Craze of 1896', *Victorian Review*, 2001, 27(2): 56–74.
91. Aldersmith, *Ringworm*, 1897, 296.
92. Walsh, D., *The Roentgen Rays in Medical Work: With an Introductory Section upon Electrical Apparatus and Methods by J. E. Greenhill*, London, Baillière & Co., 1897.
93. Anon, '"X" Rays as Depilatory', *Lancet*, 1896, i: 1296; Daniel, J., 'Depilatory Action of X-rays', *Medical Records*, 1896, 49: 595–596.
94. Report, 'The Roentgen Rays as a Depilatory', *Lancet*, 1897, i: 752; Freund, L., 'Ein mit Röntgen-Strahlen behandelter Fall von Naevus pigmentosus piliferus', *Wiener Medizinische Wochenschrift*, 1897, 47: 428–434; idem, 'Nachtrag zu dem Artikel 'Ein mit Röntgen-Strahlen behandelter Fall von Naevus pigmentosus piliferus', *Wiener Medizinische Wochenschrift*, 1897, 47: 856–860; Report, 'Depilation by High-Tension Electric Currents', *Lancet*, 1901, i: 121; Walsh, D., 'The Removal of Superfluous Hair by a Combination of X-ray Exposure and Electrolysis', *Lancet*, 1901, ii: 1191–1192.
95. Pusey, W. A., 'Roentgen-ray Therapy Twenty Years Ago', *JAMA*, 1923, 81(15): 1257–1260.
96. Pignot, M. M., 'Souvenir sur Raimond Jacques Sabouraud 1864–1938', *Mycopathologia*, 1954, 7: 348–364.
97. Guido Holzknecht, an Austrian physician, had pioneered the use of chemical monitoring in the 1890s, placing mixtures that were sensitive to radiation in pastilles between the generator and the patient. Doctors calibrated tissue damage against dosage as revealed by colour changes, largely by trial and error. Holzknecht created a unit 'H' (from his own initial) and an 'H-scale' which allowed doctors to quantify the alteration in the 'tint' of pastilles by comparison with a painted colour chart. However, he kept the formula of his pastilles secret; hence, they were expensive

and supplies were limited. Sabouraud introduced a cheaper method using barium platino-cyanide, which was the standard chemical used on X-ray plates before they were fixed photographically. These pastilles were not only cheaper, they could be reused as they returned to their original colour after exposure. Sabouraud set out detailed specifications of the distance between machine and patient, the protection of surrounding skin, generator settings, the position of the pastille and the required degree of colour change. For Holzknecht, see: Angetter, D. C., *Guido Holzknecht: Leben und Werk des österreichischen Pioniers der Röntgenologie*, Wien, Werner Eichbauer, 1998. For more, also see: Paul, W., 'A History of Radiation Detection Instrumentation', *Health Physics*, 2005, 88(6): 616; Sabouraud R. and Noiré, H., 'Traitement des teignes tondantes par les rayons X', *La Presse Mèdicale*, 1904: 12: 825–827.

98. Walker, N., 'X-rays in the Treatment of Tinea', *BMJ*, 1904, i: 868.
99. Adamson, H. G., 'On the Treatment of Ringworm of the Scalp by Means of X-rays', *Lancet*, 1905, i: 1715.
100. Bunch, 'Sabouraud's Method', 416.
101. Morris, M., 'The Harveian Lecture on Some New Therapeutic Methods in Dermatology', *BMJ*, 1905, i: 699.
102. Ibid.
103. MacLeod, J. M. H., 'The Treatment of the Scalp by X-rays', *BMJ*, 1905, ii: 14.
104. MacLeod, J. H. M., 'The Treatment of Ringworm of the Scalp by X-rays', *BMJ*, 1905, ii: 13–15. Also see: Higham Cooper, R., 'The Supposed Risks Attending X-ray Treatment of Ringworm', *BMJ*, 1909, ii: 454–457.
105. Sichel, G., 'The X-ray Treatment of Ringworm', *BMJ*, 1906, i: 256–257. Also see: Sequeira, J. H., 'The Varieties of Ringworm and Their Treatment', *BMJ*, 1906, ii: 193–196.
106. See letters in response to Sichel's article in: *BMJ*, 1906, i, 359–360, 419–420, 539–540, 840 and 1018–1020.
107. LMA, Children's Committee Report for 1905, Metropolitan Asylums Board; Ayers, G. M., *England's First State Hospitals and the Metropolitan Asylums Board, 187–1930*, London, Wellcome Institute, 1971, 171–175 and 207.
108. Report, 'The Metropolitan Asylums Board', *BMJ*, 1907, i: 1314.
109. Bulkley, L. D., 'The X-ray Treatment of Ringworm of the Scalp', *JAMA*, 1911, 56: 1706–1709.
110. Macleod, J. H. M., *Diseases of the Skin: A Text-book for Students and Practitioners*, London, H. K. Lewis, London, 1920.
111. Report, 'Children's Committee, Metropolitan Asylums Board', *BMJ*, 1907, i: 1314.
112. *Times*, 9 December 1908, 6c.
113. Prior, J. R., 'X-ray Treatment of Ringworm', *Public Health*, 1910–1911, 24: 153–154.
114. Adam, T., 'The Control of Ringworm in School', *Public Health*, 1912–1913, 26: 3–8; Bernard Shaw, A. F., 'The Diagnosis of Ringworm in School Children', *Public Health*, 1912–1913, 26: 366–369.
115. *Times*, 31 March 1909, 12d.
116. *Times*, 1 April 1909, 18e.
117. Letter H. M. Harris, 18 March 1910, LMA, PH/SHS/2/9.
118. Letter from Walter Longley, 8 April 1910, LMA, PH/SHS/2/9.
119. Letter from Henry Carter, 29 May 1910, LMA, PH/SHS/2/9.

120. Cates, J., 'The Administrative Control of Ringworm', *Public Health*, 1910–1911, 24: 226–233.
121. On the continuing controversies about the treatment see: Anon, 'Favus and Ringworm among Schoolchildren', *Lancet*, i: 1909: 1636.
122. Anon, 'The Lancet Commission of Ringworm: Its Prevalence, Influence and Treatment', *Lancet*, 1910, i: 51–56.
123. Ibid., 55.
124. *Daily Mirror*, 5 November 1901, 16; 8 February 1912, 15c-d; 7 December 1922, 14 a–b.
125. Reported in Cates, 'The Administrative Control', 232.
126. Ernest Dore, S., 'The Present Position of the X-ray Treatment of Ringworm', *Lancet*, 1911, i: 432.
127. Ibid.
128. *Annual Report for 1908 of the Chief Medical Officer of the Board of Education*, BPP, 1910, Cd. 4986, XXIII: 55–57.
129. 'The Health of School Children', *Times*, 30 October 1911: 11a.
130. MOH Report for 1912.
131. Payne, J. F., 'An Address on Bacteria in Diseases of the Skin', *Lancet*, 1896, ii: 2–3.
132. MOH Report, Manchester.
133. 'Manchester and District', *BMJ*, 1913, ii: 205.
134. Walker, N., 'Fifty Years of Dermatology', *Lancet*, 1929, ii: 212.
135. LMA.
136. Adam, 'The Control of Ringworm', 3–8; Bernard Shaw, 'The Diagnosis of Ringworm', 366–369.
137. Report, 'Medicine in the Schools', *BMJ*, 1920, 2: 826.
138. Report, 'School Health in London in 1934', *Public Health*, 1935, 48(12): 403; *The Health of the School Child: Annual Report of the Chief Medical Officer of the Board of Education*, 1937, London, HMSO, 1938, 87–88.
139. Between 1922 and 1931 2,426 cases were treated there, only 200 or so per year. *The Health of the School Child: The Annual Report of the Chief Medical Officer of the Board of Education for 1925*', London, HMSO, 1926, 41.
140. *The Health of the School Child: The Annual Report of the Chief Medical Officer of the Board of Education for 1933*, London, HMSO, 1934, 9.
141. Cochrane Shanks, S., 'Vale Epilation: X-ray Epilation of the Scalp at Goldie Leigh Hospital, Woolwich (1922–1958)', *Br J Dermatol*, 19, 79(4): 237–238.
142. Walker, 'Fifty Years', 211.
143. *The Health of the School Child*, 1933, 86.
144. Walker, 'Fifty Years', 211; Percival, G. H., 'The Treatment of Ringworm of the Scalp with Thallium Acetate', *Br J Dermat*, 1930, 42(2): 59–69.
145. Editorial, 'Thallium: A Dangerous Drug', *N Engl J Med*, 1931, 204: 1117; Lewis, D. R. and Lloyd, A. W., 'Treatment of Ringworm of the Scalp with Thallium Acetate', *BMJ*, 1933, ii: 99–100.
146. *The Health of the School Child*: *The Annual Report of the Chief Medical Officer of the Board of Education for 1938*, London, HMSO, 1939. Also see: Barber, H. W., 'The Relationship of Dermatology to General Medicine', *Lancet*, 1929, ii: 363–370, 483–492 and 591–599.
147. Underwood, E. A., 'National Health and Physical Fitness', *Public Health*, 1937–1938, 51: 328–333.

2 Hygiene, Fitness and Athlete's Foot

1. Anon, 'Dermatology in 1938', *BMJ*, 1939, i: 924.
2. Majima, A., 'The Invention of "Athlete's foot": Lifestyle, cleanliness, and American leisure classes in the early twentieth century', *Seikatsugaku ronsō*, 2010, 17: 3–13.
3. Whitfield, A., 'A Note on some unusual cases of Trichophytic infection', *Lancet*, 1908, ii: 237–238.
4. Emmons, C. W., 'The Jekyll-Hydes of mycology', *Mycologia*, 1960, 52: 669–680, 671.
5. Bulmer, G. S., 'The changing spectrum of mycological education', *Mycopathologia*, 1995, 130: 127–128.
6. Robbins, W. J., 'Bernard O. Dodge, mycologist, plant pathologist', *Science*, 133, 1960: 741–742.
7. Davis, R. H. and Perkins, D. D., 'Neurospora: a model of model microbes', *Nature Reviews Genetics*, 2002, 3, 397–403.
8. Andrews, G. C., 'J Gardner Hopkins', *Arch Derm Syphilol*, 1951, 64(6): 810–812.
9. Georg, L. K., 'Rhoda Benham, 1894–1957', *Arch Dermatol*, 1957, 76(3): 363–364. Hopkins worked at the Laboratory for Medical Mycology of the College of Physicians and Surgeons, in the Department of Botany at Columbia University.
10. Kwon-Chung, K. J. and Campbell, C. C., 'Chester Wilson Emmons', *Medical Mycology*, 1986, 24(1) 89–90.
11. Emmons, 'The Jekyll-Hydes', 671.
12. Emmons, C. W., 'Dermatophytes: Natural grouping based on the form of the spores and accessory organs', *Arch Derm Syphilol*, 1934, 30: 337–362.
13. 'Review', *Arch Derm Syphilol*, 1932, 26: 956–957.
14. Rudolph, E. D., 'Carroll William Dodge, 1895–1988', *Mycologia*, 1990, 82(2): 160–164.
15. Swartz, J. H., 'The role of fungi in medicine', *N Engl J Med*, 1936, 215: 322.
16. Ibid., 323.
17. Greenwood, A., 'Fungus diseases of the skin', *N Engl J Med*, 193, 213: 363–370.
18. Adamson, H. G., 'On the treatment of scabies and some other common skin afflictions in soldiers', *Lancet*, 1917, i: 222–223.
19. MacCormac, H., 'Skin-diseases under war conditions', *Brit J Dermatol*, 1917, 29: 113–131; Adamson, H. G., 'On the Treatment of Scabies and some other common skin affections in soldiers', *Lancet*, 1917, i: 221–223.
20. MacPherson, W. G. et al, *History of the Great War Based on Official Documents: Medical Services Pathology*, London, HMSO, 1923; MacPherson, W. G. et al, *Medical Services, Diseases of the War*, London, HMSO, 1923.
21. Nickerson, J. W. et al, 'Sandals and hygiene and infections of the feet', *Arch Derm Syphilol*, 1945, 52: 365–368.
22. Ormsby, O. S. and Mitchell, J. H., 'Ringworm of the hands and feet', *JAMA*, 1916, 67: 711–717; Mitchell, J. H., 'Ringworm of the hands and feet: An historical review', *JAMA*, 1951, 146(6): 541–546.
23. *Oxford English Dictionary*, http://www.oed.com/. Accessed on line 10 February 2011.

24. 'Athlete's foot', *Literary Digest*, 22 December 1928, 17.
25. Legge, R. T. et al, 'Ringworm of the foot: Preliminary report', *JAMA*, 1929, 92: 1507–1508.
26. Legge, R. T. et al, 'Incidence of foot ringworm amongst college students: Its relation to gymnasium hygiene', *JAMA*, 1929, 93: 170.
27. 'Bears investigate athlete's foot', *Los Angeles Times*, September 27, 1931, F5. Also see Maima, 'Invention of "Athlete's foot" ', 7.
28. Gould, J. E., 'Ringworm of the feet', *JAMA*, 1931, 96: 1300–1302.
29. Anon, 'An American letter', *Public Health*, 1932–1933, 46: 59.
30. Swartz, 'The role of fungi', 322.
31. Blaisdell, J. H., 'Epidermophytosis', *N Engl J Med*, 1930, 202: 1059–1064.
32. Maima, 'Invention of "Athlete's foot" ', 7–8.
33. Gilman, R. T., 'The incidence of ringworm of the feet in a university group: Control and treatment', *JAMA*, 1933, 100: 716.
34. Underwood G. B. et al, 'Overtreatment dermatitis of the feet', *JAMA*, 1946, 130: 249.
35. White, C. J., 'Fungus disease of the skin, clinical aspects and treatment', *Arch Derm Syphilol*, 1927, 15: 387–414.
36. 'The History of Absorbine'. After Absorbine became widely available across America, farmers realised that the same liniment that helped their horses also helped their own aches and pains. Seeing the need, Wilbur and Mary Ida's son Wilbur II suggested a version for people. In 1904, Absorbine Jr. was introduced, named after Wilbur Jr. Like Absorbine Veterinary Liniment, Absorbine Jr. helps the body heal itself by increasing blood flow to the affected area. It has the same analgesic and antiseptic properties as the veterinary liniment. It works great to relieve the itch caused by athlete's foot. W.F. Young, Inc. actually coined the phrase 'athlete's foot'. Absorbine Jr. is now widely available at major mass-retailers and smaller pharmacies and stores. http://absorbine.blogspot.com/2010/06/history-of-absorbine.html. Accessed 8 October 2010.
37. Falls, A. I., 'Doing business as Falls Chemical Co. v. Scholl Mfg. Co., Inc. case to protect Solvex', *The Trade-Mark Reporter*, 27 Trademark Rep. (1937), 444.
38. Pillsbury, D. et al, *A Manual of Cutaneous Medicine*, Philadelphia, W. B. Saunders, 1961, 604. For a later view, see: Bhutani, L. K. et al, 'Tinea pedis – a penalty of civilization A sample survey of rural and urban population', *Mycoses*, 1971, 14: 335–336.
39. Fraser, P. K., 'Tinea of the foot', *BMJ*, 1938, i: 842–844; H. MacCormac, 'Ringworm of the foot', *BMJ*, 1940, i: 739–741.
40. 'Pithead baths' *BMJ*, 1931, i: 25; Morgan, W. J., 'The miners' welfare fund in Britain 1920–1952', *Social Policy & Administration*, 1990, 24: 199–211.
41. Souter, J. C., 'A Clinical note on fungus infection of the skin of the feet', *Proc Roy Soc Med*, 1937, 30: 1107–1116.
42. MacKenna, R. M. B., et al, 'Dermatological practice in war-time', in *Medicine and Pathology: History of the Second World War*, London: Her Majesty's Stationery Office, 1952, 408–419; Pillsbury, D. M. and Livingood, C. S., 'Experiences in military dermatology: Their interpretation in plans for improved general medical care', *Arch Derm Syphilol*, 1947, 55: 441–462.
43. Dewitt Mackenzie, *Men without Guns*, Philadelphia, The Blakiston Company, 1943, 15–16 and Plate 1.

44. 'Report', *JAMA*, 1941, 117: 1973.
45. De Kruif, P., 'A working cure for athlete's foot', *Reader's Digest, 1942*, 40: 46–48.
46. Summers, W. C., 'On the origins of the science in Arrowsmith: Paul De Kruif, Félix d'Hérelle and phage', *J Hist Med Allied Sci*, 1991, 46(3): 315–332.
47. See the review of de Kruif's *The Male Hormone* in *Arch Derm Syphilol*, 1945, 52(1): 71.
48. Report, 'Food and drug administration warns o Phenol Camphor mixture, *JAMA*, 1942, 119: 713. Also see: Miller, F. G., 'Poisoning by phenol', *Can Med Assoc J*, 1942; 46(6): 615–616; Phillips, B., 'The phenol-camphor treatment of dermatophytosis', *Br J Dermatol*, 1944, 56(11–12): 219–227.
49. Sanderson, P. H. and Sloper, J. C., 'Skin disease in the British Army in SE Asia', *Br J Dermatol*, 1953, 65, 252–264, 300–309 and 362–372.
50. Ainsworth, G. C., 'The medical research council's medical mycology committee (1943–1969): A chapter in the history of medical mycology in the UK', *Sabouraudia*, 1978, 16: 1–7.
51. Souter, 'A clinical note on fungus infection', 1107.
52. Knowles, R. B., 'Dermatitis in coal-miners: A survey of the factors influencing its nature and cause', unpublished M. D. Thesis, University of Sheffield, 1943; idem, 'Factors Influencing dermatitis in coal-miners', *BMJ*, 1944, ii: 430–432; H. R. Vickers, 'Arthur Rupert Hallam', *BMJ*, 1955, ii: 741–751.
53. Capel, E. H., 'A medical service for the coal mining industry', *Journal of the Royal Society for the Promotion of Health*, 68, 1948, 525–531, 526. Also see 'Royal sanitary institute congress', *BMJ,* 1948, i: 1196.
54. Hodgson, G. A., 'The history of coal miners' skin diseases', in Cule, J. ed, *Wales and Medicine: An Historical Survey from Papers Given at the Ninth British Congress on the History of Medicine*, London: British Society for the History of Medicine, 1975, 59.
55. H. R. Vickers was a lecturer at the University of Sheffield by the time of appointment with the CIE, therefore, it could be that Vickers supervised Knowles's study in 1943.
56. However, Lane resigned almost immediately after the launch of the Committee, giving his reason that 'industrial medicine was adequately represented on the Committee by Dr. Rogan'. Committee on Industrial Epidermophytosis', Minutes for the First Meeting, 13 November 1951, MRC. 51/739 CIE. Min. 1, Committee on Industrial Epidermophytosis (Foot ringworm in coal miners and other workers in Great Britain) Manuscripts, Reports, Correspondence 1950–1955. Contemporary Medical Archives Centre, GC1/1, Wellcome Library, p. 3.
57. Cochrane, A. L. and Blythe, M., *One Man's Medicine: An autobiography of Professor Archie Cochrane,* London, The British Medical Journal, 1989.
58. For a description on the relationship between the NCB and the government, see McIvor, A. and Johnston, R., *Miners' Lung: A History of Dust Disease in British Coal Mining*, Farnham, Ashgate, 2007, 146–147; Smith, J. H., 'The distribution of power in nationalized industries', *British Journal of Sociology*, 1951, 2(4), 275–293; Presthus, R. V., 'British public administration: The national coal board', *Public Administration Review*, 1949, 9(3): 200–210.
59. Committee on Industrial Epidermophytosis', Minutes for the First Meeting, 13 November 1951, MRC. 51/739 CIE. Min. 1, Committee on Industrial

Epidermophytosis (Foot ringworm in coal miners and other workers in Great Britain) Manuscripts, Reports, Correspondence 1950–1955. Contemporary Medical Archives Centre, GC1/1, Wellcome Library, p. 1.

60. Rogan, J. M., 'Epidermophytosis and the coal miners – an introductory note', 5 November 1951, MRC. 51/683 CIE. 51/1, Committee on Industrial Epidermophytosis (Foot ringworm in coal miners and other workers in Great Britain) Manuscripts, Reports, Correspondence 1950–1955. Contemporary Medical Archives Centre, GC1/1, Wellcome Library, p. 2.
61. 'Committee on industrial epidermophytosis', Minutes for the First Meeting, 13 November, 1951, MRC. 51/739 CIE. Min. 1, Committee on Industrial Epidermophytosis.
62. Holmes, J. G., 'Pilot study of epidemiology of epidermophytosis in the coal-mining industry', MRC.53/72 CIE.53/1, Committee on Industrial Epidermophytosis, p. 2.
63. Ibid.
64. Gentles, J. C. and Holmes, J. G., 'Foot ringworm in coal-miners', *Br J Indust Med*, 1957, 14: 22–29.
65. Holmes, 'Pilot study of epidemiology of epidermophytosis', 4, p. 9.
66. Duncan, J. T., 'The epidemiology of fungus diseases', *Trans R. Soc Trop Med Hyg*, 1948, 42: 207–216, 209.
67. Rosman, N., 'Infections with *Trichophyton rubrum*', *Br J Dermatol*, 1966, 78(4): 208–212.
68. Walker, J., 'The dermatophytoses of Great Britain: Report of a three year survey', *Br J Dermatol*, 1950, 62: 239–251.
69. Sproot, N. A., 'Athlete's foot', *BMJ*, 1957, ii: 1064 and 1243.
70. Holmes, J. G. and Gentles, J. C., 'Diagnosis of foot ringworm', *Lancet*, 1956, ii: 62–63.
71. Peterkin, G. A. G., 'The diagnosis and treatment of tinea pedis', *Practitioner*, 1957, 180: 543–552.
72. Cruickshank, R., 'The epidemiology of some skin infections', *BMJ*, 1956, i: 58.
73. Pillsbury, D. M. et al, *Dermatology*, Philadelphia, W. B. Saunders, 1956, 606. English, M., '*Trichophyton rubrum* infection in families', *BMJ*, 1957, i: 746 and 755.
74. G. B. Underwood et al, 'Overtreatment dermatitis of the feet', *JAMA,* 1946, 130(5): 249–256.
75. Ibid., 249.
76. Schwartz, L. et al, 'Control of the scalp amongst school children', *JAMA*, 1946, 132: 58–62; Miller, J. L. et al, 'Local treatment of tinea capitis', *JAMA*, 1946, 132: 67–70.
77. Stevens, R. J. and Lynch, F. W., 'Ringworm of the scalp: A report on the current epidemic', *JAMA*, 1947, 133: 306–309; McKee, G. M. et al, 'Treatment of tinea capitis with Roentgen rays', *Arch Derm Syphilol,* 1946, 53: 458–470.
78. Bocobo, F. C. et al, 'Epidemiologic study of tinea capitis caused by *T tonsurans* and *M audouinii*', *Public Health Rep*, 1952, 67: 53–56.
79. Modan, B. et al, 'Thyroid neoplasms in a population irradiated for scalp tinea in childhood', in De Groot, C., ed, *Radiation Associated Thyroid Carcinoma*, New York, Grune & Stratton Inc, 1977, pp. 449–459; Hempelman,

L. H. et al, 'Neoplasms in persons treated with X-rays in infancy: Fourth survey in 20 years', *J Natl Cancer Inst*, 1975, 55: 519–530.

80. Hornblum, A. M., *Acres of Skin: Human Experiments at Holmesburg Prison*, New York: Routledge, 1998.
81. Kligman, A. M., 'The pathogenesis of tinea capitis due to *Microsporum audouini* and *Microsporum canis*', *J Invest Dermatol*, 1952, 18, 231–246. Also see: Strauss, J. S. and Kligman, A. M., 'Effect of x-rays on sebaceous glands of the human face: Radiation therapy of acne', *J Invest Dermatol*, 1959, 33: 347–356.
82. Ibid., 231.
83. Kligman, A. M. and Anderson, W. W., 'Evaluation of current methods for the local treatment of tinea capitis', *J Invest Dermatol*, 1951, 16: 155–168.
84. Strauss, J. S. and Kligman, A. M., 'An experimental study of tinea pedis and onychomycosis of the Foot', *AMA Arch Derm*, 1957, 76(1): 70–79, 70.
85. Gilchrest, B. A. and Leyden, J. L., 'In memoriam: Mites and the mighty: The last work and lasting legacy of Albert M. Kligman, PhD, MD', *Journal of Investigative Dermatology*, 2011, 131, 6–7.
86. Gellene, D., Obituary, Dr Albert M. Kligman', *New York Times*, 22 Feb 2010, 26a.
87. Weyers, W., 'Medical experiments on humans and the development of guidelines governing them: The central role of dermatology', *Clinics in Dermatology*, 2009, 27(4): 384–394.
88. Georg, L. K., '*Trichophyton tonsurans* ringworm: A new public health problem', *Public Health Rep* 1952, 67: 53–56; Bronson, D. M. et al, 'An epidemic of infection with *Trichophyton tonsurans* revealed in a 20-year survey of fungal infections in Chicago', *J Am Acad Dermatol*, 1983, 8(23): 322–330; Rippon, J. W., 'Forty four years of dermatophytes in a Chicago clinic (1944–1988)', *Mycopathologia, 1992,* 119: 25–28.
89. Shockman, J. and Urbach, F., 'Tinea Capitis in Philadelphia', *Int J Dermatol*, 1983, 22(9): 522–523.
90. Jawetz, E., 'The rational use of antimicrobial agents: Reason versus emotion in chemotherapy', *Oral Surg Oral Med Oral Pathol*, 8(9): 982–987.
91. Sulzberger, M. B. and Kano, A., 'Undecylenic and propionic acids in the prevention and treatment of dermatophytosis', *Arch Derm Syphilol* 1947, 55: 391–395.
92. Hartley, F., 'Parachlorphenyl-a-glycerol as an antibacterial and antifungal agent of pharmaceutical interest', *Quarterly Journal of Pharmacy and Pharmacology*, 1947, 20: 388–395; Petrow, V. and Hartley, Sir F., 'The rise and fall of British Drug Houses, Ltd.', *Steroids*, 1996, 61: 476–482.
93. Anon, 'Treatment of ringworm of the feet', *Lancet*, 1946, I; 95.
94. Peterkin, G. A. G., The diagnosis and treatment of tinea pedis', *Practitioner*, 1957, 180: 551.
95. Ibid., 550.
96. The development of the drug by Glaxo and its commercial exploitation is discussed in detail in Chapter 9 of a company history of Glaxo, see: Davenport-Hines, R. P. T. and Slinn, J., *Glaxo: A History to 1962*, Cambridge, Cambridge University Press, 1992, 200–222. The chapter is entitled – 'The development and commercial exploitation of griseofulvin'.
97. Oxford, A. E. et al, 'Griseofulvin, $C_{17}H_{17}O_6Cl$, a metabolic product of *Penicillium griseo-fulvum* Dierckx, *Biochem J*, 33, 1939: 240–248.

98. Bud, R., *Penicillin: Triumph and Tragedy*, Oxford, Oxford University Press, 2007, 26–29; Birkinshaw, J. H., 'Harold Raistrick, 1890–1971', *Biogr Mems Fell R. Soc,* 1972, 18: 488–509.
99. Brian, P. W., 'Studies on the biological activity of Griseofulvin', *Annals of Botany*, 1949, 13: 59–77.
100. The work of A. R. Martin at ICI's Pharmaceutical Division at Alderley Park is discussed in Anon, 'The symposium', *Transactions of the St John's Dermatological Society*, 1960, 45: 1.
101. Anon, 'Fungicide by mouth', *Lancet*, 1958, ii: 1216.
102. This paragraph is based on the chapter on griseofulvin in Davenport-Hines and Slinn, *Glaxo*, 200–222.
103. Gentles, J. C., 'Experimental ringworm in guinea pigs: Oral treatment with Griseofulvin', *Nature*, 1958, 182: 476–477.
104. Paget, G. E. and Walpole, A. L., 'Some cytological effects of griseofulvin', Nature, 1958, 182, 1320–132; idem, 'The experimental toxicology of griseofulvin', *Arch Dermatol,* 1960, 81: 750–757.
105. Quintal, D. and Jackson, R., 'The development of 20th century dermatologic drugs', *Clinics in Dermatology*, 1989, 7 (3), 42–43.
106. Williams, D. I. et al, 'Oral treatment of ringworm with Griseofulvin', *Lancet*, 1958, ii: 1212–1213.
107. Ibid., 1212.
108. Quoted in Davenport-Hines, *Glaxo,* 209.
109. Gentles, J. C., 'Experimental ringworm in guinea pigs: Oral treatment with griseofulvin', *Nature*, 1958, 182: 476–477.
110. Ibid., 476.
111. Gentles, J. C., 'The treatment of ringworm with Griseofulvin', *Br J Dermatol*, 1959, 71: 427–433.
112. Williams, D. I. et al, 'Griseofulvin', *Br J Dermatol*, 1959, 71: 434.
113. Ibid., 434 and 442.
114. Ibid., 442.
115. Blank, H. and Roth, J. F., 'The treatment of dermatomycoses with orally administered Griseofulvin', *Arch Dermatol*, 1960, 81: 259–267.
116. Pillsbury, D. M., 'Griseofulvin therapy in dermatophytic infections', *Trans Am Clin Climat Assoc*, 1959, 71: 52–57.
117. Blank, H., 'Symposium on Griseofulvin', *Arch Dermatol*, 1960, 51: 649. The full proceedings were published as 'Griseofulvin and dermatomycoses: An international symposium sponsored by University of Miami, October 26–27, 1959', *Arch Dermatol*, 1960, 81: 649–789.
118. Maibach, H. I. and Kligmann A. M., 'Short-term treatment of onychomycosis with Griseofulvin', *Arch Derm Syphilol*, 1960, 81: 733–734; Dillaha, C. J. and Jansen, G., 'Dosage requirements of Griseofulvin in Onychomycosis Due to Trichophyton Rubrum. Preliminary Report', Ibid., 790–766.
119. Report, 'Oral treatment of fungus infections with griseofulvin: An international symposium', *Transactions of the St John's Dermatological Society*, 1960, 45: 1–145.
120. The figure given was £21 for six month's treatment, which would be £300 in 2013. This would not be that expensive today, which says something about drug price inflation.
121. Anon, 'The symposium', *Transactions of the St John's Dermatological Society*, 1960, 45: 1.

122. Frain Bell, W., and Stevenson, J. C., 'Report on a clinical trial', *Transactions of the St John's Dermatological Society*, 1960, 45: 47–53. Russell, B. et al, 'Chronic ringworm infection of the skin and nails treated with griseofulvin: Report of a therapeutic trial', *Lancet*, 1960, i: 1141–1147.
123. Russell, B. F., 'Correlation of clinical and laboratory findings and the criteria of cure', *Transactions of the St John's*, 1960, 45: 141.
124. Davenport-Hines and Slinn, *Glaxo*, 219.
125. Ibid.
126. Anon, 'Griseofulvin', *Lancet*, 1960, i: 1175–1176.
127. English, M. P., 'Some controversial aspects of tinea pedis', *Br J Dermatol*, 1962, 74: 50–56; idem, *BMJ*, 1961, i: 1086.
128. Anon, 'Tinea pedis', *Lancet*, 1962, i: 785–786.
129. Blank, H., 'Antifungal and other effects of griseofulvin', *Am J Med*, 1965, 39(5): 831–838; Davies, R. R. and Everall, J. D., 'Mycological and clinical evaluation of griseofulvin for chronic onychomycosis', *BMJ*, 1967, ii: 464–468; Anon, 'Today's drugs: Griseofulvin', *BMJ*, 1967, iv: 608–609.
130. Anon, 'Today's drugs: Fungal antibiotics', *BMJ*, 1963, i: 1659–1660; Anon, 'Antibiotics in dermatology', *BMJ*, 1963, ii: 981–982.
131. Blank, H., 'Antifungal and other effects of Griseofulvin', *Am J Med*, 1965, 39: 831–838; Report, 'Today's drugs: Griseofulvin', *BMJ*, 1967, ii: 608–609.
132. Weston Hurst, A., 'Protoporphyrin, cirrhosis and hepatomata in the livers of mice given griseofulvin', *Br J Dermatol*, 1963, 75(3): 105–112; Anderson, D. W., 'Griseofulvin: Biology and clinical usefulness, a review', *Ann Allergy*, 1965, 23: 103–110.
133. Conte, N. F. et al, 'Prophylactic Griseofulvin against *Trichophyton mentagrophytes* infections', in H. M. Robinson, ed, *The Diagnosis and Treatment of Fungal Infections*, Springfield: Charles C. Thomas, Inc., 1974, 543.
134. Allen, A. M., *Internal Medicine in Vietnam: Volume 1, Skin Disease in Vietnam, 1965–1972*, Washington DC, Office of the Surgeon General, 1972, 59–82. For a summary, see: Allen, A. M. et al, 'Skin infections in Vietnam', *Military Medicine*, 1972, 137: 295–301.
135. Maertens, J. A., 'History of the development of azole derivatives', *Clin Microbiol Infect*, 2004, 10, Suppl 1: 1.
136. Cartwright, R. Y., 'Use of antibiotics: Antifungals', *BMJ*, 1978, ii: 108–111.
137. Montgomery, B. J., 'Belgian oral antifungal agent looks promising', *JAMA*, 1980, 243(1): 12.
138. Check, W. A., 'Oral antifungal agent effective even for widespread infections', *JAMA*, 1980, 244: 2019–2020.
139. Restrepo, A. et al, 'Introduction', *Reviews of Infectious Diseases*, 1980, 2(4): 519.
140. Dismukes, W. E. et al, 'Criteria for evaluation of therapeutic response to antifungal drugs', *Rev Infect Dis*, 1980, 2(4): 535–545.
141. Borelli, D. et al, 'Ketoconazole, an oral antifungal: Laboratory and clinical assessment of imidazole drugs', *Postgraduate Medical Journal*, 1979, 55: 657–661.
142. Dismukes, W., 'Concluding remarks', *Rev Infect Dis*, 1980, 2(4): 688.
143. Robertson, M. H. et al, 'Oral therapy with ketoconazole for dermatophyte infections unresponsive to griseofulvin', *Rev Infect Dis*, 1980, 2(4): 578–581.

144. Hay, R. J., 'A comparative double blind study of ketoconazole and griseofulvin in dermatophytosis', *Br J Dermatol,* 112, 1985: 691–696.
145. Lambert, D. R. et al, 'Griseofulvin and ketoconazole in the treatment of dermatophyte infections', *Int J Dermatol,* 1989, 28: 300–304.

3 An Integrated Study of Antibiotics and Candida

1. Macfarlane, G., *Alexander Fleming: The Man and the Myth,* Oxford, Oxford University Press, 1984.
2. Christensen, C. M., *The Molds and Man: An Introduction to the Fungi,* Minneapolis, University of Minnesota Press, 1951.
3. The Oxford English Dictionary dates the first use of the term for a disease to none other than Samuel Pepys and a diary entry for 17 June 1665, when he wrote of someone: 'He hath a fever – a thrush and a Hickup', OED online. Accessed 8 August 2012.
4. Vogel, M. J. and Rosenberg, C. E., eds, *The Therapeutic Revolution: Essays in the Social History of American Medicine,* Philadelphia, University of Pennsylvania Press, 1979.
5. Li, J. W.-H and Vederas, J. C., 'Drug discovery and natural Products: End of an era or an endless frontier?' *Science,* 2009, 325: 161–165.
6. Medical Research Council, 'Treatment of pulmonary tuberculosis with streptomycin and para-aminosalicylic acid', *BMJ,* 1950, ii: 1073–1085; Medical Research Council, 'Various combinations of isoniazid with streptomycin or with PAS in the treatment of pulmonary tuberculosis', *BMJ,* 1955, ii: 435–445.
7. Jawetz, E., 'Infectious diseases: Problems of antimicrobial therapy', *Ann Rev Med,* 1954, 5: 6.
8. Earlier in the century, *M. albicans* had been known as *Oidium albicans.*
9. Kane, R. L., 'Iatrogenesis: Just what the doctor ordered', *Journal of Community Health,* 1980, 5(3): 149–158; Whorton, J., 'Antibiotic abandon: The resurgence of therapeutic rationalism', in Parascandola, J., ed, *The History of Antibiotics: A Symposium,* Madison, Wis, American Institute of the History of Pharmacy, 1980, 125–136.
10. Sáez-Gómez, J. M. and Romero-Maroto, M., 'Scientific ideas on muguet (Thrush) in the XVIII century', *Journal of Dental Research,* 2010, 89: 571–574.
11. Goodhart, J. F., *The Diseases of Children,* 6th Edn, London, J. & A. Churchill, 1899, 114.
12. West Walker, J., 'On diphtheria', *BMJ,* 1863; i: 504, 551 and 660.
13. Stuart Wilkinson, J., 'Some remarks upon the development of epiphytes: With the description of a new vegetable formation found in connexion with the human uterus', *Lancet,* 1849, ii: 448–451.
14. Pelling, M., *Cholera, Fever and English Medicine,* Oxford, Clarendon Press, 1976.
15. Wilkinson, 'Some remarks', 450.
16. Bashford, A., *Purity and Pollution: Gender, Embodiment and Victorian Medicine,* Palgrave, 1998.
17. Hewitt, G., 'Lectures on the diagnosis and treatment of diseases of women', *BMJ,* 1862, i: 54.

18. Hurley, R., 'Candidal vaginitis', *Proc R. Soc Med*, 1977, 70(Suppl 4): 1–2; Also see: Hurley R., and de Louvois, J., '*Candida* vaginitis', *Postgrad Med J*, 1979, 55: 645–647.
19. Plass, E. P. et al, 'Monilial vulvovaginitis', *Am J Obstet Gynecol*, 1931, 21: 320.
20. Semon, H. C., 'The non-venereal affections of the genitalia', *Br J Vener Dis*, 1929, 5: 114–127.
21. Harkness, A. H., 'Non-gonococcal urethritis', *Br J Vener Dis,* 1933(3), 173–186 and 187–191.
22. Sharp, B. B., 'Vulvo-vaginitis', *Br J Vener Dis*, 1930(6): 301.
23. Sharman, A., 'The significance of leucorrhoea', *BMJ*, 1935, ii: 1199–1201: Bland, P. D. et al, 'Vaginal trichomoniasis in the pregnant woman', *JAMA*, 1931, 96: 157–163; Solomon, E. and Dockeray, G. C., 'Vaginal discharges', *Irish Journal of Medical Science* 1936–1937, 11, 548–551.
24. See Chapter 2.
25. Georg, L. K., 'Rhoda Benham, 1894–1957', *Arch Dermatol*, 1957, 76(3): 363–364.
26. Benham, R., 'Certain *Monilias* parasitic on man: Their identification by morphology and by agglutination', *J Infect Dis*, 1931, 49: 183–215.
27. Ibid., 212. Sprue was a tropical disease of the small intestine.
28. Berkhout, M. C., *De schimmelgeslachten Monilia, Oidium, Oospora en Torula, Scheveningen*, Edauwe & Johanssen, 1923; Shrewsbury, J. D., 'The genus *Monilia*', *J Path Bact*, 1934, 38: 213–254,
29. Skinner, C. F., 'The yeast-like fungi: *Candida* and Brettomyces', *Bacteriol Rev*, 1947, 11(4): 227–274.
30. Martin, D. S. et al, 'A practical classification of the Monilias', *J Bacteriol* 34, 1937: 99–129; Martin, D. S. and Jones, C. P., 'Further studies on the practical classification of the Monilias', *J Bacteriol*, 1940, 39: 609–630.
31. Gay, F. P., *Agents of Disease and Host Resistance*, Baltimore, Charles C. Thomas: 1935, 1118–1123.
32. Cruickshank, R. and Sharman, A., 'Hormones and vaginitis', *J Obst Gynecol*, 1934, 41: 190.
33. Bland, P. D. et al, 'Experimental vaginal and cutaneous moniliasis: Clinical and laboratory studies of certain monilias associated with vaginal, oral and cutaneous thrush', *Arch Derm Syphilol*, 1937, 36: 760.
34. Tattersall, R., *Diabetes: A Biography*, Oxford, Oxford University Press, 2009, 82–85.
35. Hesseltine, H. C., 'Diabetic and mycotic vulvovaginitis: Preliminary report', *JAMA*, 1933; 100(3): 177–178.
36. Feudtner, C., *Bittersweet: Diabetes, Insulin, and the Transformation of Illness*, Chapel Hill, NC, University of North Carolina Press, 2003,
37. Woodruff, P. and Hesseltine, H. C., 'Relationship of oral thrush to vaginal mycosis and the incidence of each', *Am J Obstet Gynecol*, 1938, 36: 467.
38. Liston, G. and Cruickshank, L. G., 'On thrush, with special reference to vaginal thrush', *Edin Med J*, 1940, 47: 369–390; Liston, G. and Cruickshank, L. G., 'Leucorrhoea in pregnancy: A study of 200 cases', *Br J Obstet Gynaecol*, 1940, 47: 109–129.
39. Comment, 'Vaginal thrush', *Lancet*, 1940, i: 1174; Editorial, 'Vaginal discharge', *Lancet*, 1940, ii: 300. Also see: Bland, P. B. and Rakoff, A. E.,

'Leukorrea: Clinical and therapeutic aspects', *JAMA*, 1940, 115(12): 1013–1018.
40. Editorial, 'Vaginal discharge', 300.
41. Cregor, F. W. and Gastineau, F. M., 'Stovarsol in the treatment of syphilis: A preliminary report', *Arch Derm Syphilol,* 1927, 15(1): 43–53.
42. *The Medical Annual 1941: A Year Book of Treatment and Practitioner's Index*, Bristol, John Wright, 1941.
43. Ludlam, G. B. and Henderson, J. L., 'Neonatal thrush in a maternity hospital', *Lancet*, 1942, i: 64–70.
44. Menzies, M. F., 'Hospital or domiciliary confinement?', *Lancet*, 1942, ii: 35–38 and 201.
45. McNeil, C., 'Death in the first month and the first year', *Lancet*, 1940, i: 819–821.
46. 'Thrush in infants', *BMJ*, ii: 1950: 1430–1431.
47. Wagner, J. M. and Kessel, I., 'Complications of *C. albicans* infection in infancy', *BMJ*, 1958, ii: 362–366.
48. Donald, I., 'Aetiology and investigation of vaginal discharge', *BMJ*, 1952, ii: 1223–1226.
49. Russell, C. S., 'Leucorrhoea', *BMJ*, 1953, ii: 91–93. Also see: Anon, 'Any questions? Vaginitis', *BMJ*, 1952, ii: 813–815 and 1954, i: 59.
50. Collins, J. H., 'Vulvovaginitis', *Obstet Gynecol Surv*, 1952, 7(2): 224–227; Thomas, H. H., 'Candidal vulvovaginitis: Treatment with mycostatin', *Obstet Gynecol*, 1957, 9(2): 163–166.
51. Smith, G., 'The Subway grate scene in the seven year itch: "The staging of an appearance-as-disappearance" ', *Cinémas: Journal of Film Studies*, 2004, 14(2–3): 213–244.
52. Report, 'Council on pharmacy and medicine', *JAMA*, 1951, 145: 1267.
53. Bud, R., *Penicillin: Triumph and Tragedy,* Oxford, Oxford University Press, 2007, 105–107.
54. Smith, L. W. and Walker, A. D., *Penicillin Decade 1941–1951: Sensitizations and Toxicities*, Washington, Arundel Press, 1951.
55. Scales, I. K. et al, 'Oral fungus infection: Candidiasis albicans', *Oral Surg Oral Med Oral Pathol*, 1956, 9: 970–977.
56. Colgan, M. T., 'The bacterial flora of the intestinal tract: Changes in diarrheal disease and following antimicrobial therapy', *Journal of Pediatrics*, 1956, 49: 214–228; Editorial, 'Antibiotics and monilial infection', *Lancet*, ii, 532.
57. Hirst, H. L. et al, 'Methods of administration of penicillin', *J Lab Clin Med*, 1947, 32: 32.
58. Lane, S. L., 'A review of current opinion on the hazards of indiscriminate antibiotic therapy in dental practice', *Oral Surg Oral Med Oral Pathol*, 1956, 9: 952–961.
59. Hussar, A. E. and Holley, H. L., *Antibiotics and Antibiotic Therapy*, New York, Macmillan, 1954, 12–34. Also see: Binns, T. B., 'Gastro-intestinal complications of oral antibiotics', *Lancet*, 1956, i: 336–338.
60. Harris, H. J., 'Aureomycin and chloramphenicol in Brucellosis: With special reference to side effects', *JAMA*, 1950, 142: 161–165.
61. Woods, J. W. et al, 'Monilial infections complicating the therapeutic use of antibiotics', *JAMA*, 1951, 145: 207–211.

62. Joekes, T. H. and Simpson, R. H., 'Bronchomoniliais', *Lancet*, 1923, ii: 108–111; Anon, 'An investigation into bronchomoniliais', *Lancet*, 1924, i: 714.
63. Greer, A. E., 'The synergism between mycotic and tuberculous infections of the lungs', *Dis Chest*, 1948, 14: 33–40; Brown, T. G., Pulmonary mycosis, *Edin Med J*, 1947, 54: 414–422.
64. Oblath, R. W. et al, 'Pulmonary moniliasis', *Ann Intern Med*, 1951, 35: 97–116.
65. Editorial, 'A danger of the newer antibiotics', *BMJ*, 1951, i: 1196.
66. Editorial, 'Fungus infection complicating antibiotic therapy', *JAMA*, 1952, 149: 762–763.
67. Kligman, A. M., 'Are fungus infections increasing as a result of antibiotic therapy', *JAMA*, 1952, 149: 979–983.
68. Huppert, M. D. et al, 'Pathogenesis of *C. albicans* infection following antibiotic therapy. I. The effect of antibiotics on the growth of *C. albicans*', *J Bacteriol,* 1953, 65: 171–176.
69. Kligman, 'Are fungus infections', 979.
70. Ibid., 983; Editorial, 'Antibiotic therapy and fungous infections', *N Engl J Med*, 1952, 247, 491–492.
71. Jawetz, 'Infectious diseases', 6.
72. Finland, M. and Weinstein, L., 'Complications induced by antimicrobial agents', *N Engl J Med*, 1953, 248, 220–226.
73. Weinstein, L. et al, 'Infections occurring during chemotherapy', *N Engl J Med*, 1954, 251: 251–259.
74. Sharp, J. L., 'The growth of *Candida* albicans during antibiotic therapy', *Lancet*, 1954, i: 390–392.
75. Cannon, P. R., 'The changing pathologic picture of infection since the introduction of chemotherapy and antibiotics', *Bull N Y Acad Med*, 1955, 31: 89–91.
76. Kozinn, P. J. et al, 'Candida albicans: Saprophyte or pathogen? A diagnostic guideline', *JAMA*, 1966, 198(2): 170–172.
77. Baldwin, R. S., *The Fungus Fighters: Two Women Scientists and Their Discovery*, Ithaca, Cornell University Press, 1981.
78. Ibid., 75.
79. Hazen, E. L. and Brown, R., 'Two antifungal agents produced by a soil actinomycete', *Science*, 1950, 112: 423; idem, 'Fungicidin, an antibiotic produced by a soil actinomycete', *Exp Biol Med*, 1951, 76: 93–97.
80. Hazen, E. L. and Brown, R., 'Nystatin', *Ann N Y Acad Sci,* 1960, 27, 89: 258–266.
81. Waksman, S. et al, 'Antifungal antibiotics', *Bull World Hlth Org*, 1952, 6: 163–172.
82. Garrod, L. P., 'The sensitivity of actinomyces to antibiotics', *BMJ*, 1952, i: 263; Hussar and Holley, *Antibiotics*, 366–369.
83. Espinel-Ingroff, A. V., *Medical Mycology in the United States: A Historical Analysis (1894–1996)*, Dordrecht, Kluwer Academic Publishers, 2003, 86 and 94–96.
84. The powder was also used in laboratories as an antifungal agent, to suppress the contamination of sera, tissue cultures, culture plates, and other in vitro media. See: Report, 'Mycostatin available for laboratories', *Journal of the Franklin Institute*, 1956, 261: 285.

85. Brabander, J. O. W. et al, 'Intestinal moniliasis in adults', *Canad Med Assoc J*, 1957, 77: 478–483.
86. Shrand, H., 'Thrush in the newborn', *BMJ*, 1961, ii: 1530–1533, i: 186 and 567.
87. Sternberg, T. H. and Newcomer, V. D., *Therapy of Fungal Diseases: An International Symposium*, Boston, Little Brown & Company, 1956.
88. Ibid., 'Contents'.
89. Sloane, M. B. 'New antifungal antibiotic: Mycostatin (Nystatin) of the treatment of moniliasis: A preliminary report', *J Invest Dermat*, 1955, 24: 569–571.
90. Chesney, J., ' "Nystatin" ("Mycostatin")', *BMJ*, 1956, i: 1043–1044.
91. Pace, H. and Schantz, S., 'Nystatin (Mycostatin) in the treatment of monilial and nonmonilial vaginitis', *JAMA*, 162, 1956: 268–271.
92. Lang, W. R. et al, 'Nystatin vaginal tablets in the treatment of *Candida*l vulvovaginitis', *Obstet Gynecol*, 1956, 8: 364–367.
93. Wright, E. T. et al, 'Treatment of moniliasis with nystatin', *JAMA*, 1957, 163: 92–94.
94. Barr, W., 'Nystatin', *Practitioner*, 1957, 178: 616–617.
95. Baldwin, *Fungus Fighters*, 99–101.
96. Loh, W. P. and Baker, E. E., 'Fecal flora of man after oral administration of chlortetracycline or oxytetracycline', *Arch Intern Med*, 1955, 95(1): 74–82; McGovern, J. J. et al, 'The effect of aureomycin and chloramphenicol on the fungal and bacterial flora of children', *N Engl J Med*, 1953, 248(10): 397–403.
97. Sharp, 'The growth of *Candida*', 392; Sakewitz, A. B., 'Treatment of genitourinary moniliasis with orally administered nystatin', *Ann Intern Med*, 1955, 42(6): 1187–1199.
98. Childs, A. J., 'Effect of nystatin on growth of *C. albicans* during antibiotic therapy', *BMJ*, 1956, i: 660–662; Gimble A. I. et al, 'Nystatin and tetracycline in the treatment of bacterial infections', *Antibiot Annu*, 1955–1956; 3: 676–680. Lederle introduced a version number the brand 'Lederstatin'. Anon, 'Gastrointestinal complications of treatment by broad spectrum antibiotics', *Drugs and Therapeutic Bulletin*, 1964, 2: 69–71; Anon, 'Old and new tetracyclines', *Drugs and Therapeutic Bulletin*, 1967, 5: 77–80.
99. Another practice that reinforced the idea was antibiotic 'sterilisation' of the colon before surgery with the antibiotic neomycin and nystatin. See: Cohen, I. and Longacre, A. B., 'Neomycin-Nystatin preoperative preparation of the colon', *Am Surg*, 1956, 22: 301–307.
100. Report, 'Fixed combinations of antimicrobial agents. national academy of sciences – national research council division of medical sciences drug efficacy study', *N Engl J Med*, 1969, 280: 1149–1154.
101. McMahon, F. G., 'Drug combinations: A critique of proposed new federal regulations', *JAMA*, 1971, 216: 1008–1010.
102. Report, 'Council on drugs', *JAMA*, 1962, 182(1): 63–66.
103. Silverman, M., and Lee, P. R., *Pills, Profits and Politics*, Berkeley, University of California Press, 1974; Anon, 'Ebert and Squibb', *Harvard Crimson*, 6 December 1972. http://www.thecrimson.com/article/1972/12/6/ebert-and-squibb-pbwbhat-are-the/. Accessed 1 March 2013.
104. Butler, W. T., 'Pharmacology, toxicity, and therapeutic usefulness of amphotericin B', *JAMA*, 1966, 195: 371–375.

105. Oura, M. et al, 'A new antifungal antibiotic, amphotericin B', *Antibioc Annu*, 1955–1956, 3: 566–573; Dutcher, J. D., 'The discovery and development of amphotericin B', *Chest*, 1968, 54: 296–298. The soil came from the Orinoco Basin in Venezuela, which illustrates the breadth of the search for new antibiotic compounds.
106. Newcomer, V. D. et al, 'Current status of amphotericin B. in the treatment of the systemic fungus infections', *J Chron Dis*, 1959, 9: 354–374; Newcomer, V. D. et al, 'The treatment of systemic fungus infections with amphotericin B', *Ann N Y Acad Sci*, 1960, 89: 221–239.
107. Crounse, R. G. et al, 'Cryptococcosis; case with unusual skin lesions and favorable response to amphotericin B. therapy', *Arch Derm*, 1958, 77(2): 210–215; Derbes, B. and Krafchuk, J. D., 'Response of North American blastomycosis to amphotericin', *Bull Tulane Univ Med Fac,* 1958, 17(3): 157–163; Littman, B. et al, 'Coccidioidomycosis and its treatment with amphotericin B', *Am J Med*, 1958, 24(4): 568–592; Baum, B. and Schwarz, J., 'Clinical experiences with amphotericin B', *Antibiot Annu,* 1959–1960, 7: 638–643.
108. Hurley, R. and Morris, E. D., 'The pathogenicity of Candida species in the human vagina', *Br J Obstet Gynaecol*, 1964, 71(5): 692–695.
109. Hurley, R., 'General discussion', *Proc R Soc Med*, 1977, 70, Suppl 4: 30. On Hurley, see: Duerden, B., 'Obituary, Dame Rosalinde Hurley', *BMJ,* 2004, ii: 516.
110. Winner and Hurley, *Candida*, 139.
111. Hurley, 'Candidal vaginitis', 2.
112. Sobel, J. D. et al, 'Clotrimazole treatment of recurrent and chronic Candida vulvovaginitis', *Int J Gynecol Obstet*, 1989, 29(4): 386.
113. Elewski, B. et al, 'Long-term outcome of patients with interdigital tinea pedis treated with terbinafine or clotrimazole', *J Am Acad Dermatol*, 1995, 32(2–1): 290–292.
114. Winner, H. I. and Hurley, R., *Candida albicans,* London, Churchill 1964.
115. Duerden, B., 'Obituary: Rosalinde Hurley', *BMJ*, 2004, 329: 516. Also see: *J Obstet Gynaecol*, 2004, 24(7): 847. Howard Winner was Professor of Bacteriology at Charing Cross from 1965 to 1982. Wright, D. J. M., 'Obituary: H. I. Winner', *BMJ*, 1993, 306: 1335.
116. Winner and Hurley, *Candida*, 56–61.
117. Winner and Hurley, *Candida*, 59.
118. Hussar and Holley, *Antibiotics*, 367.
119. Winner and Hurley, *Candida*, 59–60.
120. Newcomer, V. D. et al, 'Current status of Amphotericin B in the treatment of the systemic fungus infections', *J Chron Dis*, 1959, 9: 353–374.
121. Winner, H. I. and Hurley, R., *A Symposium on Candida Infections*, Edinburgh, E. & S. Livingstone, 1966, 221–244.
122. Seelig, M. S., 'The role of antibiotics in *Candida* infection', *Amer J Med*, 1966, 40: 887–917; Downing, J. G. and Conant, N., 'Mycotic infections', *N Engl J Med*, 233, 153 and 181.
123. Cantor, D., 'Cortisone and the politics of drama, 1949–1955', in Pickstone, J. V., ed, *Medical Innovation in Historical Perspective*, Basingstoke, Macmillan, 1992, 225–245.
124. Wikler, A. et al, 'Mycotic endocarditis: Report of a case', *JAMA*, 119, 1942: 33; Caplan, H., 'Monilia (*Candida*) endocarditis following treatment with

antibiotics', *Lancet,* 1955, ii: 95; Utz, J. P. and Roberts, W. C. '*Candida* endocarditis', *Ann Intern Med,* 1961, 54: 1058.

125. Sanger, P. et al, '*Candida* infection as a complication of heart surgery: Review of the literature and report of two cases', *JAMA,* 1962, 181: 108.
126. Birt, A. R., 'The increasing problem of drug reactions', *Can Med Assoc J,* 1957; 77: 709–715; Smith, T. J., 'Antibiotic-induced disease', in R. H. Moser, ed, *Diseases of Medical Progress,* Springfield, Ill, Charles C. Thomas, 1963.
127. Plummer, N. S., '*Candida* infection in the lung', in Winner and Hurley, *Symposium,* 214.
128. Cohen, A. C., 'Pulmonary moniliasis', *Amer J Med Sci,* 1953, 226: 16–23; Seelig, 'Role of antibiotics', 903–906.
129. Cohen, A. C., 'Pulmonary', 23.
130. Winner and Hurley, 110–113.
131. Borel, J. F. et al, 'The history of the discovery and development of cyclosporine (Sandimmun®)' in Vincent, J. et al, eds, *The Search for Anti-inflammatory Drugs,* Boston, O. Birkhauser 1995; Amor, K. T. et al, 'The use of cyclosporine in dermatology: Part I', *J Am Acad Dermatol,* 2010, 63: 925–946.
132. Gottlieb, H. S. et al, 'Pneumocystitis carinii pneumonia and mucosal candidiasis in previously healthy homosexual men: evidence of a new acquired cellular immunodeficiency', *N Engl J Med,* 1981; 305: 1425–1431; Waterson, A., 'Acquired immune deficiency syndrome', *BMJ,* (Clin Res Ed) 1983; 286: 743–746; Seligmann, M. et al, 'AIDS – An immunologic re-evaluation', *N Engl J Med,* 1984; 311: 1286–129.
133. Klein, R. S. et al, 'Oral candidiasis in high-risk patients as the initial manifestation of the acquired immunodeficiency syndrome', *N Engl J Med,* 1984; 311: 354–358; Pranatharhti, H. and Molinari, J. A., 'Oral candidiasis: Forerunner of acquired immunodeficiency syndrome (AIDS)?' *Oral Surg Oral Med Oral Path,* 1985, 60: 532–534.
134. McCarthy, G. M., 'Host factors associated with HIV-related oral candidiasis: A review', *Oral Surg Oral Med Oral Path,* 1992, 73: 181–186.
135. 'Fluconazole: A major advance for cryptococcal meningitis and other systemic fungal infections?' *AIDS Treatment News,* 1987, 41.
136. Maertens, J. A., 'History of the development of azole derivatives', *Clin Microbiol Infect,* 2004, 10 Suppl 1: 3–4.
137. Troke, P. F., 'Efficacy of UK-49,858 (Fluconazole) against *Candida* albicans experimental infections in mice', *Antimicrob Agents Chemother,* 1985, 28(6): 815–818; Odds, F. C. et al, 'Antifungal effects of fluconazole (UK-49858), a new triazole antifungal, in vitro', *Antimicrob Agents Chemother,* 1986, 18: 473–478; Hay, R. J., 'Fluconazole', *J Infect,* 1990, 21: 1–6; Richardson, K. et al, 'Discovery of fluconazole, a novel antifungal agent', *Clin Infect Dis,* 1990, 12: S267–271.
138. de Wit, S. et al, 'Comparison of fluconazole and ketoconazole for oropharyngeal candidiasis in AIDS', *Lancet,* 1989, i: 746–748.
139. *Lancet,* 1989, i: 1130–1131.
140. Anon, 'Products in development: Progress continues in search for AIDS-related drugs', *Aids Patient Care,* August 1988, 2(4): 28–33; Williams, R. D., 'Living with AIDS: New treatments give hope', *FDA Consumer,* January-February 1992, 26; Lindemann, E., 'Importing AIDS drugs: Food and drug

administration policy and its limitations', *George Washington Journal of International Law and Economics*, 1994, 28: 133–170.
141. British Society for Antimicrobial Chemotherapy Working Party, 'Antifungal chemotherapy in patients with acquired immunodeficiency syndrome', *Lancet* 1992: 648–651. Coleman, D. C. et al, 'Oral *Candida* in HIV infection and AIDS: New perspectives/new approaches', *Crit Rev Microbial,* 1993; 19: 61–82.
142. McNeill, M. et al, 'Mortality in the United States, 1980–1997, due to candidiasis, aspergillosis, and other mycoses in persons infected and persons not infected with HIV trends in mortality due to invasive mycotic diseases in the United States, 1980–1997', *Clin Infect Dis*, 2001, 33(5): 641–647.
143. Odds, *Candida*, 1988, 5.
144. Fisher-Hoch, S. P. and Hutwanger, L., 'Opportunistic candidiasis: an epidemic of the 1980s', *Infect Dis*, 1995, 21(4): 897–904.
145. Dismukes, W. E., 'Antifungal therapy: Lessons learned over the past 27 years', *Clin Infect Dis*, 2006, 42: 1289–1330.
146. Ibid., 1290.
147. Bennett, J. E. et al, 'A comparison of amphotericin B. alone and combined with flucytosine in the treatment of cryptococcal meningitis', *N Engl J Med*, 1979, 301(3): 126–131.
148. Dismukes, W. E. et al, 'Criteria for evaluation of therapeutic response to antifungal drugs', *Rev Infect Dis*, 1980, 2(4): 535–545; idem, 'Antifungal Therapy', passim. Flucocystine, had been developed as an anti-cancer compound in the 1950s, however, it proved ineffective and it was only in the 1960s that its antifungal properties were recognised. It was effective against cryptococcosis and candidiasis, but its value was limited by the development of resistance, hence combined usage, and toxicity, though it was less so than amphotericin B. J. E. Bennett, 'Flucocystine', *Ann Intern Med*, 1977, 86(3): 319–321.
149. Ayliffe, G. and English, M., *Hospital Infection: from Miasmas to MRSA*, Cambridge, Cambridge University Press, 2003.
150. Pfaller, M. A., 'Nosocomial fungal infections: Epidemiology of candidiasis', *Journal of Hospital Infection*, 1995, 30 (Suppl): 329–338.
151. Ibid., 330–333.
152. Odds, F. C., 'Epidemiological shifts in opportunistic and nosocomial *Candida* infections: mycological aspects', *Int J Antimicrob Agents*, 1996, 6: 141–144.
153. For a popular account of the 'yeast connection', see Barrett, S., 'Unproven "Allergies": An Epidemic of Nonsense "Environmental illness" and the "yeast connection" ', in Barrett S. and Jarvis, J. T., eds, *The Health Robbers; A Close Look at Quackery in America*, New York, Prometheus Press, 1993.
154. Odds, *Candida* (1988), 233.
155. Crook, W. G., *The Yeast Connection: A Medical Breakthrough*, Jackson, T., Professional Books, 1983; O. Truss, *The Missing Diagnosis*, Birmingham, The Missing Diagnosis, Inc., 1983.
156. Crook, W. G., *Answering Parent's Questions*, Jackson, Professional Books, 1963; idem, *Your Allergic Child: A Pediatrician's Guide to Normal Living for Allergic Adults and Children*, New York, Medcom Pres, 1973; idem, *Can Your Child Read? Is He Hyperactive?: A Pediatrician's Suggestions for Helping the*

Child with Hyperactivity, Behavior and Learning Problems, Jackson, Tenn, Professional Books 1975; idem, *Are You Allergic?: A Guide to Normal Living for Allergic Adults and Children*, Jackson, Tenn, Professional Press, 1977.

157. Truss, C. O., 'The role of Candida Albicans in human illness', *Orthomolecular Psychiatry*, 1981, 8: 228–238; Truss, C. O., 'Tissue injury induced by *C. albicans*: Mental and neurologic manifestations', *J Orthomol Psychiatr*, 1978, 1, 17–37.
158. Brief details of Truss's career are given at http://www.trussmd.com/about.html. Accessed 26 April 2012.
159. Goertzl, T. and Goertzl, B., *Linus Pauling: A Life in Science and Politics*, New York, HarperCollins, 1995; Hager, T., *Linus Pauling and the Chemistry of Life*, New York: Oxford University Press, 1998.
160. Pauling, L., 'Orthomolecular psychiatry: Varying the concentrations of substances normally present in the human body may control mental disease', *Science*, 1968, 160: 265–271; Pauling, L. et al, 'On the orthomolecular environment of the mind: orthomolecular theory', *Am J Psychiatry*, 1974, 131: 1251–1267. Orian Truss was born on 1 December 1922 and died in Birmingham, Alabama on 10 September 2009.
161. Task Force Report 7, *Megavitamin and Orthomolecular Therapy in Psychiatry*, Washington, DC, APA, 1973; Editorial, 'Molecules and mental health', *BMJ*, 1975, i: 296.
162. Williams, R. J. and Wright, D. K., *A Physician's Handbook on Orthomolecular Medicine*, New York Pergamon Press, 1977.
163. Hess, D. J., *Evaluating Alternative Cancer Therapies: A Guide to the Science and Politics of An Emerging Medical Field*, New Brunswick, NJ, Rutgers University Press, 1999; idem, *Can Bacteria Cause Cancer?: Alternative Medicine Confronts Big Science*, New York, New York University Press, 1997.
164. Truss, C. O., 'Tissue injury induced by *Candida albicans*: Mental and neurologic manifestations', *J Orthomol Psychiatr*, 1978, 7(1): 17: 37; idem, 'Restoration of immunologic competence to *C. albicans*', *J Orthomol Psychiatr*, 1980, 9: 287.
165. Ibid., 289.
166. Truss, C. O., 'Restoration of immunologic competence to Candida Albicans', *J Orthomol Psychiatr*, 1980, 9: 290.
167. Randolph, T. G., *Human Ecology and Susceptibility to the Chemical Environment*, Springfield, Ill: Thomas, 1962; Buscher, D., 'Obituary: Theron G. Randolph, MD, 1906–1995', *Journal of Nutritional & Environmental Medicine*, 1996, 6: 245–246.
168. Task Force on Clinical Ecology, 'Clinical ecology – a critical appraisal', *West J Med*, 1986, 144: 239–245.
169. Crook, W. G., 'Letters depression associated with *C. albicans* Infections', *JAMA*, 1984: 51: 2928–2929.
170. Crook, *Yeast Connection*, vi.
171. Crook summarises the meeting in Chapter 37 of *The Yeast Connection*.
172. Ibid., vi and Crook, W. G., 'The coming revolution in medicine', *Journal of the Tennessee Medical Association*, 1983, 76: 145–149.
173. Crook, *Yeast Connection*, viii.
174. Quinn, J. P. et al, Ketoconazole and the yeast connection, *JAMA*, 1986, 255, 3250.

175. Morgan, P. P., 'Should scientists study "20th-century disease"?', *Can Med Assoc J*, 1985, 133: 961–962; Zimmerman, B. and Weber, E., '*Candida* and "20th-century disease" ', Ibid., 1985 133: 965–966; Maclennan, J. G., '*Candida* and "20th-century disease" ', Ibid., 1986 134: 1112–1113; Lornzani, S., *Candida: A Twentieth Century Disease*, New Canaan, Conn, Keats Publishing, 1986; Murphy, M., *Sick Building Syndrome and the Problem of Uncertainty: Environmental Politics, Technoscience, and Women Workers*, Durham, NC, Duke University Press, 2006.
176. For a popular presentation see: Rovner, S., 'HEALTHTALK: The yeast theory', *Washington Post*, Mar 9, 1984: D5.
177. Haas, A. et al, 'The "Yeast Connection" meets chronic mucocutaneous candidiasis', *N Engl J Med*, 314: 854–855, 1986.
178. Coleman, III, W. P. and Edwards, D. E., 'Letters depression and *Candida* – Reply', *JAMA*, 1985, 253: 3400.
179. Anderson, J. A. et al, 'Position statement on candidiasis hypersensitivity', *J Allergy Clin Immunol*, 1986, 78: 271–273.
180. Edwards, J. E., 'Systemic symptoms from *Candida* in the gut: Real or imaginary?', *Bull N. Y. Acad Med,* 1988, 64(6): 544–549.
181. Ibid., 548.
182. Infectious Diseases and Immunization Committee of the Canadian Paediatric Society, 'Candidiasis: current misconceptions', *Can Med Assoc J*, 1988, 139: 729; Blonz, E. R., 'Is there an epidemic of chronic candidiasis in our midst?', *JAMA*, 1986, 256: 3138–3139.
183. Aronowitz, R., 'From myalgic encephalitis to yuppie flu: a history of chronic fatigue syndromes', in Rosenberg, C. and Golden, J., eds, *Framing Disease: Studies in Cultural History*, New Brunswick, NJ: Rutgers University Press, 1992, 155–181; Jenkins, R. and Mowbray, J. F., eds, *Post-viral Fatigue Syndrome: (myalgic encephalomyelitis)*, Chichester: John Wiley & Sons, 1992.
184. Finlay, S., 'An illness doctors don't recognise', *Observer*, 1 June 1986, 43. Also see follow up article: Finlay, S., 'Voice for sufferers', *Observer*, 2 August 1987, 39; Chaitlow, L., *Candida Albicans: Could Yeast be Your Problem?*, Wellingborough, Thorsons, 1985.
185. Collings, J., 'The quiet epidemic that is ruining modern lifestyle', *Guardian*, 4 February 1988, 13.
186. Crook, *The Yeast Connection*, v–vi.
187. Mildenhall, R., '*Candida* views', *Observer*, 26 June 1988, 37.
188. Renfro, L. et al, 'Yeast Connection among 100 patients with chronic fatigue', *Amer J Med*, 1989, 86, 165–168.
189. Ibid., 168.
190. Dismukes, W. E. et al, 'A randomized double-blind trial of nystatin therapy for the candidiasis hypersensitivity syndrome', *N Engl J Med*, 1990, 323: 1717–1723.
191. Ibid., 1723.
192. Correspondence from Crooks, W., Truss, C. O. et al, W. J. Ledger et al, and M. Crandall, *N Engl J Med*, 1991, 324: 1592–1594.
193. Kay, A. B. and Lessor, M. H., *Allergy: Conventional and Alternative Concepts*, London, Royal College of Physicians of London, 1992.

194. Downing D. and Davies, S., '"Allergy: Conventional and Alternative Concepts": A critique of the Royal College of Physicians of London's Report', *Journal of Nutritional Medicine*, 1992, 3: 331–349.
195. Kay, A. B., 'Alternative allergy and the general medical council', *BMJ*, 1993, i: 122–124, 328–331 and 582.
196. Mumby, K., 'Science or flat earthers? The clinical ecologist replies', *BMJ*, 1993, ii: 1055–1056.
197. Eisenberg, D. M. et al, 'Trends in alternative medicine use in the United States, 1990–1997:Results of a follow-up national survey', *JAMA*, 1998, 280: 1569–1575.
198. Hyams, K., 'Developing case definitions for symptom-based conditions: The problem of specificity', *Epidemiologic Reviews*, 1998, 20(2): 148–156.
199. Crook, W. G., *Nature's Own Candida Cure*, Alive Books, 2003; Crook, W. G. et al, *The Yeast Connection and Women's Health*, Square One, 2007; Crook, W. G., *Tired So Tired: and the Yeast Connection*, Square One, 2007.
200. Weig, M. et al, 'Clinical aspects and pathogenesis of *Candida* infection', *Trends in Microbiology*, 2012, 20(8): 468.

4 Regionally Specific Fungal Infections

1. Reiss, F., ed, 'Medical mycology', *Ann N Y Acad Sci*, 1950, 50: 1209–1404.
2. Conant, N. F., 'Future developments in mycological investigative methods', *Ann N Y Acad Sci*, 1950, 50: 1245–1249.
3. Jackson, M., *Asthma: The Biography*, Oxford, Oxford University Press, 2009.
4. Smith, D. T., 'The diagnosis and therapy of mycotic infections', *Bull N Y Acad Med*, 1953, 29(10): 778.
5. Jillson, O. F., 'Mycology', *N Engl Med J*, 1953, 249: 523–530 and 561–566.
6. Salvin, S. B., 'Public health aspects of fungus infections', *Ann N Y Acad Sci*, 1950, 50: 1217.
7. Nickerson, W. J., 'Medical mycology', *Ann Rev Microbiol*, 1953, 7: 245–272.
8. *Vital Statistics of the United States, 1950*, Volume 3, Mortality Data, Washington: US Depart of Health, Education and Welfare, 1953, Table 51, 62, *Vital Statistics of the United States, 1960*, Volume 2 – Mortality, Part A., Washington: US Department of Health, Education and Welfare, 1963, Table 5–6, 5–16.
9. Nickerson, 'Medical mycology', 246.
10. Henrici, A. T., 'Characteristics of fungous diseases', *J Bacteriol*, 1940, 39: 113–138.
11. Fildes, P., 'Richard Friedrich Johannes Pfeiffer, 1858–1945', *Biog Mem Fell R Soc*, 1956, 2: 237–247; Jackson, M., *Allergy: The History of a Modern Malady*, London, Reaktion Books, 2006, 87–88.
12. Smith, 'The diagnosis and therapy', 782.
13. Schwarz, J. and Baum, G. L., 'A critical review of medical mycology in the United States, 1946–1956', *Mycopatholgia et Mycologia Applicata*, 1957, 8: 271–326.
14. Espinel-Ingroff, A. V., *Medical Mycology in the United States: A Historical Analysis (1894–1996)*, Dordrecht, Kluwer Academic Publishers, 2003, 73–78.
15. Smith, 'The diagnosis and therapy', 782.

16. Emmons, C. W., 'Mycology and medicine', *Mycologia*, 1961, 53: 1.
17. Haynes, D. M., *Imperial Medicine: Patrick Manson and the Conquest of Tropical Disease,* Philadelphia, University of Pennsylvania Press, 2001.
18. Harden, V. A., *Rocky Mountain Spotted Fever: History of a Twentieth-Century Disease,* Baltimore, Johns Hopkins University Press, 1990.
19. Hirschmann, J. V., 'The early history of coccidioidomycosis: 1892–1945', *Clin Infect Dis*, 2007: 44: 1202–1207.
20. Dickson, E. C., 'Valley fever', *Calif West Med,*1937, 47: 151–155; idem, 'Coccidioidomycosis', *JAMA*, 1938, 111: 1362–1364; Smith, C. E., 'Epidemiology of acute coccidioidomycosis with *Erythema nodosum* ("San Joaquin" or "Valley Fever")', *Am J Publ Health*, 1940, 40: 600–611.
21. Saubolle, M. and Sutton, J., 'Coccidioidomycosis: Centennial year on the North American continent', *Clinical Microbiology Newsletter*, 1994, 16(18): 137–144.
22. Hirschmann, 'The early history', 1206; Espinel-Ingroff, *Medical Mycology*', 40–41.
23. Dowling, H. F., 'The emergence of the cooperative clinical trial', *Transactions and Studies of the College of Physicians of Philadelphia*, 1975, 43: 22–23; Marks, H. M., *The Progress of Experiment: Science and Therapeutic Reform in the United States, 1900–1990*, Cambridge, Cambridge University Press, 1997, 115–128; Tucker, W. B., 'The evolution of the cooperative studies in the chemotherapy of tuberculosis of the Veterans Administration and Armed Forces of the USA: An account of the evolving education of the physician in clinical pharmacology', *Bibl Tuberc*, 1960, 15: 1–68.
24. Comstock, G. W., 'In memoriam: Carroll Edwards Palmer, 1903–1972', *J Epidemiol*, 1972, 95: 305–307.
25. Joffe, B., 'An epidemic of Coccidioidomycosis probably related to soil', *N Engl Med J.,* 1960, 262: 720–722.
26. Espinel-Ingroff, *Medical Mycology*, 39–41, 62–68, 91–92.
27. Fiese, M. J., *Coccidioidomycosis*, Springfield, Ill, Thomas, 1958. Fiese was killed in a train crash in Bakersfield in March 1960.
28. For an accessible introduction to coccidioidomycosis see: Odds, F. C., 'Coccidioidomycosis: Flying conidia and severed heads', *Mycologist*, 2003, 17: 37–40.
29. Ajello, L., 'Coccidioidomycosis and histoplasmosis: A review of the epidemiology and geographical distribution', *Mycopathologia et Mycologia Applicata*, 1971, 45, 221–230.
30. Stevens, D. A., 'Coccidioidomycosis', *N Engl Med J*, 1995, 332: 1077.
31. Pappagianis, D. and Einstein, H., 'Tempest from Tehachapi takes toll or coccidioides conveyed aloft and afar', *West J Med*, 1978, 129: 527–530.
32. Ibid., 528–529.
33. Pappagianis, D., 'Epidemiology of coccidioidomycosis', in Stevens, D. A., ed, *Coccidioidomycosis: A Text*, New York: Plenum Book Company, 1980.
34. Pappagianis, D., 'Marked increase in cases of coccidioidomycosis in California: 1991, 1992, and 1993', *Clin Infect Dis*, 1994, 19, Supplement 1: S14–S18; Johnson, R. H. et al, 'The great coccidioidomycosis epidemic: Clinical features', in Einstein, H. E., and Catanzaro, A., eds, *Coccidioidomycosis: Proceedings of the 5th International Conference*, Washington, National Foundation for Infectious Diseases, 1996: 77–87.

35. Pappagianis, 'Marked increase', S16–18.
36. Rothstein, N. E. et al, 'Risk factors for severe pulmonary and disseminated coccidioidomycosis: Kern County, California, 1995–1996', *Clin Infect Dis.*, 2001, 32(5): 708–714.
37. Ibid., 713.
38. Kirkland, T. N. and Fierer, J., 'Coccidioidomycosis: A reemerging infectious disease', *Emerg Infect Dis* [serial on the Internet]. 1996, Sep. Available from www.nc.cdc.gov/ncidod/eid/vol2no3/kirkland.htm DOI: 10.3201/eid0203.960305.
39. Schneider, E. et al, 'A coccidioidomycosis outbreak following the Northridge, California, earthquake', *JAMA*, 1997, 277; Jibson, R. W. et al, 'An outbreak of coccidioidomycosis (Valley Fever) caused by landslides triggered by the 1994 Northridge, California earthquake', in Welby, C. W. and Gowan, M. E., *A Paradox of Power: Voices of Warning and Reason in the Geosciences*: Geological Society of America, Reviews in Engineering Geology, 1998, 53–61; Pappagianis, D., 'Epidemiology of coccidioidomycosis', McGinnis, M. R., ed, *Current Topics in Medical Mycology, Vol 2*, New York: Springer-Verlag, 1988: 199–238.
40. Bronnimann, D. A. et al, 'Coccidioidomycosis in the acquired immunodeficiency syndrome', *Ann Intern Med*, 1987, 106: 372–379.
41. Galgiani, J. N., 'Coccidioidomycosis: A regional disease of national importance: rethinking approaches for control', *Ann Intern Med*, 1999, 130 (4 Part 1): 293–300.
42. Kirkland, T. N., and Fierer, J., 'Coccidioidomycosis: A reemerging infectious disease', *Emerg Infect Dis.*, 1996, 2(3): 192–199.
43. Ibid., 194–195.
44. Deresinski, S. C. et al, 'Soluble antigens of mycelia and spherules in the *in vitro* detection of immunity to *Coccidioides immitis*', *Infection and Immunity*, 1977, 10 (4): 700–704; Stevens, D. A. et al, 'Dermal sensitivity to different doses of spherulin and coccidioidin', *Chest*, 1974, 65: 530–533; Stevens, D. A. et al, 'Immunotherapy in recurrent coccidioidomycosis', *Cell Immunol*, 1974, 12: 37–48.
45. Stevens, D. A. et al, 'Miconazole in coccidioidomycosis-II: Therapeutic and pharmacologic studies in man', *Am J Med*, 1976, 60: 191–202; Levine, H. B., 'Miconazole in coccidioidomycosis', *Proc R Soc Med*, 1977, 70 (Suppl 1): 13–17; Cartwright, R Y, 'Antifungal drugs', *J Antimicrob Chemother*, 1975, 1: 148–151.
46. Stevens, D. A., *Coccidioidomycosis: A text*, 1980, New York, Plenum Medical Book Co., 1980.
47. *Proceedings of symposium on coccidioidomycosis, held at Phoenix, Arizona, February 11–13, 1957*, Atlanta, Ga., CDC, 1957; Ajello, L., *Coccidioidomycosis: Current Clinical and Diagnostic Status: A Comprehensive Reference for the Clinician and Investigator: Selected Papers from the Third International Coccidioidomycosis Symposium*, Tucson, Arizona, Miami, Fla., Symposia Specialists, 1977.
48. Galgiani, J. N., 'Coccidioidomycosis: Changing perceptions and creating opportunities for its control', *Ann N Y Acad Sci*, 2007, 1111: 5–10.
49. Ampel, N. N. et al, 'Coccidioidomycosis: Clinical update', *Clin Infect Dis*, 1989, 11(6): 897–911.

50. Pappagianis, D. et al, 'Evaluation of the protective efficacy of the killed *Coccidioides immitis* spherule vaccine in humans', *Am Rev Respir Dis*, 1993, 148: 656–660.
51. Sievers, M. L., 'Coccidioidomycosis and race', *Am Rev Respir Dis*, 1979, 119(5): 839; Pappagianis, D. 'Epidemiology of coccidioidomycosis', *Current Topics in Medical Mycology*, 1988, 2: 199–238.
52. Vaughan, J. E. and Ramirez, H., 'Coccidioidomycosis as a complication of pregnancy', *Calif Med*, 1951, 74(2): 121–125; Wack, E. E. et al, 'Coccidioidomycosis during pregnancy: An analysis of ten cases among 47, 120 pregnancies', *Chest*, 1988, 94: 376–379.
53. Galgiani, J. N. et al, 'Infectious diseases society of America: Practice guideline for the treatment of coccidioidomycosis', *Clin Infect Dis*, 2000, 30: 658–661.
54. Gilchrist, T. C. and Stokes, R. W., 'A case of pseudolupus vulgaris caused by Blastomyces', *J Exp Med,* 1898, 3: 53.
55. Curtis, A. C. and Bocobo, F. C., 'North American blastomycosis', *J Chron Dis,* 1957, 5(4): 404.
56. Conant, N. and Howell, A. F., 'The similarity of the fungi causing South American blastomycosis (paracoccidioidal granuloma) and North American blastomycosis (Gilchrist's disease)', *J Invest Dermatol*, 1942, 5 (6): 353–370.
57. Tenenbaum, M. J. et al, 'Blastomycosis', *Crit Rev Microbiol*, 1982, 9(3): 158–160.
58. Furcolow, M. L. et al, 'Blastomycosis: An important medical problem in the Central United States', *JAMA*, 1966, 198: 115–118; Chin, D. D. Y., 'The Kansas city field station', 1950–1973, *Public Health Reports*, 1999, 114, 377–380.
59. Tenenbaum, 'Blastomycosis', 160.
60. Pappas, P. G. et al, 'Blastomycosis in immunocompromised patients', *Medicine*, 1993, 72: 311–325.
61. Chapman, S. W. et al, 'Endemic blastomycosis in Mississippi: Epidemiological and clinical studies', *Semin Respir Infect*, 1997, 12(3): 219–228: Quillen, J. H. et al, 'Blastomycosis in North Tennessee', *Chest*, 1998, 114(2): 436–443.
62. The condition was also known as cave disease, Darling's disease, Reticuloendotheliosis, Spelunker's Lung, and Caver's disease.
63. Ajello, L. et al, eds, *Histoplasmosis: Proceedings of the Second National Conference*, Springfield, Ill, Charles C. Thomas Publisher, 1971; Ajello, 'Coccidioidomycosis and histoplasmosis', 221–230.
64. Daniel, T. M. and Baum, G. L., *Drama and Discovery: The Story of Histoplasmosis*, Greenwood, 2002. A version of the earlier chapters was published as Baum, G. L. and Schwarz, J., 'The history of histoplasmosis 1906–1956', *N Engl Med J*, 1957, 256: 253–258.
65. Darling, S. T., 'A Protozoan general infection producing pseudotuberculosis in the lungs and focal necrosis in the liver, spleen, and lymph nodes', *JAMA*, 1906, 46: 1283–1285.
66. Daniel and Baum, *Drama*, 32–36.
67. 'Histoplasmosis cooperative study. I. frequency of histoplasmosis among adult hospitalized males: Veterans administration cooperation study on histoplasmosis', *Amer Rev Resp Dis*, 1961, 84: 663–668.

68. Furcolow, M. L. et al, 'Serologic evidence of histoplasmosis in sanatoriums in the U.S.', *JAMA*, 1962, 180: 109–114.
69. Daniel and Baum, *Drama*, 1–5.
70. Rubin, H. et al, 'The course and prognosis of histoplasmosis', *Am Med J*, 1959, 27(2): 278–288; Schwarz J. and Baum, G. L., 'Histoplasmosis', 1962', *Arch Intern Med*, 1963, 111(6): 710–718.
71. Daniel and Baum, *Drama*, 79–83.
72. Wheat, J., 'Endemic mycoses in AIDS: A clinical review', *Clin Microbiol Rev*, 1995, 8(1): 146–153.
73. Rothwell, T. A., Aspergillosis, MD Thesis, Victoria University, Manchester, 1899; Mettam, A. E., 'Aspergillosis – Aspergillar mycosis', *Transactions of the Royal Academy of Medicine in Ireland*, 1911, 29: 484–494; Lapham, M. E., 'Aspergillosis of the lungs and its association with tuberculosis', *JAMA*, 1926, 87: 1031–1033.
74. Henrici, A. T., *Molds, Yeasts and Actinomycetes: A Handbook for Students of Bacteriology*, New York: J. Wiley & Sons, 1930. Also see similar treatment in Jacobson, H. P., *Fungous Diseases: A Clinic-Mycological Text*, London, Baillière, Tindall & Cox, 1932.
75. Taylor, F., ed, *The Practice of Medicine*, London: J. & A. Churchill, 1936, 103–104.
76. Fawcitt, R., 'Fungoid conditions of the lungs – Part I', *Br J Radiol*, 1936, 9: 172–195; idem, 'Fungoid conditions of the lungs – Part II', *Br J Radiol*, 1936, 9: 354–378.
77. Campbell, M., 'Acute symptoms following work with hay', *BMJ*, 1932, ii: 1143–1144.
78. Historians have emphasised how new technologies collected 'dust' and made it more visible, but ignored the fact that cleaning of all types also spread dust and perhaps it was the finer particles that eluded the duster and vacuum cleaner. Schwartz Cowan, R., *More Work for Mother: The Ironies of Household Technology from the Open Hearth to the Microwave*, New York: Basic Books, 1983; Steadman, C., *Dust*, Manchester, Manchester University Press, 2002.
79. Jackson, *Asthma*, 118–136; Jackson, *Allergy*, 139–147.
80. Brown, G. T., 'Hypersensitiveness to fungi', *J Allergy*, 1936, 7(5): 455–470.
81. Thom, C. and Church, M. B., *The Aspergilli*, Baltimore, Williams and Wilkins, 1926.
82. Meier, F. C. with field notes and material by Lindberg, C. A., 'Collecting micro-organisms from the Arctic atmosphere', *Scientific Monthly*, 1935, 40: 5–20.
83. Koerth, C. J. et al, 'Fungus disease of the lung', *Texas State Journal of Medicine*, 1942, 38: 1–58; Morrow, M B et al, 'Mold fungi in the etiology of respiratory allergic diseases. I. A survey of air-borne molds', *J Allergy*, 1942, 13: 215–226 and 231–247.
84. Duncan, J. T., 'Survey of fungous diseases in Great Britain: Results from the first eighteenth months', *BMJ*, 1945, ii: 716.
85. Ibid.
86. Studdert, T. C., 'Farmer's lung', *BMJ*, 1953, i: 1308.
87. Ibid., 1309. Also see: *Lancet*, 1953, i: 933.

88. *Farmer's Lung: Report by the Industrial Injuries Advisory Council*, BPP, 1963–1964, Cmnd 2403: 863–878.
89. Ibid., 869.
90. Pickworth, K. H., 'Farmer's lung', *Lancet*, 1961, ii: 660; Emanuel, D. A. et al, 'Farmer's lung: Clinical, pathologic and immunologic study of twenty-four patients', *Am J Med*, 1961, 37: 392–401.
91. Hinson, K. W. F et al, 'Broncho-pulmonary aspergillosis: A review and a report of eight new cases', *Thorax*, 1952: 7: 317–333.
92. Williams Jr, M. H. and Serff, N. S., 'Chronic obstructive pulmonary disease: An analysis of clinical, physiologic and roentgenologic features', *Am J Med*, 1963, 35: 20–30; Report, 'Chronic obstructive pulmonary disease', *Lancet*, 1964, ii: 1438–1439.
93. Meiklejohn, A., 'The development of compensation for occupational diseases of the lungs in Great Britain', *Br J Ind Med*, 1954, 11: 198–212; Tweedale, G. and Hansen, P., 'Protecting the Workers: The Medical Board and the Asbestos Industry, 1930s–1960s', *Medical History*, 1998, 42: 439–457.
94. Pepys, J. et al, 'Clinical and immunological significance of *Aspergillus fumigatus* in sputum', *Am Rev Respir Dis*, 1959, 80: 167.
95. Pepys, J., 'Allergic broncho-pulmonary aspergillosis', *Clin Allergy*, 1971, 1: 261–286.
96. Slavin, R. G., 'Allergic bronchopulmonary aspergillosis – A north American rarity', *Am J Med*, 1969, 47: 306–313.
97. Rosenberg M. and Paterson, R., 'Allergic bronchopulmonary aspergillosis: An emerging disease', *J Chron Dis*, 1977, 30: 193–194; R. G. Slavin and P. Winzenberger, 'Epidemiologic aspects of allergic aspergillosis', *Ann Allergy,* 1977, 38(3): 215–218.
98. Schwartz, H. J. et al, A comparison of the prevalence of sensitization to *Aspergillus* antigens among asthmatics in Cleveland and London, *J Allergy Clin Immunol*, 1978, 62: 9–14; Slavin, R. G., 'What does fungus among us really mean?', *J Allergy Clin Immunol*, 1978, 62: 1–2.
99. Greenberger, P. A., 'Allergic bronchopulmonary aspergillosis', *J Allergy Clin Immunol*, 1982, 74: 645–652; Slavin, R. G., 'Allergic bronchopulmonary aspergillosis', *Clin Rev Allergy Immunol*, 1985, 3(2): 167–182.
100. Greenberger, 'Allergic bronchopulmonary aspergillosis', 645.
101. Wang, J. L. et al, 'The management of allergic bronchopulmonary aspergillosis', *Am Rev Respir Dis*, 1979, 120(1): 87–92.
102. Denning, D. W. et al, 'The link between fungi and severe asthma: A summary of the evidence', *Europ Respir J*, 2006, 27: 615–626.
103. Novey, H., 'Epidemiology of allergic bronchopulmonary aspergillosis', *Immunol Allergy Clin N Amer*, 1998, 18: 641–653.
104. Batten, J., 'Cystic fibrosis: A review', *Br J Dis Chest*, 1965, 59: 1–9; Brueton, M. J. et al, 'Allergic bronchopulmonary aspergillosis complicating cystic fibrosis in childhood', *Arch Dis Child*, 1980, 55: 348.
105. Nelson, L. et al, 'Aspergillosis and atopy in cystic fibrosis', *Am Rev Respir Dis*, 1979, 120: 863; Laufer, P. et al, 'Allergic bronchopulmonary aspergillosis in cystic fibrosis', *J Allergy Clin Immunol*, 1984, 73: 44–48.
106. See recent reviews: Foweraker, J., 'Recent advances in the microbiology of respiratory tract infection in cystic fibrosis', *Br Med Bull*, 2009, 89: 93–110;

LiPuma, J. J., 'The changing microbial epidemiology of cystic fibrosis', *Clin Microbiol Rev*, 2010, 23: 299–323.

107. Gilligan, P. H., 'Microbiology of airway disease in patients with cystic fibrosis', *Clin Microbiol Rev*, 1991, 4(10): 35–51; Mroueh, S. and Spock, A., 'Allergic bronchopulmonary aspergillosis in patients with cystic fibrosis', *Chest*, 1994, 105(1): 32–36.
108. Stevens, D. A. et al, 'Allergic bronchopulmonary aspergillosis in cystic fibrosis – state of the art: Cystic fibrosis foundation consensus conference', *Clin Infect Dis* 2003, 37 (Suppl 3): S225–S264.
109. McNeill, M. M. et al, 'Trends in mortality due to invasive mycotic diseases in the United States, 1980–1997', *Clin Infect Dis*, 2001, 33: 641–647.
110. Ibid., 644.
111. Ibid.
112. Ampel, N. M. et al, 'Coccidioidomycosis in Arizona: Increase in incidence from 1990 to 1995', *Clin Infect Dis*, 1998, 27: 1528–1530.
113. McNeill, 'Trends in mortality', 644–645.

5 Technology and Aspergillosis

1. Bennett, J. W., 'Aspergillus: A primer for the novice', *Medical Mycology*, 2009, 47 (Suppl 1): S5–12; idem, 'An overview of the genus *Aspergillus*', in Machida, M. and Gomi, K., eds, *Aspergillus: Molecular Biology and Genomics*, Norfolk, Caister Academic Press, 2010, 1–18.
2. Al-Doory, Y. and Wagner, G. E., eds, *Aspergillosis*, Springfield, Ill.: Thomas, 1985.
3. de Haller, R. and Suter, F., *Aspergillosis and farmer's lung in man and animal: Proceedings of the 4th International Symposium*, 7th–9th October 1971, Davos, Bern, Hans Huber, 1974.
4. Warnock, D. W., 'Trends in the epidemiology of invasive fungal infections', *Jpn J Med Mycol*, 2007, 48: 1–12.
5. Richard, J. L., 'Discovery of aflatoxins and significant historical features', *Toxin Reviews*, 2008, 27: 171–201.
6. Alexander, D. J., 'Newcastle disease', *British Poultry Science*, 2001, 42(1), 5–22. In 1959–1960, 5.2 million birds were slaughtered to control fowl pest and £3.3 million paid in compensation.
7. BPP, *Report of the Committee on Fowl Pest Policy*, Parl. Papers, 1961–1962, Cmnd.1664, VIII, 271.
8. Blount, W. P., 'Turkey "X" disease', *Turkeys*, March–April 1961: 52–60.
9. Spensley, P. C., 'Aflatoxin, the active principle in turkey "X" disease', *Endeavour*, 1963, 22: 75–79.
10. Sargeant, K. et al, 'Toxicity associated with certain samples of groundnuts', *Nature*, 1961, 192: 1096–1097; *Toxicity Associated with Certain Batches of Groundnuts-Report of the Interdepartmental Working Party on Groundnut Toxicity Research*, Department of Scientific and Industrial Research, 1962.
11. Wogan, G. N., 'Aflatoxin as a human carcinogen', *Hepatology*, 1999, 30: 573–575.
12. See, for example, Shurtleff, William and Akiko Aoyagi, 'History of Koji – Grans and/or soybeans enrobed with a mold culture (300 BCE to 2012)',

17 July 2012, http://www.soyinfocenter.com/books/154. Accessed 3 May 2013; Sakaguchi, Kin'ichiro, *Nihon no sake*, Tokyo, Iwanami Shoten, 2007. Also, for Kikkoman Corporation, of the internationally renowned Japanese soy sauce brand Kikkoman, its proprietary koji culture has been the most valued item essential for its global success. Yates, Ronald E., *The Kikkoman Chronicles: A Global Company with a Japanese Soul*, New York, McGraw Hill, 1998, 60–61.

13. Quoted at: The Tokyo Foundation, http://www.tokyofoundation.org/en/topics/japanese-traditional-foods/vol.-10-koji-an-aspergillus. Accessed 27 May 2012.
14. Editorial, 'Toxic product in groundnuts', *BMJ*, 1962, i: 309.
15. Diener, U. L. et al, 'Toxin-producing *Aspergillus* isolated from domestic peanuts', *Science*, 1963, 142: 1491–1492.
16. Wilson, B. J. and Wilson, C. H., 'Toxin from *Aspergillus flavus*: Production on food materials of a substance causing tremors in mice', *Science*, 1964, 144: 177–178. The OED states that the first use of the term 'mycotoxin' was in 1962.
17. Editorial, 'Aflatoxin', *Lancet*, 1964, i: 1090.
18. Stoloff, L., 'Molds and mycotoxins: What FDA is doing about the mycotoxin problem', *Farm Technol. Agri-Fieldman*, 1972, 28: 60a.
19. Maggon, K. K. et al, 'Biosynthesis of aflatoxins', *Bacteriol. Rev.*, 1977, 41: 822–855.
20. Wogan, G. N., 'Chemical nature and biological effects of the Aflatoxins', *Bacteriol Rev*, 1966, 30: 468.
21. Heathcote, J. and Hibbert, J. R., *Aflatoxins: Chemical and Biological Aspects*, Oxford, Elsevier, 1978, 2.
22. Epstein, S. S., 'Environmental determinants of human cancer', *Cancer Res*, 1974, 34: 2425–2435.
23. Higginson, J., 'The geographic pathology of primary liver cancer', *Cancer Research*, 1963, 23: 1624–1633.
24. Hutt, M. S. R. and Burkitt, D., 'Geographical distribution of cancer in East Africa: A new clinicopathological approach', *BMJ*, 1965, 2: 719–722. Also see: Korobkin, M. and Williams, E. H., 'Hepatoma and groundnuts in the West Nile district of Uganda', *Yale J Biol Med*, 1968, 41(1): 69–78. Epstein, A., 'Burkitt, Denis Parsons (1911–1993)', *Oxford Dictionary of National Biography*, Oxford University Press, 2004 [http://www.oxforddnb.com/view/article/57333, accessed 15 August 2011].
25. Doll, R. et al, *Cancer Incidence in Five Continents*, Genève, International Union against Cancer, 1966. On Richard Doll's work see: Peto, R. and Beral, V., 'Doll, Sir (William) Richard Shaboe (1912–2005)', *Oxford Dictionary of National Biography*, Oxford University Press, January 2009, http://www.oxforddnb.com/view/article/95920, accessed 23 May 2013].
26. Higginson, J., 'Epidemiology of cancer', *Proc R Soc Med*, 1968, 61: 724.
27. Ibid., 725.
28. Wogan, 'Chemical nature', 465–466.
29. Heathcote and Hibbert, *Aflatoxins*, 83.
30. *Food Safety Policy: Scientific and Societal Considerations, Part 2, Committee for a Study of Saccharin and Food Safety Policy*, Washington, National Academy of Science, 1979.

31. de la Peña, C., *Empty Pleasures: The Story of Artificial Sweeteners from Saccharin to Splenda*, Chapel Hill, University of North Carolina Press, 2010.
32. Smith, R. J., 'Institute of medicine report recommends complete overhaul of food safety laws', *Science*, 1979, 203: 1221–1223.
33. Food safety, S. 3–4.
34. Ibid., S-4.
35. Park, D. L. and Stoloff, 'Aflatoxin control – How a regulatory Agency managed risk from an unavoidable natural toxicant in food and feed', *Regulatory Toxicology and Pharmacology*, 1989, 9(2): 109–130.
36. Smith, D. F., 'Food panics in history: Corned beef, typhoid and "risk society" ', *J Epidemiol Community Health*, 2007, 61(7): 566–570.
37. Bruce, R. D., 'Risk assessment for aflatoxin: II. Implications of human epidemiology data', *Risk Anal,* 1990, 10: 561–569 and 1994, 14: 896–897.
38. Salmon, D. E., *The Diseases of Poultry*, G. E. Howard & Co., 1899, 75; Taylor, F., *A Manual of the Practice of Medicine*, London, J. & A. Churchill, 1898, 472.
39. Daison, R. W., *Practical Poultry Culture: A Concise and Practical Treatise on the Management of Poultry for Profit*, Indianapolis, Ind., The Epitomist, 1898, 63.
40. Dieulafoy, G. et al, 'Une pseudo-tuberculose mycosique', *Gaz Hosp Paris*, 1890, 63: 821.
41. *Lancet*, 1898, i: 149; Reports, 'Pseudo-tuberculosis', *BMJ*, 1899, i: 471–472.
42. Bryder, L., *Below the Magic Mountain: A Social History of Tuberculosis in Twentieth-Century Britain*, Oxford, Clarendon Press, 1988.
43. *Lancet*, 1899, i: 1363.
44. Rénon, L., *Etude Sur L'*aspergillose *Chez Les Animaux Et Chez L'homme*, Paris, Masson et Cte. 1897.
45. Rothwell, T. A., *Aspergillosis*, MD Thesis, Victoria University, Manchester, 1899.
46. Delepine, S., 'A case of melanomycosis of the skin', *Trans Path Soc Lond*, 1891, 58: 131; Worboys, M., 'Delépine, Auguste Sheridan (1855–1921)', Oxford Dictionary of National Biography, Oxford University Press, 2004 [http://www.oxforddnb.com/view/article/57113, accessed 5 August 2011].
47. Gradmann, C., *Laboratory Disease: Robert Koch's Medical Bacteriology*, Baltimore, Johns Hopkins University Press, 2009.
48. Kohn, H., 'Ein Fall von Pneumonomycosis aspergillina', *Deutsche Medicinische Wochenschrift*, 1893, 50: 1332–1333; Podack, M., 'Zur Kenntniss der Aspergillusmykosen im menschlichen Respirationsapparat', *Virchow's Archiv*, 1895, 139(2): 260–281.
49. Rénon, L., *Recherches Cliniques et Experimentales sur las pseudo-tuberculose aspergillarie*, Paris, G. Steinheil, 1893.
50. Rolleston, H. D., 'Pulmonary aspergillosis', in C. Allbutt, ed, *A System of Medicine*, London, Macmillan, 1898.
51. Worboys, M., 'Unsexing gonorrhoea: Bacteriologists, gynaecologists and suffragists in Britain, 1860–1920', *Soc Hist Med*, 17(1), 31–59.
52. Mettam, A. E., 'Aspergillosis – Aspergillar mycosis', *Trans R Acad Med Irel*, 1911, 29: 484–494.
53. Lapham, M. E., 'Aspergillosis of the lungs and its association with tuberculosis', *JAMA*, 1926, 87(13): 1031–1033.
54. Bud, R., *The Uses of Life: A History of Biotechnology*, Cambridge, Cambridge University Press, 1993.

55. Wells, P. A. and Herrick, H. T., 'Citric acid industry', *Ind Eng Chem*, 1938, 30(3): 255–262.
56. Hines, S., *Pfizer...An Informal History*, New York, Pfizer, 1978; Anon, *The Pasteur Fermentation Centennial: 1857–1957*, New York, 1958.
57. Bud, R., *Penicillin: Triumph and Tragedy*, Oxford, Oxford University Press, 2007, 34–35.
58. Neushul, P., 'Science, government and the mass production of penicillin', *J Hist Med Allied Sci*, 1993, 48(4): 371–395.
59. Waksman, S. A. and Schatz, A., 'Strain specificity and production of antibiotic substances', *PNAS*, 1943, 29(2): 74–79.
60. Benedict, R. G. and Langlykke, A. F., 'Antibiotics', *Annual Review*, 205–206; Tobie, W. C., 'Aspergillin: A name misapplied to several different antibiotics', *Nature*, 1946, 158, 709.
61. Dulaney, E. L., 'Penicillin production by the *Aspergillus nidulans* group', *Mycologia*, 1947, 39: 582–586; Raper, K. B., 'The development of improved penicillin producing molds', *Ann N Y Acad Sci*, 1946, 48: 41–56; Sheehan, J. C., *The Enchanted Ring: The Untold Story of Penicillin*, Cambridge, Mass, MIT Press, 1982.
62. Downing, J. G. and Conant, N. F., 'Medical progress: Mycotic infections', *N Engl J Med*, 1945, 233: 153–161 and 181–188.
63. Jillson, O. F., 'Medical progress: Mycology', *N Engl J Med*, 1953, 249: 527.
64. Duncan, J. T., 'Survey of fungous diseases in Great Britain: Results from the first eighteenth months', *BMJ*, 1945, ii: 716.
65. Monod, O. et al, 'New form of pulmonary aspergillosis: Aspergilloma causing bronchiectasis', *Bull Acad Natl Med*. 1951, 135(29–30): 508–511; Pesle, G. D. and Monod, O., 'Bronchiectasis due to aspergilloma', *Chest*, 1954, 25(2): 172–183. Also see: Gerstl B. et al, 'Pulmonary aspergillosis: Report of two cases', *Ann Intern Med*, 1948, 28: 662–665.
66. Ramires, J., 'Pulmonary aspergilloma: Endobronchial treatment', *N Engl J Med*, 1964, 271: 1281–1285; Higgins, I. T. T., 'The epidemiology of chronic respiratory disease', *Preventive Medicine*, 1973, 2 (1): 14–33.
67. British Tuberculosis Association, '*Aspergillus* in persistent lung cavities after tuberculosis: A report from the research committee of the British tuberculosis association', *Tubercle*, 1968, 49: 1–11.
68. British Thoracic and Tuberculosis Association, 'Aspergilloma and residual tuberculosis cavities – The results of a resurvey', *Tubercle*, 1970, 51: 227–245.
69. Ikemoto, H. B., 'Treatment of pulmonary aspergilloma with amphotericin B', *Arch Intern Med.*, 1965, 115: 598–601; Varkey, H. B. and Rose, H. D., 'Pulmonary aspergilloma: A rational approach to treatment', *Am J Med*, 1976, 61: 626–631.
70. Jewkes, J. et al, 'Pulmonary aspergilloma: Analysis of prognosis in relation to haemoptysis and survey of treatment', *Thorax*, 1983, 38: 572–578.
71. Asper, S. P. and Heffernan, A. G. A., 'Insidious fungal disease', *Trans Am Clin Climatol Assoc*, 1965, 76: 99–105.
72. Ibid., 99.
73. Ibid., 101.
74. Fraumeni, F. J. and Miller, R. W., 'Epidemiology of human leukaemia: Recent observations', *J Natl Cancer Inst*, 1967, 38: 593–605.
75. Asper, 'Insidious fungal', 102.

76. Gruhn, J. G. and Sansom, J., 'Mycotic infection of leukemia patients at autopsy', *Cancer*, 1963, 16: 61.
77. Ibid., 68–71; Bodey, G. P., 'Fungal infections complicating acute leukemia', *J Chron Dis*, 1966, 19: 667–687.
78. Gruhn, 'Mycotic infection', 72.
79. Sidransky, H. and Friedman L., 'The effect of cortisone and antibiotic agents on experimental pulmonary aspergillosis', *Amer J Path*, 1959, 35: 169; Sidransky, H. et al, 'Experimental pulmonary aspergillosis', *Arch Path*, 1965, 79: 299.
80. Bodey, 'Fungal infections', 667.
81. Young, R. C., 'Aspergillosis: The spectrum of disease in 98 patients', *Medicine*, 1970, 49(2): 147–173.
82. Meyer, R. et al, 'Aspergillosis complicating neoplastic disease', *Am J Med*, 1973, 54: 6–15.
83. Mirsky, H. S. and Cuttner, J., 'Fungal infection in acute leukemia', *Cancer*, 1972, 30: 348–352.
84. Degregorio, M. et al., 'Fungal infections in patients with acute leukemia', *Am J Med*, 1982, 73: 543–548.
85. Meyer, 'Aspergillosis complicating', 12.
86. Campbell, J. et al, 'Bronchopulmonary aspergillosis: A correlation of the clinical and laboratory findings in 272 patients investigated for bronchopulmonary aspergillosis', *Am Rev Resp Dis*, 1964, 89: 186.
87. Report, 'Mycoses', *BMJ*, 1970, i: 185.
88. Peitzman, S., *Dropsy, Dialysis, Transplant: A Short History of Failing Kidneys*, Baltimore, Johns Hopkins University Press, 2007.
89. Gallis, H. A. et al, 'Fungal infection following renal transplantation', *Arch Intern Med*, 1975, 135: 1163–1172; Walker, P. R. and Moorhead, J. F., 'Infection in the renal transplant patient', *J R Soc Med*, 1978, 71: 84–85; Howard, R. J. et al, 'Fungal infections in renal transplant recipients', *Ann Surg*, 1978, 188: 598–605.
90. Report, 'Fungus infection identified', *Guardian*, 19 August 1969: 18; Roper, J., 'Heart graft Briton dies', *Times*, 1 September 1969: 1a.
91. For a review of rent work see: Bennett, J. E., 'Salvage therapy for aspergillosis', *Clin Infect Dis*, 2005, 41 (Suppl 6): S387–8.
92. St Clair Symmers, W., 'Amphotericin pharmacophobia', *BMJ*, 1973, iv: 460–463.
93. Ibid., 463.
94. Forgan-Smith, R. and Darrell, J. H., 'Amphotericin pharmacophobia and renal toxicity', *BMJ*, 1974, i: 244.
95. Malo, J. L. et al, 'Studies in chronic pulmonary aspergillosis', *Thorax*, 1977, 32: 254–261.
96. Odds, F. C., 'Laboratory evaluation of antifungal agents: A comparative study of five imidazole derivatives of clinical importance', *J Antimicrob Chemother*, 1980, 6: 749–761.
97. Van Cutsem, J. et al, 'Itraconazole, a new triazole in that is orally active in aspergillosis', *Antimicrob Agents Chemother*, 1984, 26: 527–534.
98. Cauwenburgh, G. et al, 'Itraconazole in the treatment of human mycoses: Review of three years of clinical experience', *Rev Infect Dis*, 1987, 9: S146–52.

99. Hay, R. J., The First International Symposium on Itraconazole was held in Oaxaca, Mexico in October 1985, *Rev Inf Dis*, 1987, 9: S1–152.
100. Bennett, J. E., 'Fluconazole: A novel advance in therapy for systemic fungal infections: Overview of the symposium', *Rev Infect Dis*, 1990, 12 (Suppl): S263–266.
101. Epstein, S., *Impure Science: AIDS, Activism, and the Politics of Knowledge*, Berkeley, University of California Press, 1998.
102. Patterson, T. F. et al, 'Efficacy of fluconazole in experimental invasive aspergillosis', *Rev Infect Dis*, 1990, 12 (Suppl): S281–S285.
103. Richardson, K. et al, 'Discovery of fluconazole: A novel antifungal agent', *Rev Infect Dis*, 1990, 12: S267–271.
104. Hay, R. J., 'The azole antifungals', *J Antimicrob Chemother*, 1987, 20: 5.
105. Vanden Bossche, H. et al, eds, *Aspergillus and Aspergillosis*, New York, Plenum Press, 1978. The meeting was also the Second International Symposium in Topics in Mycology.
106. Seeliger, H. P. R., 'Summary and outlook', in Vanden Bossche, *Aspergillus*, 300.
107. Ibid., 301.
108. Denning, D. W. et al, 'Treatment of invasive aspergillosis with itraconazole', *Am J Med*, 1989, 86: 791–800; Tucker, R. M. et al, 'Adverse events associated with itraconazole in 189 patients on chronic therapy', *J Antimicrob Chemother*, 1990, 26: 561–566; Denning, D. W. and Stevens, D. A., 'Antifungal and surgical treatment of invasive aspergillosis: Review of 2,121 published cases', *Rev Inf Dis*, 1990, 12: 1147–1201.
109. Hay, 'The azole antifungals', 1–5.
110. Graybill, J. R., 'Lipid formulations of Amphotericin B: Does the emperor need new clothes?', *Ann Intern Med*, 1996, 124: 921–923.
111. Denning, D. W., 'Therapeutic outcome of invasive aspergillosis', *Clin Inf Dis*, 1996, 23: 607–615.
112. Denning, D., 'Early diagnosis of invasive aspergillosis', *Lancet*, 2000, i: 423.
113. Richardson, M. D., 'Changing patterns and trends in systemic fungal infections', *J Antimicrob Chemother*, 2005, 56: S1, i5–i11.
114. Groll, A. H. et al, 'Trends in the post-mortem epidemiology of invasive fungal infections at a university hospital', *J Infect*, 1996, 33: 23–32, 25.
115. Denning, D. W. et al, *Report on a European Science Foundation Workshop on Invasive* aspergillosis, 21–28 October 1998. http://www.aspergillus.org.uk. Accessed 4 December 2011.
116. Patterson, T. F. et al, 'Invasive aspergillosis: Disease spectrum, treatment practices, and outcomes', *Medicine*, 2000, 79(4): 250–260.
117. Ibid., 258.
118. Barlett, J. G., '*Aspergillus* Update', *Medicine*, 2000, 79: 282.
119. Hitchcock, C. A. et al, 'UK-109,496. 'A novel wide-spectrum triazole derivative for the treatment of fungal infections: antifungal activity and selectivity in vitro', in *Proceedings and Abstracts of the 35th Intersciences Conference on Antimicrobial Agents and Chemotherapy*. Washington DC: American Society for Microbiology, 1995, 125.
120. Cuenca-Estrella, M. et al, 'Comparison of the in vitro activity of voriconazole (UK-109,496), itraconazole and amphotericin B against clinical isolates of *Aspergillus* fumigatus', *J Antimicrob Chemother*, 1998, 42: 531–533.

121. Martin, M. V., 'Comparison of voriconazole (UK-109,496) and itraconazole in prevention and treatment of *Aspergillus* fumigatus endocarditis in guinea pigs', *Antimicrob Agent Chemother*, 1997, 41: 13–16.
122. Also see: Denning, D. W., 'Invasive aspergillosis: The state of the art', *Clin Infect Dis*, 1998, 26: 786.
123. Ahmad, K., 'Voriconazole victory versus amphotericin', *Lancet Infect Dis*, 2002, 2(10): 588.
124. Denning, D. W. et al, 'Efficacy and safety of voriconazole in the treatment of acute invasive aspergillosis', *Clin Infect Dis*, 2002, 34(5): 563–571; Ghannoum, M. W. and Kuhn, D. M., 'Voriconazole: Better chances for patients with invasive mycoses', *Eur J Med Res*, 2002, 7(5): 242–256; Enoch, D. A., 'Invasive fungal infections: A review of epidemiology and management options', *J of Medical Microbiology*, 2006, 55: 809–818; Walsh, T. J., 'Treatment of aspergillosis: Clinical practice guidelines of the infectious diseases society of America', *Clin Infect Dis*, 2008, 46: 327–360; Denning, D. W., 'Echinocandin antifungal drugs', *Lancet*, 2003, 362: 1142–1151; Nailor, M. D. and Sobel, J. D., 'Progress in antifungal therapy: Echinocandins versus azoles', *Drug Discovery Today: Therapeutic Strategies*, 2006, 3(2): 221–226.
125. Office of National Statistics, *Mortality statistics: Deaths registered in 2010* (Series DR) Table 5. http://www.ons.gov.uk/ons/publications/re-reference-tables.html?edition=tcm per cent3A77–230730. Accessed 28 May 2012; *CDC Underlying Causes of Death, 1999–2009*, http://wonder.cdc.gov/controller/datarequest/D76. Accessed 28 May 2012.
126. Bazan, E. and Waks, L. J., 'The iatrogenic body and beyond: The illich-duden research program', *Bull Sci Tech Soc*, 1986, 6: 17–18.

Summary and Reflections

1. Worboys, M., *Spreading Germs: Disease Theories and Medical Practice in Britain, 1865–1900*, Cambridge, Cambridge University Press, 2000, 193–223.
2. Such assessments have proved controversial, see Wilson, L. G., 'The historical decline of tuberculosis in Europe and America: Its causes and significance', *J Hist Med Allied Sci*, 1990, 45(3): 366–396; Bryder, L., 'Correspondence', *J Hist Med Allied Sci*, (1991) 46(3): 358–362.
3. McKeown, T. and Record, R. G., 'Reasons for the decline of mortality in England and Wales during the nineteenth century', *Population Studies*, 1964, 16(2): 94–122; McKeown, T., *The Role of Medicine: Dream, Mirage, or Nemesis?* Oxford, Blackwell, 1979; Rosenberg, C. E., 'Pathologies of progress: The idea of civilization as risk', *Bull Hist Med*, 1998, 72(4): 725–726.
4. Anderson, W., 'Natural histories of infectious disease: Ecological vision in twentieth-century biomedical science', *Osiris*, 2004, 19: 39–61.
5. Johnson, N. P. A. S. and Mueller, J., 'Updating the accounts: Global mortality of the 1918–1920 "Spanish" influenza pandemic', *Bull Hist Med*, 2002, 76(1): 108–115.
6. Taubenberger, J. K. and Morens, D. M. '1918 Influenza: The mother of all pandemics', *Rev Biomed*, 2006, 17; 69–79.
7. Mulkay, M. J., *The Social Process of Innovation*, London, Macmillan, 1972.

8. Gieryn, T. F. and Hirsh, R. F., 'Marginality and innovation in science', *Social Studies of Science*, 1983, 13(1): 87–106 and responses *Soc Stud Sci*, 1984, 14(4): 612–614.
9. On the history of laboratory and clinic see Study, S., 'Looking for trouble: Medical science and clinical practice in the historiography of modern medicine', *Soc Hist Med*, 2011, 24(3): 739–757.
10. Reverby S. M. and Rosner D., ' "Beyond the great doctors" revisited: a generation of the "new" social history in medicine', in Huisman F. and Warner J. H., eds, *Locating Medical History: Stories and Their Meanings*, Baltimore, Johns Hopkins University Press, 2004, 167–193; Linker, B., 'Resuscitating the "Great Doctor": The career of biography in medical history', in Söderqvist, T., ed, *Poetics of Biography in Science, Technology, and Medicine*, Aldershot, Ashgate Press, 2007, 221–239.
11. Cooter, R., 'The life of a disease?', *Lancet*, 2010, i: 111–112.
12. Ibid., 112.

Bibliography

Ainsworth, G. C., *Introduction to the History of Medical and Veterinary Mycology*, Cambridge, Cambridge University Press, 1987.

Ainsworth, G. C., *Introduction to the History of Mycology*, Cambridge, Cambridge University Press, 1976.

Ainsworth, G. C., *Introduction to the History of Plant Pathology*, Cambridge, Cambridge University Press, 1981.

Ajello, L., *Coccidioidomycosis: Current Clinical and Diagnostic Status: A Comprehensive Reference for the Clinician and Investigator: Selected Papers from the Third International Coccidioidomycosis Symposium*, Tucson, Arizona, Miami, Fla., Symposia Specialists, 1977.

Ajello, L. et al, eds, *Histoplasmosis: Proceedings of the Second National Conference*, Springfield, Ill, Charles C Thomas Publisher, 1971.

Alder Smith, H., *Ringworm: Its Diagnosis and Treatment*, London, H. K. Lewis & Co. Ltd, 1880, 2nd Edition, 1882, 3rd Edition, 1885.

Aldersmith, H., *Ringworm and Alopecia Areata*, 4th Edition, London, H. K. Lewis & Co. Ltd, 1897.

Al-Doory, Y. and Wagner, G. E., eds, *Aspergillosis*, Springfield, Ill., Thomas, 1985.

Allan, G. A. T., *Christ's Hospital*, London, Town and County, 1984.

Allbutt, C., ed, *A System of Medicine*, Vol., London, Macmillan, 1898.

Allen, A. M., *Internal Medicine in Vietnam: Volume 1, Skin Disease in Vietnam, 1965–72*, Washington DC, Office of the Surgeon General, 1972.

Arcieri, G. P., *Agostino Bassi in the History of Medical Thought*, Florence, L. S. Olschki, 1956.

Ayers, G. M., *England's First State Hospitals*, Berkeley, University of California Press, 1971.

Ayliffe, G. and English, M., *Hospital Infection: From Miasmas to MRSA*, Cambridge, Cambridge University Press, 2003.

Baldwin, R. S., *The Fungus Fighters: Two Women Scientists and Their Discovery*, Ithaca, Cornell University Press, 1981.

Bashford, A., ed, *Medicine at the Border: Disease, Globalization, and Security, 1850 to the Present*, Basingstoke, Palgrave, 2006.

Bashford, A., *Purity and Pollution: Gender, Embodiment and Victorian Medicine*, Basingstoke, Palgrave, 1998.

Beeton, I., *Beeton's Book of Household Management*, London, S O Beeton, 1861.

Berkhout, M. C., *De schimmelgeslachten Monilia, Oidium, Oospora en Torula, Scheveningen*, Edauwe & Johanssen, 1923.

British Association of Dermatologists, *A Biographical History of British Dermatology*, London, British Association of Dermatologists, 1995.

Brown, H., *Ringworm and Some Other Scalp Affections: Their Cause and Cure*, London, J. & A. Churchill, 1899.

Bryder, L., *Below the Magic Mountain: A Social History of Tuberculosis in Twentieth-Century Britain*, Oxford, Clarendon Press, 1988.

Bud, R., *Penicillin: Triumph and Tragedy*, Oxford, Oxford University Press, 2007.

Bud, R., *The Uses of Life: A History of Biotechnology*, Cambridge, Cambridge University Press, 1993.

Burnett, J. C., *Ringworm: Its Constitutional Nature and Cure*, Philadelphia, Boericke & Tafel, c1892.

Bynum, H., *Spitting Blood: The History of Tuberculosis*, Oxford, Oxford University Press, 2012.

Chaitlow, L., *Candida Albicans: Could Yeast Be Your Problem?*, Wellingborough, Thorsons, 1985.

Christensen, C. M., *The Molds and Man: An Introduction to the Fungi*, Minneapolis, University of Minnesota Press, 1951.

Cochrane, A. L. and Blythe, M., *One Man's Medicine. An Autobiography of Professor Archie Cochrane,* London, The British Medical Journal, 1989.

Codell Carter, K., *The Rise of Causal Concepts of Disease*, Aldershot, Ashgate, 2003.

Collings, J., 'The quiet epidemic that is ruining modern lifestyle', *Guardian*, 4 February 1988, 13.

Conant, N. F. et al, *Manual of Clinical Mycology*, Philadelphia, W. B. Saunders, 1944 and 1954.

Crissey, J. T. and Parish, L. C., *The Dermatology and Syphilology of the Nineteenth Century,* New York, Praeger, 1981.

Crook, W. G. et al, *The Yeast Connection and Women's Health*, Square One, 2007.

Crook, W. G., *Answering Parent's Questions*, Jackson, Professional Books, 1963.

Crook, W. G., *Are You Allergic? A Guide to Normal Living for Allergic Adults and Children*, Jackson, Tenn, Professional Press, 1977.

Crook, W. G., *Can Your Child Read? Is He Hyperactive?: A Pediatrician's Suggestions for Helping the Child with Hyperactivity, Behavior and Learning Problems*, Jackson, Tenn, Professional Books, 1975.

Crook, W. G., *Nature's Own Candida Cure*, Alive Books, 2003.

Crook, W. G., *The Yeast Connection: A Medical Breakthrough*, Jackson, T., Professional Books, 1983.

Crook, W. G., *Tired So Tired: and the Yeast Connection*, Square One, 2007.

Crook, W. G., *Your Allergic Child:A Pediatrician's Guide to Normal Living for Allergic Adults and Children*, New York, Medcom Pres, 1973.

Daison, R. W., *Practical Poultry Culture: A Concise and Practical Treatise on the Management of Poultry for Profit*, Indianapolis, Ind., The Epitomist, 1898.

Daniel, T. M. and Baum, G. L., *Drama and Discovery: The Story of Histoplasmosis*, Westport, Conn, Greenwood, 2002.

Davenport-Hines, R. P. T. and Slinn, J., *Glaxo: A History to 1962*, Cambridge, Cambridge University Press, 1992.

de Haller, R. and Suter, F., *Aspergillosis and Farmer's Lung in Man and Animal: Proceedings of the 4th International Symposium 7th–9th October 1971*, Davos, Bern, Hans Huber, 1974.

de la Peña, C., *Empty Pleasures: The Story of Artificial Sweeteners from Saccharin to Splenda*, Chapel Hill, University of North Carolina Press, 2010.

Digby, A., *Making A Medical Living: Doctors and Patients in the English Market for Medicine, 1720–1911*, Cambridge, Cambridge University Press, 1994.

Digby, A. and Searby, P., eds, *Children, School and Society in Nineteenth-Century England*, London, Macmillan, 1981.

Doll, R. et al, *Cancer Incidence in Five Continents,* Genève, International Union against Cancer, 1966.

Epstein, S., *Impure Science: AIDS, Activism, and the Politics of Knowledge,* Berkeley, University of California Press, 1998.

Erichsen, J. E., *The Science and Art of Surgery*, London, J. Walton, 186.

Espinel-Ingroff, A. V., *Medical Mycology in the United States: A Historical Analysis (1894–1996),* Dordrecht, Kluwer Academic Publishers, 2003.

Evans, R. J., *Death in Hamburg: Society and Politics in the Cholera Years, 1830–1910,* Cambridge, Cambridge University Press, 1987.

Farley, J., *Bilharzia: A History of Imperial Tropical Medicine*, Cambridge, Cambridge University Press, 1991.

Feudtner, C., *Bittersweet: Diabetes, Insulin, and the Transformation of Illness*, Chapel Hill, NC, University of North Carolina Press, 2003.

Fiese, M. J., *Coccidioidomycosis*, Springfield, Ill, Thomas, 1958.

Gay, F. P., *Agents of Disease and Host Resistance.* Baltimore, Charles C. Thomas, 1935.

Goertzl, T. and Goertzl, B., *Linus Pauling: A Life in Science and Politics,* New York, HarperCollins, 1995.

Goodhart, J. F., *The Diseases of Children*, 6th Edition, London, J & A Churchill, 1899.

Gradmann, C., *Laboratory Disease: Robert Koch's Medical Bacteriology,* Baltimore, Johns Hopkins University Press, 2009.

Hager, T., *Linus Pauling and the Chemistry of Life,* New York, Oxford University Press, 1998.

Hamlin, C., *Cholera: The Biography*, Oxford, Oxford University Press, 2009.

Harden, V. A., *Rocky Mountain Spotted Fever: History of a Twentieth-Century Disease,* Baltimore, Johns Hopkins University Press, 1990.

Harris, B., *The Health of the Schoolchild: A History of the School Medical Service in England and Wales*, Buckingham, Open University Press, 1995.

Haynes, D. M., *Imperial Medicine: Patrick Manson and the Conquest of Tropical Disease,* Philadelphia, University of Pennsylvania Press, 2001.

Heathcote, J. and Hibbert, J. R., *Aflatoxins: Chemical and Biological Aspects*, Oxford, Elsevier, 1978.

Henrici, A. T., *Molds, Yeasts and Actinomycetes: A Handbook for Students of Bacteriology*, New York, J. Wiley & Sons, 1930.

Hess, D. J., *Can Bacteria Cause Cancer?: Alternative Medicine Confronts Big Science,* New York, New York University Press, 1997.

Hess, D. J., *Evaluating Alternative Cancer Therapies: A Guide to the Science and Politics of An Emerging Medical Field*, New Brunswick, NJ: Rutgers University Press, 1999.

Hines, S., *Pfizer... An Informal History*, New York, Pfizer, 1978.

Hogg, J., *Parasitic or Germ Theory of Disease: The Skin, Eye, and Other Affections,* London, Baillière, Tindall and Cox, 1876.

Hopkins, D. R., *The Greatest Killer: Smallpox in History*, Chicago, University of Chicago Press, 2002.

Hornblum, A. M., *Acres of Skin: Human Experiments at Holmesburg Prison,* New York, Routledge, 1998.

Hussar, A. E. and Holley, H. L., *Antibiotics and Antibiotic Therapy,* New York, Macmillan, 1954.

Inglis, B., *The Diseases of Civilization*, Chicago, Academy Chicago Publishers, 1981.
Jackson, M., *Allergy: The History of a Modem Malady*, London, Reaktion Books, 2006.
Jackson, M., *Asthma: The Biography*, Oxford, Oxford University Press, 2009.
Jackson, M., *The Age of Stress: Science and the Search for Stability*, Oxford, Oxford University Press, 2013.
Jacobson, H. P., *Fungous Diseases: A Clinic-Mycological Text*, London, Baillière, Tindall & Cox, 1932.
Jenkins R. and Mowbray, J. F., eds, *Post-Viral Fatigue Syndrome: (myalgic encephalomyelitis)*, Chichester, John Wiley & Sons, 1992.
Jones, S. D., *Death in a Small Package: A Short History of Anthrax*, Baltimore, Johns Hopkins University Press, 2010.
Kay, A. B. and Lessor, M. H., *Allergy: Conventional and Alternative Concepts*, London, Royal College of Physicians of London, 1992.
Kraut, A. M., *Silent Travelers: Germs, Genes, and the Immigrant Menace*, New York, Basic Books, 1994.
Lailler, C.-P., *Leçons cliniques sur les teignes, faites à l'hôpital Saint-Louis, par le Dr C. Lailler*, Paris, V-A Delahaye, 1878.
Lawrence, C., *Medical Theory, Surgical Practice: Studies in the History of Surgery*, London, Routledge, 1992.
Lornzani, S., *Candida: A Twentieth Century Disease*, New Canaan, Conn, Keats Publishing, 1986.
M'Call Anderson, T., *On the Parasitic Affections of the Skin,* London, Churchill, 1861.
Macfarlane, G., *Alexander Fleming: The Man and the Myth*, Oxford, Oxford University Press, 1984.
Macleod, J. H. M., *Diseases of the Skin: A Text-book for Students and Practitioners*, London, H. K. Lewis, London, 1920.
MacPherson, W. G. et al, *History of the Great War Based on Official Documents: Medical Services Pathology*, London, HMSO, 1923.
MacPherson, W. G. et al, *Medical Services, Diseases of the War*, London, HMSO, 1923.
Mansell, K., *Christ's Hospital in the Victorian Era*, Whitton, Ashwater Press, 2011.
Marks, H. M., *The Progress of Experiment: Science and Therapeutic Reform in the United States, 1900–1990*, Cambridge, Cambridge University Press, 1997.
Mayne, R. G., *An Expository Lexicon of the Terms, Ancient And Modern, in Medical and General Science*, Pt 2, London, J Churchill, 1854.
McIvor, A. and Johnston, R., *Miners' Lung: A History of Dust Disease in British Coal Mining*, Farnham, Ashgate, 2007.
Morris, M., *Ringworm in the Light of Recent Research*, London, Cassell and Co., 1898.
Moser, R. H., ed, *Diseases of Medical Progress*, Springfield, Ill, Charles C Thomas, 1963.
Mulkay, M. J., *The Social Process of Innovation*, London, Macmillan, 1972.
McKeown, T., *The Role of Medicine: Dream, Mirage, or Nemesis?*, Oxford, Blackwell, 1979.

Murphy, M., *Sick Building Syndrome and the Problem of Uncertainty: Environmental Politics, Technoscience, and Women Workers*, Durham, NC, Duke University Press, 2006.

Nasaw, D., *Schooled to Order: A Social History of Public Schooling in the United States*, New York, Oxford University Press, 1979.

Neill, D. J., *Networks in Tropical Medicine: Internationalism, Colonialism, and the Rise of a Medical Specialty, 1890–1930*, Stanford, Stanford University Press, 2012.

O. Truss, *The Missing Diagnosis*, Birmingham, The Missing Diagnosis, Inc., 1983.

Odds, F. C., *Candida and Candidosis,* Leicester, Leicester University Press, 1979.

Odds, F. C., *Candida and Candidosis,* London, Bailliere Tindall 1988.

Packard, R. M., *The Making of a Tropical Disease: A Short History of Malaria,* Baltimore, Johns Hopkins University Press, 2007.

Peitzman, S., *Dropsy, Dialysis, Transplant: A Short History of Failing Kidneys,* Baltimore, Johns Hopkins University Press, 2007.

Pelling, M., *Cholera, Fever and English Medicine, 1830–1865*, Oxford, Clarendon Press, 1976.

Pernick, M. J., *A Calculus of Suffering: Pain, Professionalism and Anaesthesia in Nineteenth Century America*, New York, Columbia University Press, 1985.

Picard, A., *Making the American Mouth: Dentists and Public Health in the Twentieth Century*, New Brunswick, NJ: Rutgers University Press, 2009.

Pillsbury, D. et al, *A Manual of Cutaneous Medicine*, Philadelphia, W. B. Saunders, 1961.

Pillsbury, D. M. et al, *Dermatology*, Philadelphia, W B Saunders, 1956.

Plumbe, S., *An Address to the Governors of Christ's Hospital, on the Causes and Means of Prevention of Ring-Worm in That Establishment; To Which Is Attached, a Few Rules for the Domestic Management of the Scholars during Their Vacations*, London, 1834.

Proceedings of Symposium on Coccidioidomycosis, held at Phoenix, Arizona, February 11–13, 1957, Atlanta, Ga., CDC, 1957.

Pusey, W. A., *The History of Dermatology*, Sprinagfield, Ill., C.C. Thomas, 1933.

Randolph, T. G., *Human Ecology and Susceptibility to the Chemical Environment*,. Springfield, Ill, Thomas. 1962.

Rénon, L., *Etude Sur L'aspergillose Chez Les Animaux Et Chez L'homme*, Paris, Masson et Cte. 1897.

Rénon, L., *Recherches Cliniques et Experimentales sur las pseudo-tuberculose aspergillarie*, Paris, G Steinheil, 1893.

Richardson, N., *Typhoid in Uppingham: Analysis of a Victorian Town and School in Crisis, 1875–7,* London, Pickering & Chatto, 2008.

Rosen, G., *The Specialization of Medicine with Particular Reference to Ophthalmology*, New York, Froben Press, 1944.

Russell, B. F., ed, *St. John's Hospital for Diseases of the Skin, 1863–1963*, Edinburgh, E. & S. Livingstone, 1963.

Sabouraud, R., *Les Trichophyties humaines,* Paris, Rueff and Cie, 1894.

Sabouraud, R., *Maladies Cryptogamiques, Les Teigne*, Paris, Masson & Cie, 1910.

Sakaguchi, Kin'ichiro, *Nihon no sake* (Tokyo, Iwanami shoten, 2007).

Salmon, D. E., *The Diseases of Poultry*, G. E. Howard & Co., 1899.

Sanderson, M., *Education, Economic Change and Society in England 1780–1870*, Cambridge, Cambridge University Press, 1995.
Schwartz Cowan, R., *More Work for Mother: The Ironies of Household Technology from the Open Hearth to the Microwave*, New York, Basic Books, 1983.
Sheehan, J. C., *The Enchanted Ring: The Untold Story of Penicillin*, Cambridge, MA, M.I.T. Press, 1982.
Silverman, M., and Lee, P. R., *Pills, Profits and Politics*, Berkeley, University of California Press, 1974.
Simon, B., *Studies in the History of Education*, London, Lawrence and Wishart, 1966.
Smith, L. W. and Walker, A. D., *Penicillin Decade 1941–1951. Sensitizations and Toxicities*, Washington, Arundel Press, 1951.
Steadman, C., *Dust*, Manchester, Manchester University Press, 2002.
Sternberg T. H. and Newcomer, V. D., *Therapy of Fungal Disease: An International Symposium*, Boston, Little brown & Company, 1956.
Stevens, D. A., *Coccidioidomycosis: A Text*, New York, Plenum Medical Book Co., 1980.
Stevens, R., *Medical Practice in Modern England: The Impact of Specialization and State Medicine*, New Haven, Yale University Press, 1966.
Tattersall, R., *Diabetes: A Biography*, Oxford, Oxford University Press, 2009.
Taylor, F., *A Manual of the Practice of Medicine*, London, J & A Churchill, 1898.
The Medical Annual 1941: A Year Book of Treatment and Practitioner's Index. Bristol, John Wright, 1941.
The Pasteur Fermentation Centennial, 1857–1957, New York, 1958.
Thom, C. and Church, M. B., *The Aspergilli*, Baltimore, Williams and Wilkins, 1926.
Tilbury Fox, G., *Skin Diseases of Parasitic Origin*, London, Robert Hardwicke, 1863.
Tilles, G. and Tilles, *G, Teignes et Teigneux: Histoire Medicale et Sociale*, Paris, Springer, 2008.
Turner, J. P., *Ringworm and Its Successful Treatment*, Philadelphia, F.A. Davis, 1921.
Vanden Bossche, H. et al, eds, *Aspergillus and Aspergillosis*, New York, Plenum Press, 1978.
Vogel, M. J. and Rosenberg, C. E., eds, *The Therapeutic Revolution: Essays in the Social History of American Medicine*, Philadelphia, University of Pennsylvania Press, 1979.
Walsh, D., *The Roentgen Rays in Medical Work: With an Introductory Section upon Electrical Apparatus and Methods by J. E. Greenhill*, London, Baillière & Co., 1897.
Weisz, G., *Divide and Conquer: A Comparative History of Medical Specialization*, New York, Oxford University Press, 2006.
Williams, R. J. and Wright, D. K., *A Physician's Handbook on Orthomolecular Medicine*, New York, Pergamon Press, 1977.
Wilson, D. J., *Living with Polio: The Epidemic and Its Survivors*, Chicago, University of Chicago Press, 2005.
Wilson, J. W., *Clinical and Immunologic Aspects of Fungous Diseases*, Springfield, Charles C. Thomas, 1957.
Winner, H. I. and Hurley, R., *A Symposium on Candida Infections*, Edinburgh, E. & S. Livingstone, 1966.
Winner, H. I. and Hurley, R., *Candida albicans*, London, Churchill 1964.

Worboys, M., *Spreading Germs: Disease Theories and Medical Practice in Britain, 1865–1900*, Cambridge, Cambridge University Press, 2000.

Yates, Ronald E., *The Kikkoman Chronicles: A Global Company with a Japanese Soul*, New York: McGraw Hill, 1998.

Unpublished PhD Theses

Jamieson, A., *An Intolerable Affliction: A History of Lupus vulgaris in Late 19th and Early 20th Century Britain*, Unpublished PhD Thesis, University of Leeds, 2010.

Knowles, R. B., *Dermatitis in Coal-miners: A Survey of the Factors Influencing Its Nature and Cause*, Unpublished MD Thesis, University of Sheffield, 1943.

Newson Kerr, M., *Fevered Metropolis: Epidemic Disease and Isolation in Victorian London*, Unpublished PhD Thesis, University of Southern California, 2007.

Rothwell, T. A., *Aspergillosis*, MD Thesis, Victoria University, Manchester, 1899.

Russell, R., *Nausea and Vomiting: A History of Signs, Symptoms and Sickness in Nineteenth-Century Britain*, Unpublished PhD Thesis, University of Manchester, 2012.

Stark, J., *Industrial Illness in Cultural Context: 'La maladie de Bradford' in Local, National and Global Settings, 1878–1919*, Unpublished PhD Thesis, University of Leeds, 2011.

Government Publications

Annual Report for 1908 of the Chief Medical Officer of the Board of Education, Parl. Papers, 1910, Cd. 4986, XXIII: 1.

Farmer's Lung: Report by the Industrial Injuries Advisory Council, BPP, 1963–1964, Cmnd 2403: 863–878.

Food Safety Policy: Scientific and Societal Considerations, Part 2, Committee for a Study of Saccharin and Food Safety Policy, Washington, National Academy of Science, 1979.

Mortality Statistics: Deaths Registered in 2010 (Series DR) Table 5. Office of National Statistics, http://www.ons.gov.uk/ons/publications/re-reference-tables.html?edition=tcm%3A77-230730. Accessed 28 May 2012.

Megavitamin and Orthomolecular Therapy in Psychiatry, Washington, DC, APA, 1973.

Report of the Committee on Fowl Pest Policy, Parl. Papers, 1961–1962, Cmnd.1664, VIII, 271.

The Health of the School Child: Annual Report of the Chief Medical Officer of the Board of Education, 1937, London, HMSO, 1938.

The Health of the School Child: The Annual Report of the Chief Medical Officer of the Board of Education for 1925, London, HMSO, 1926.

The Health of the School Child: The Annual Report of the Chief Medical Officer of the Board of Education for 1933, London, HMSO, 1934.

The Health of the School Child: The Annual Report of the Chief Medical Officer of the Board of Education for 1938, London, HMSO, 1939.

Toxicity Associated with Certain Batches of Groundnuts-Report of the Interdepartmental Working Party on Groundnut Toxicity Research, Department of Scientific and Industrial Research, London, HMSO, 1962.

Underlying Causes of Death, 1999–2010, Atlanta, CDC, http://wonder.cdc.gov/wonder/help/ucd.html. Accessed 2 August 2013.

Vital Statistics of the United States, 1950, Volume 3, Mortality Data, Washington: US Depart of Health, Education and Welfare, 1953.

Vital Statistics of the United States, 1960, Volume 2 – Mortality, Part A, Washington: US Depart of Health, Education and Welfare, 1963.

Articles and Book Chapters

Abraham, P. S. and Eddowes, A., 'Contagious skin diseases in schools', *Lancet*, 1894, ii: 275.

Adam, T., 'The control of ringworm in school', *Public Health*, 1912–1913, 26: 3–8.

Adamson, H. G., 'On the treatment of ringworm of the scalp by means of X-rays', *Lancet*, 1905, i: 1715.

Adamson, H. G., 'On the treatment of scabies and some other common skin affections in soldiers', *Lancet*, 1917, i: 221–223.

Ahmad, K., 'Voriconazole victory versus amphotericin', *Lancet Infect Dis*, 2002, 2(10): 588.

Ainsworth, G. C., 'The medical research council's medical mycology committee (1943–1969): A chapter in the history of medical mycology in the UK', *Sabouraudia*, 1978, 16: 1–7.

Ajello, L., 'Coccidioidomycosis and histoplasmosis: A review of the epidemiology and geographical distribution', *Mycopathologia et Mycologia Applicata*, 1971, 45: 221–230.

Alexander, D. J., 'Newcastle disease', *British Poultry Science*, 2001, 42(1): 5–22.

Allen, A. M. et al, 'Skin infections in Vietnam', *Military Medicine*, 1972, 137: 295–301.

Allen, S. K. and Semba, R. D., 'The trachoma "Menace" in the United States, 1897–1960', *Survey of Ophthalmology*, 2002, 47(5): 500–599.

Amor, K. T. et al, 'The use of cyclosporine in dermatology: Part I', *J Am Acad Dermatol*, 2010, 63: 925–946.

Ampel, N. M. et al, 'Coccidioidomycosis in Arizona: Increase in incidence from 1990 to 1995', *Clin Infect Dis*, 1998, 27: 1528–1530.

Ampel, N. N. et al, 'Coccidioidomycosis: Clinical update', *Clin Infect Dis*, 1989, 11(6): 897–911.

Anderson, D. W., 'Griseofulvin: Biology and clinical usefulness, a review', *Ann Allergy*, 1965, 23: 103–110.

Anderson, J. A. et al, 'Position statement on candidiasis hypersensitivity', *J Allergy Clin Immunol*, 1986, 78: 271–273.

Anderson, W., 'Natural histories of infectious disease: Ecological vision in twentieth-century biomedical science', *Osiris*, 2004, 19: 39–61.

Andrews, G. C., 'J Gardner Hopkins', *Arch Derm Syphilol*, 1951, 64(6): 810–812.

Armengol, C. E., 'A historical review of *Pneumocystis carinii*', *JAMA*, 1995, 273(9): 747, 750–751.

Aronowitz, R., 'From myalgic encephalitis to yuppie flu: A history of chronic fatigue syndromes', in Rosenberg, C. and Golden, J., eds, *Framing Disease: Studies in Cultural History*, New Brunswick, NJ: Rutgers University Press, 1992, 155–181.

Arthur Whitfield, 'A note on some unusual cases of Trichophytic infection', *Lancet*, 1908, ii: 237–238.

Asherson, G. L., 'Fox, William Tilbury (1836–1879)', *Oxford Dictionary of National Biography*, Oxford University Press, 2004. [http://www.oxforddnb.com/view/article/10048, accessed 15 August 2008].

Asper, S. P. and Heffernan, A. G. A., 'Insidious fungal disease', *Trans Am Clin Climatol Assoc*, 1965, 76: 99–105.

Banham, R., 'Certain *Monilias* parasitic on man: Their identification by morphology and by agglutination', *J Infect Dis*, 1931, 49: 183–215.

Barber, H. W., 'The relationship of dermatology to general medicine', *Lancet*, 1929, ii: 363–370, 483–492 and 591–599.

Barlett, J. G., '*Aspergillus* Update', *Medicine*, 2000, 79: 282.

Barr, W., 'Nystatin', *Practitioner*, 1957, 178: 616–617.

Barrett, S., 'Unproven "Allergies": an epidemic of nonsense "environmental illness" and the "yeast connection" ', in Barrett, S and Jarvis, J. T., eds, *The Health Robbers: A Close Look at Quackery in America*, New York, Prometheus Press, 1993.

Batten, J., 'Cystic fibrosis: A review', *Br J Dis Chest*, 1965, 59: 1–9.

Baum, B. and Schwarz, J., 'Clinical experiences with amphotericin B', *Antibiot Annu*, 1959–1960, 7: 638–643.

Baum, G. L. and Schwarz, J., 'The history of histoplasmosis 1906–1956', *N Engl J Med*, 1957, 256: 253–258.

Baxter Forman, E., 'A lecture on medical London', *Lancet*, 1899, i: 213.

Bazan, E. and Waks, L. J., 'The iatrogenic body and beyond: The Illich-Duden research program', *Bull Sci Tech Soc*, 1986, 6: 17–18.

Benedict, R. G. and Langlykke, A. F., 'Antibiotics', *Annual Review of Microbiology*, 1947, 1: 193–236.

Benham, R., 'Certain *Monilias* parasitic on man: Their identification by morphology and by agglutination', *J Infect Dis*, 1931, 49: 183–215.

Benham, R. W., 'Manual of clinical mycology', *Am J Public Health*, 1945, 35: 1091.

Bennett, J. E., 'Flucocystine', *Ann Intern Med*, 1977, 86(3): 319–321.

Bennett, J. E., 'Fluconazole: A novel advance in therapy for systemic fungal infections: Overview of the symposium', *Rev Infect Dis*, 1990, 12, Suppl.: S263–266.

Bennett, J. E., 'Salvage therapy for aspergillosis', *Clin Infect Dis*, 2005, 41, Suppl 6: S387–388.

Bennett, J. W., 'An overview of the genus *Aspergillus*', in Machida, M. and Gomi, K., eds, *Aspergillus: Molecular Biology and Genomics*, Norfolk, Caister Academic Press, 2010, 1–18.

Bennett, J. W., 'Aspergillus: A primer for the novice', *Medical Mycology*, 2009, 47 Suppl. 1: S5–12.

Bennett, J. E. et al, 'A comparison of amphotericin B alone and combined with flucytosine in the treatment of cryptoccal meningitis', *N Engl J Med*, 1979, 301(3): 126–131.

Bernard Shaw, A. F., 'The diagnosis of ringworm in school children', *Public Health*, 1912–1913, 26: 366–369.

Bhutani, L. K. et al, 'Tinea pedis – a penalty of civilization A sample survey of rural and urban population', *Mycoses*, 1971, 14: 335–336.

Binns, T. B., 'Gastro-intestinal complications of oral antibiotics', *Lancet*, 1956, i: 336–8.

Birkinshaw, J. H., 'Harold Raistrick, 1890–1971', *Biogr Mems Fell R Soc*, 1972, 18: 488–509.

Birt, A. R., 'The increasing problem of drug reactions', *Can Med Assoc J*, 1957, 77: 709–715.

Blaisdell, J. H., 'Epidermophytosis', *N Engl J Med*, 1930, 202: 1059–1064.

Bland, P. B. and Rakoff, A. E., 'Leukorrea: Clinical and therapeutic aspects', *JAMA*, 1940, 115(12): 1013–1018.

Bland, P. D. et al, 'Experimental vaginal and cutaneous moniliasis: Clinical and laboratory studies of certain monilias associated with vaginal, oral and cutaneous thrush', *Arch Derm Syphilol*, 1937, 36: 760–780.

Bland, P. D. et al, 'Vaginal trichomoniasis in the pregnant woman', *JAMA*, 1931, 96: 157–163.

Blank, H., 'Antifungal and other effects of griseofulvin', *Am J Med*, 1965, 39(5): 831–838.

Blank, H., 'Symposium on griseofulvin', *Arch Dermatol*, 1960, 51: 649.

Blank, H. and Roth, J. F., 'The treatment of dermatomycoses with orally administered Griseofulvin', *Arch Derm Syphilo*, 1959, 81: 259–267.

Blount, W. P., 'Turkey "X" disease', *Turkeys*, March–April 1961: 52–60.

Blonz, E. R. 'Is there an epidemic of chronic candidiasis in our midst?', *JAMA*, 1986, 256: 3138–3139.

Bocobo, F. C. et al, 'Epidemiologic study of tinea capitis caused by *T tonsurans* and *M audouinii*', *Public Health Rep*, 1952, 67: 53–56.

Bodey, G. P., 'Fungal infections complicating acute leukemia', *J Chronic Dis*, 1966, 19: 667–687.

Borel, J. F. et al, 'The History of the discovery and development of cyclosporine (Sandimmun®)', in Vincent, J et al, eds, *The Search for Anti-inflammatory Drugs*, Boston, O Birkhauser 1995.

Borelli, D. et al, 'Ketoconazole, an oral antifungal: Laboratory and clinical assessment of imidazole drugs', *Postgrad Med J*, 1979, 55: 657–661.

Boseley, S., 'Are you ready for a world without antibiotics?', *Guardian*, 12 August 2010.

Brabander, J. O. W. et al, 'Intestinal moniliasis in adults', *Can Med Assoc J*, 1957, 77: 478–83.

Brandt, A. M. and Gardner, M., 'The golden age of medicine', in Cooter, R. and Pickstone, J. V., eds, *Medicine in the Twentieth Century*, Amsterdam, Harwood, 2000: 21–37.

Brian, P. W., 'Studies on the biological activity of griseofulvin', *Annals of Botany*, 1949, 13: 59–77.

British Society for Antimicrobial Chemotherapy Working Party, 'Antifungal chemotherapy in patients with acquired immunodeficiency syndrome', *Lancet*, 1992: 648–651.

British Thoracic and Tuberculosis Association, 'Aspergilloma and residual tuberculosis cavities – The results of a resurvey', *Tubercle*, 1970: 51: 227–245.

British Tuberculosis Association, '*Aspergillus* in persistent lung cavities after tuberculosis: A report from the Research Committee of the British Tuberculosis Association', *Tubercle*, 1968, 49: 1–11.

Bronnimann, D. A. et al, 'Coccidioidomycosis in the acquired immunodeficiency syndrome', *Ann Intern Med*, 1987, 106: 372–379.

Bronson, D. M. et al, 'An epidemic of infection with *Trichophyton* tonsurans revealed in a 20-year survey of fungal infections in Chicago', *J Amer Acad Dermatol*, 1983, 8(23): 322–330.

Brown, G. T., 'Hypersensitiveness to fungi', *J Allergy*, 1936, 7(5): 455–470.

Brown, T. G., 'Pulmonary mycosis', *Edin Med J*, 1947, 54: 414–422.

Bruce, R. D., 'Risk assessment for Aflatoxin: II. Implications of human epidemiology data', *Risk Analysis*, 1990, 10: 561–569 and 1994, 14: 896–897.

Brueton, M. J. et al, 'Allergic bronchopulmonary aspergillosis complicating cystic fibrosis in childhood', *Arch Dis Child*, 1980, 55: 348–353.

Brunton, D., 'Willan, Robert (1757–1812)', *Oxford Dictionary of National Biography*, Oxford University Press, 2004. Accessed 8 February 2013, http://www.oxforddnb.com/view/article/29438.

Bryder, L., 'Correspondence', *J Hist Med Allied Sci*, 1991, 46(3): 358–362.

Bulkley, L. D., 'The X-ray treatment of ringworm of the scalp', *JAMA*, 1911, 56: 1706–1709.

Bulmer, G. S., 'The changing spectrum of mycological education', *Mycopathologia*, 1995, 130: 127–128.

Bunch, J. L., 'Sabouraud's method of ringworm treatment' *Lancet*, 1905, i: 414–416.

Burnham, J. C., 'American medicine's golden age: What happened to it?', *Science*, 1982, 215: 1474–1479.

Buscher, D., 'Obituary: Theron G Randolph, M. D., 1906–1995', *Journal of Nutritional & Environmental Medicine*, 1996, 6: 245–246.

Butler, W. T., 'Pharmacology, toxicity, and therapeutic usefulness of amphotericin B', *JAMA*, 1966, 195: 371–375.

Campbell, J. et al, 'Bronchopulmonary aspergillosis.a correlation of the clinical and laboratory findings in 272 patients investigated for bronchopulmonary aspergillosis, *Am Rev Resp Dis*, 1964, 89: 186.

Campbell, M., 'Acute symptoms following work with hay', *BMJ*, 1932, ii: 1143–1144.

Cannon, P. R., 'The changing pathologic picture of infection since the introduction of chemotherapy and antibitoics', *Bull N Y Acad Med*, 1955, 31: 89–91.

Cantor, D., 'Cortisone and the politics of drama, 1949–55' in Pickstone, J. V., ed, *Medical Innovation in Historical Perspective*, Basingstoke, Macmillan, 1992, 225–245.

Capel, E. H., 'A Medical Service for the Coal Mining Industry', *Journal of the Royal Society for the Promotion of Health*, 1948, 68: 525–531.

Caplan, H., 'Monilia (*Candida*) endocarditis following treatment with antibiotics', *Lancet* 1955, ii: 95.

Carlet, J. et al, 'Ready for a world without antibiotics? The pensières antibiotic resistance call to action', *Antimicrobial Resistance and Infection Control*, 2012, 1(1): 1–11.

Cartwright, R. Y., 'Antifungal drugs', *J Antimicrob Chemother*, 1975, 1: 148–151.

Cartwright, R. Y., 'Use of antibiotics: Antifungals', *BMJ*, 1978, ii: 108–111.

Cates, J., 'The administrative control of ringworm', *Public Health*, 1910–1911, 24: 226–233.

Cauwenburgh, G. et al, 'Itraconazole in the treatment of human mycoses: Review of three years of clinical experience', *Rev Infect Dis*, 1987, 9: S146–152.

Chapman, S. W. et al, 'Endemic blastomycosis in Mississippi: epidemiological and clinical studies', *Semin Respir Infect,* 1997, 12(3): 219–228.

Check, W. A., 'Oral antifungal agent effective even for widespread infections', *JAMA*, 1980, 244: 2019–2020.

Chesney, J., ' "Nystatin" ("Mycostatin")', *BMJ*, 1956, i: 1043–1044.

Childs, A. J., 'Effect of Nystatin on growth of *C. albicans* during antibiotic therapy', *BMJ*, 1956, i: 660–662.

Chin, D. D. Y., 'The Kansas city field station', 1950–1973, *Public Health Reports*, 1999, 114: 377–380.

Civatte, A., 'Obituary: Raymond Sabouraud', *Br J Dermatol*, 1938, 50: 206–210.

Cochrane Shanks, S., 'Vale Epilation: X-ray epilation of the scalp at Goldie Leigh Hospital, Woolwich (1922–1958)', *Br J Dermatol*, 1967, 79(4): 237–238.

Cohen, A. C., 'Pulmonary moniliasis', *Am J Med Sci*, 1953, 226: 16–23.

Cohen, I and Longacre, A. B., 'Neomycin-Nystatin preoperative preparation of the colon', *Am Surg*, 1956, 22: 301–307.

Colan, T., 'Parasitic vegetable fungi and the diseases induced by them', *Lancet*, 1874, ii: 755–757 and 832–833.

Colcott Fox, T. and Blaxall, F. R., 'An enquiry into the plurality of fungi causing ringworm in human beings, as met with in London', *Br J Dermatol*, 1896, 8: 241.

Coleman, D. C. et al, 'Oral *Candida* in HIV infection and AIDS: new perspectives/new approaches', *Critical Reviews in Microbiology,* 1993, 19: 61–82.

Coleman III, W. P. and Edwards, D. E., 'Letters depression and *Candida*-reply', *JAMA*, 1985, 253: 3400.

Colgan, M. T., 'The bacterial flora of the intestinal tract: Changes in diarrheal disease and following antimicrobial therapy', *Journal of Pediatrics*, 1956, 49: 214–228.

Collins, J. H., 'Vulvovaginitis', *Obstet Gynecol Surv*, 1952, 7(2): 224–227.

Comstock, G. W., 'In memoriam: Carroll Edwards Palmer, 1903–1972', *J Epidemiol*, 1972, 95: 305–307.

Conant, N and Howell, A. F., 'The similarity of the fungi causing South American blastomycosis (paracoccidioidal granuloma) and North American blastomycosis (Gilchrist's disease)', *J Invest Dermatol*, 1942, 5(6): 353–370.

Conant, N. F., 'Future developments in mycological investigative methods', *Ann N Y Acad Sci*, 1950, 50: 1245–1249.

Condrau, F., 'The patient's view meets the clinical gaze', *Soc Hist Med*, 2007, 20: 525–540.

Conte, N. F. et al, 'Prophylactic griseofulvin against *Trichophyton mentagrophytes* infections', in H. M. Robinson, ed, *The Diagnosis and Treatment of Fungal Infections,* Springfield: Charles C. Thomas, Inc., 1974, 543.

Cooper, J., 'Anderson, Sir Thomas McCall (1836–1908)', revised. J O'D Alexander, *Oxford Dictionary of National Biography*, Oxford University Press, 2006. Accessed 6 October 2008, http://www.oxforddnb.com/view/article/30414.

Cooter, R., 'The life of a disease?', *Lancet*, 2010, i: 111–112.

Cregor, F. W. and Gastineau, F. M., 'Stovarsol in the treatment of syphilis: A preliminary report, *Arch Derm Syphilol,* 1927, 15(1): 43–53.

Crook, W. G., 'Letters depression associated with *C. albicans* infections', *JAMA*, 1984, 51: 2928–2929.

Crook, W. G., 'The coming revolution in medicine', *Journal of the Tennessee Medical Association*, 1983, 76: 145–149.
Crounse, R. G. et al, 'Cryptococcosis: case with unusual skin lesions and favorable response to amphotericin B therapy', *Arch Dermatol*, 1958, 77(2): 210–215.
Cruickshank, R., 'The epidemiology of some skin infections', *BMJ*, 1956, i: 58.
Cruickshank, R. and Sharman, A., 'Hormones and vaginitis', *J Obstet Gyneacol*, 1934, 41: 190.
Cuenca-Estrella, M. et al, 'Comparison of the in vitro activity of voriconazole (UK-109,496), itraconazole and amphotericin B against clinical isolates of *Aspergillus* fumigatus, *J Antimicrob Chemother*, 1998, 42: 531–533.
Curtis, A. C. and Bocobo, F. C., 'North American blastomycosis', *J Chron Dis*, 1957, 5(4): 404.
Daniel, J., 'Depilatory action of X-rays', *Medical Records*, 1896, 49: 595–596.
Darling, S. T., 'A protozoan general infection producing pseudotuberculosis in the lungs and focal necrosis in the liver, spleen, and lymph nodes', *JAMA*, 1906, 46: 1283–1285.
Davies, R. R. and Everall, J. D., 'Mycological and clinical evaluation of griseofulvin for chronic onychomycosis', *BMJ*, 1967, ii: 464–468.
Davis, R. H. and Perkins, D. D., 'Neurospora: A model of model microbes', *Nature Reviews Genetics*, 2002, 3: 397–403.
De Kruif, P., 'A working cure for athlete's foot', *Reader's Digest*, 1942, 40: 46–48.
de Wit, S. et al, 'Comparision of fluconazole and ketoconazole for oropharyngeal candidiasis in AIDS', *Lancet*, 1989, i: 746–748.
Degregorio, M. et al, 'Fungal infections in patients with acute leukemia', *Am J Med*, 1982, 73: 543–548.
Delepine, S., 'A case of melanomycosis of the skin', *Transactions of the Pathological Society of London*, 1891, 58: 131.
Denning, D., 'Early diagnosis of invasive aspergillosis', *Lancet*, 2000, i: 423.
Denning, D. W., 'Echinocandin antifungal drugs', *Lancet*, 2003, 362: 1142–1151.
Denning, D. W., 'Invasive aspergillosis: The state of the art', *Clin Infect Dis*, 1998, 26: 781–803, 786.
Denning, D. W., 'Therapeutic outcome of invasive aspergillosis', *Clin Infect Dis*, 1996, 23: 607–615.
Denning, D. W. and Stevens, D. A., 'Antifungal and surgical treatment of invasive aspergillosis: Review of 2, 121 published cases', *Rev Infect Dis*, 1990, 12: 1147–1201.
Denning, D. W. et al, 'Efficacy and safety of voriconazole in the treatment of acute invasive aspergillosis', *Clin Infect Dis*, 2002, 34(5): 563–571.
Denning, D. W. et al, 'The link between fungi and severe asthma: A summary of the evidence', *Europ Respir J*, 2006, 27: 615–626.
Denning, D. W. et al, 'Treatment of invasive aspergillosis with itraconazole', *Am J Med*, 1989, 86: 791–800.
Denning, D. W. et al, *Report on a European Science Foundation Workshop on Invasive* Aspergillosis, 21–28 October 1998. http://www.aspergillus.org.uk. Accessed 4 December 2011.
Derbes, B. and Krafchuk, J. D., 'Response of North American blastomycosis to amphotericin', *Bulletin of the Tulane University Medical Faculty*, 1958, 17(3): 157–163.

Deresinski, S. C. et al, 'Soluble antigens of mycelia and spherules in the *in vitro* detection of immunity to coccidioides immitis', *Infection and Immunity*, 1977, 10(4): 700–704.
Dickson, E. C., 'Coccidioidomycosis', *JAMA*, 1938, 111: 1362–1364.
Dickson, E. C., 'Valley Fever', *California and Western Medicine,* 1937, 47: 151–155.
Diener, U. L. et al, 'Toxin-producing *Aspergillus* isolated from domestic peanuts', *Science*, 1963, 142: 1491–1492.
Dieulafoy, G. et al, 'Une pseudo-tuberculose mycosique', *Gazette Hospital de Paris*, 1890, 63: 821.
Dillaha, C. J. and Jansen, G., 'Dosage requirements of griseofulvin in onychomycosis due to *Trichophyton rubrum*. Preliminary Report', *Arch Dermatol*, 1960, 81: 790–796.
Dismukes, W. E., 'Antifungal Therapy: Lessons Learned over the Past 27 Years', *Clin Infect Dis*, 2006, 42: 1289–1330.
Dismukes, W. E. et al, 'A randomized double-blind trial of nystatin therapy for the candidiasis hypersensitivity syndrome', *N Engl J Med*, 1990, 323: 1717–1723.
Dismukes, W. E. et al, 'Criteria for evaluation of therapeutic response to antifungal drugs', *Rev Infect Dis*, 1980, 2(4): 535–545.
Dolan, B., 'Conservative politicians, radical philosophers and the aerial remedy for the diseases of civilization', *History of the Human Sciences*, 2002, 15: 35–54.
Donald, I., Aetiology and Investigation of Vaginal Discharge', *BMJ*, 1952, ii: 1223–1226.
Dore, E. S., 'The present position of the X-ray treatment of ringworm', *Lancet*, 1911, i: 432.
Dorman, S. E. and Chaisson, R. E., 'From magic bullets back to the magic mountain: The rise of extensively drug-resistant tuberculosis', *Nature Medicine*, 2007, 3: 295–298.
Dowling, H. F., 'The emergence of the cooperative clinical trial', *Transactions and Studies of the College of Physicians of Philadelphia*, 1975, 43: 20–29.
Downing, D. and Davies, S., ' "Allergy: Conventional and Alternative Concepts": A critique of the royal college of physicians of London's report', *Journal of Nutritional Medicine*, 1992, 3: 331–349.
Downing, J. G. and Conant, N. F., 'Medical progress: Mycotic infections', *N Engl J Med*, 1945, 233: 153–161 and 181–198.
Dubos, R., 'The diseases of civilization', *Milbank Memorial Fund Quarterly*, 1969, 47(3): 327–339.
Duerden, B., 'Obituary, Dame Rosalinde Hurley', *BMJ,* 2004, ii: 516.
Duerden, B., 'Obituary: Rosalinde Hurley', *BMJ*, 2004, 329: 516.
Dulaney, E. L., 'Penicillin production by the *Aspergillus* nidulans group', *Mycologia*, 1947, 39: 582–586.
Duncan, J. T., 'Survey of fungous diseases in Great Britain: Results from the first eighteenth months', *BMJ*, 1945, ii: 716.
Duncan, J. T., 'The epidemiology of fungus diseases', *Transactions of the Royal Society of Tropical Medicine and Hygiene*, 1948, 42: 207–216, 209.
Dutcher, J. D., 'The discovery and development of Amphotericin B', *Chest*, 1968, 54: 296–298.
Eddowes, A., 'Treatment of ringworm', *BMJ*, 1893, i: 785–786.
Editorial, 'A danger of the newer antibiotics', *BMJ*, 1951, i: 1196.

Editorial, 'Aflatoxin', *Lancet*, 1964, i: 1090.
Editorial, 'Antibiotic therapy and fungous infections', *N Engl J Med*, 1952, 247: 491–492.
Editorial, 'Antibiotics and monilial infection', *Lancet*, ii: 532.
Editorial, 'Fungus infection complicating antibiotic therapy', *JAMA*, 1952, 149: 762–763.
Editorial, 'Molecules and mental health', *BMJ*, 1975, i: 296.
Editorial, 'Thallium: A dangerous drug', *N Engl J Med*, 1931, 204: 1117.
Editorial, 'The parasites of ringworm', *Lancet*, 1893, i: 1204.
Editorial, 'Thrush', *JAMA*, 1927, 89: 1429–1430.
Editorial, 'Toxic product in groundnuts', *BMJ*, 1962, i: 309.
Editorial, 'Vaginal discharge', *Lancet*, 1940, ii: 300.
Edman, J. C. et al, 'Ribosomal RNA sequence shows *Pneumocystis carinii* to Be a Member of the Fungi', *Nature*, 1988, 334: 519–522.
Edwards, J. E., 'Systemic symptoms from *Candida* in the gut: Real or Imaginary?', *Bull N Y Acad Med*, 1988, 64(6): 544–549.
Eisenberg, D. M. et al, 'Trends in alternative medicine use in the United States, 1990–1997: Results of a follow-up national survey', *JAMA*, 1998, 280: 1569–1575.
Elewski, B. et al, 'Long-term outcome of patients with interdigital tinea pedis treated with terbinafine or clotrimazole', *J Amer Acad Dermatol*, 1995, 32(2–1): 290–292.
Emanuel, D. A. et al, 'Farmer's lung: Clinical, pathologic and immunologic study of twenty-four patients', *Am J Med*, 1961, 37: 392–401.
Emmons, C. W., 'Dermatophytes: Natural grouping based on the form of the spores and accessory organs', *Arch Derm Syphilol*, 1934, 30: 337–362.
Emmons, C. W., 'Mycology and medicine', *Mycologia*, 1961, 53: 1.
Emmons, C. W., 'The Jekyll-Hydes of mycology', *Mycologia*, 1960, 52: 669–680, 671.
English, M. P., 'Some controversial aspects of tinea pedis', *Br J Dermatol*, 1962, 74: 50–56.
English, M. P., 'William Tilbury fox and dermatological mycology', *Br J Dermatol*, 1977, 97: 100–112.
English, M., '*Trichophyton rubrum* infection in families', *BMJ*, 1957, i: 746 and 755.
Enoch, D. A., 'Invasive fungal infections: A review of epidemiology and management options', *J Med Microbio*, 2006, 55: 809–818.
Epstein, A., 'Burkitt, Denis Parsons (1911–1993)', *Oxford Dictionary of National Biography*, Oxford University Press, 2004 [http://www.oxforddnb.com/view/article/57333, accessed 15 August 2011].
Epstein, S. S., 'Environmental determinants of human cancer', *Cancer Res*, 1974, 34: 2425–2435.
Espinel-Ingroff, A 'History of medical mycology in the United States', *Clinical Microbiology Reviews*, 1996, 9(2): 235–272.
Falls, A. I., 'Doing business as falls chemical Co. v. Scholl Mfg. Co., Inc. case to protect Solvex', *The Trade-Mark Reporter*, 27 Trademark Rep., 1937, 444.
Fawcitt, R., 'Fungoid conditions of the lungs – Part I and Part II', *Br J Radiol*, 1936, 9: 172–195 and 354–378.
Fiese, M. J., *Coccidioidomycosis*, Springfield, IL, Charles C. Thomas, 1958.

Finland, M. and Weinstein, L., 'Complications induced by antimicrobial agents', *N Engl J Med*, 1953, 248, 220–246.

Finlay, S., 'An illness doctors don't recognise', *Observer*, 1 June 1986, 43.

Finlay, S., 'Voice for sufferers', *Observer*, 2 August 1987, 39.

Fisher-Hoch, S. P. and Hutwanger, L., 'Opportunistic candidiasis: An epidemic of the 1980s', *Infect Dis*, 1995, 21(4): 897–904.

Forgan-Smith, R. and Darrell, J. H., 'Amphotericin pharmacophobia and renal toxicity', *BMJ*, 1974, i: 244.

Foweraker, J., 'Recent advances in the microbiology of respiratory tract infection in cystic fibrosis', *British Medical Bulletin*, 2009, 9: 93–110.

Frain Bell, W. and Stevenson, J. C., 'Report on a clinical trial', *Transactions of the St John's Dermatological Society*, 1960, 45: 47–53.

Fraser, P. K., 'Tinea of the foot', *BMJ*, 1938, i: 842–844.

Fraumeni, F. J. and Miller, R. W., 'Epidemiology of human leukaemia: recent observations', *Journal of the National Cancer Institute,* 1967, 38: 593–605.

Freund, L., 'Ein mit Röntgen-Strahlen behandelter Fall von Naevus pigmentosus piliferus', *Wiener Medizinische Wochenschrift*, 1897, 47: 428–434.

Freund, L., 'Nachtrag zu dem Artikel 'Ein mit Röntgen-Strahlen behandelter Fall von Naevus pigmentosus piliferus', *Wiener Medizinische Wochenschrift*, 1897, 47: 856–860.

Furcolow, M. L. et al, 'Blastomycosis: An important medical problem in the Central United States', *JAMA*, 1966, 198: 115–118.

Furcolow, M. L. et al, 'Serologic evidence of histoplasmosis in sanatoriums in the U.S.', *JAMA*, 1962, 180: 109–114.

Galgiani, J. N., 'Coccidioidomycosis: A regional disease of national importance: Rethinking approaches for control', *Ann Intern Med*, 1999, 130 (4 Part 1): 293–300.

Galgiani, J. N., 'Coccidioidomycosis: Changing perceptions and creating opportunities for its control', *Ann N Y Acad Sci*, 2007, 1111: 1–18.

Galgiani, J. N. et al, 'Infectious diseases society of America: Practice guideline for the treatment of coccidioidomycosis', *Clin Infect Dis*, 2000, 30: 658–661.

Gallis, H. A. et al, 'Fungal infection following renal transplantation', *Arch Intern Med*, 1975, 135: 1163–1172.

Garrod, L. P., 'The sensitivity of *Actinomyces* to antibiotics', *BMJ*, 1952, i: 263.

Gellene, D., Obituary, 'Dr Albert M Kligman', New York Times, 22 Febuary 2010.

Gentles, J. C., 'Experimental ringworm in guinea pigs: Oral treatment with griseofulvin', *Nature*, 1958, 182: 476–477.

Gentles, J. C., 'The treatment of ringworm with Griseofulvin', *Br J Dermatol*, 1959, 71: 427–433.

Gentles, J. C. and Holmes, J. G., 'Foot ringworm in coal-miners', *Br J Indust Med*, 1957, 14: 22–29.

Georg, L. K., 'Rhoda Benham, 1894–1957', *Arch Dermatol*, 1957, 76(3): 363–364.

Georg, L. K., '*Trichophyton tonsurans* ringworm: A new public health problem', *Public Health Rep* 1952, 67: 53–56.

Gerstl, B. et al, 'Pulmonary aspergillosis: Report of two cases', *Ann Intern Med*, 1948, 28: 662–665.

Ghannoum, M. W. and Kuhn, D. M., 'Voriconazole: Better chances for patients with invasive mycoses', *Eur J Med Res*, 2002, 7(5): 242–256.

Gieryn, T. F. and Hirsh, R. F., 'Marginality and innovation in science', Social studies of science, 1983, 13(1): 87–106 and responses', *Soc Stud Sci*, 1984, 14(4): 612–614.

Gilchrest, B. A. and Leyden, J. L., 'In memoriam: Mites and the mighty: The last work and lasting legacy of Albert M Kligman, PhD, MD', *J Invest Dermatol*, 2011, 131: 6–7.

Gilchrist, T. C. and Stokes, R. W., 'A case of pseudolupus vulgaris caused by Blastomyces', *J Exp Med,* 1898, 3: 53.

Gilligan, P. H., 'Microbiology of airway disease in patients with cystic fibrosis', *Clinical Microbiology Reviews*, 1991, 4(10): 35–51.

Gilman, R. T., 'The incidence of ringworm of the feet in a university group: Control and treatment', *JAMA*, 1933, 100: 716.

Gimble, A. I. et al, 'Nystatin and tetracycline in the treatment of bacterial infections', *Antibiot Annu*, 1955–1956, 3: 676–680.

Gordon Taylor, G., 'Sir William Fergusson, FRCS, FRS', *Medical History*, 1961, 5: 1–14.

Gottlieb, H. S. et al, 'Pneumocystitis carinii pneumonia and mucosal candidiasis in previously healthy homosexual men: Evidence of a new acquired cellular immunodeficiency', *N Engl J Med* 1981; 305: 1425–1431.

Gould, J. E., 'Ringworm of the feet', *JAMA*, 1931, 96: 1300–1302.

Graybill, J. R., 'Lipid formulations of Amphotericin B: Does the emperor need new clothes?', *Annals of Internal Medicine*, 1996, 124: 921–923.

Greenberger, P. A., 'Allergic bronchopulmonary aspergillosis', *J Allerg Clin Immun*, 1982, 74: 645–652.

Greer, A. E., 'The synergism between mycotic and tuberculous infections of the lungs', *Diseases of the Chest* 1948, 14: 33–40.

Groll, A. H. et al, 'Trends in the post-mortem epidemiology of invasive fungal infections at a university hospital', *J Infection*, 1996, 33: 23–32, 25.

Gruhn, J. G. and Sansom, J., 'Mycotic infection of leukemia patients at autopsy', *Cancer*, 1963, 16: 61–73.

Haas, A et al, 'The "Yeast Connection" meets chronic mucocutaneous candidiasis', *N Engl J Med*, 1986, 314: 854–855.

Hadley, R. M., 'The life and works of Sir William James Erasmus Wilson, 1809–1884', *Medical History*, 1959, 3: 215–247.

Hagen, J. B., 'Five Kingdoms, more or less: Robert Whittaker and the broad classification of organisms', *Bioscience*, 2012, 62(1): 67–74.

Hamilton, D. and Lamb, M., 'Surgeons and surgery', in O. Checkland and M. Lamb, eds, *Health Care as Social History*, Aberdeen, Aberdeen University Press, 74–80.

Hanlon, P. and Carlisle, S., 'Do we face a third revolution in human history? If so, how will public health respond?' *J of Publ Health*, 2008, 30(4): 355–361.

Harkness, A. H., 'Non-gonococcal urethritis', *Br J Vener Dis*, 1933, 3: 173–186 and 187–191.

Harris, H. J., 'Aureomycin and cloramphenicol in Brucellosis: With special reference to side effects', *JAMA*, 1950, 142: 161–165.

Hartley, F., 'Parachlorphenyl-a-glycerol as an antibacterial and antifungal agent of pharmaceutical interest', *Quarterly Journal of Pharmacy and Pharmacology*, 1947, 20: 388–395.

Hawksworth, D. L., 'Geoffrey Clough Ainsworth (1905–1998): Mycological scholar, campaigner, and visionary', *Mycological Research,* 2000, 104(1): 110–116.
Hay, R. J., 'A comparative double blind study of ketoconazole and griseofulvin in dermatophytosis', *Br J Dermatol,* 1985, 112: 691–696.
Hay, R. J., 'Fluconazole', *J Infect,* 1990, 21: 1–6.
Hay, R. J., 'The azole antifungals', *J Antimicrob Chemother,* 1987, 20: 1–5.
Hay, R. J., 'The first international symposium on Itraconazole', *Rev Infect Dis,* 1987, 9: S1–152.
Hazen, E. L. and Brown, R., 'Fungicidin, an antibiotic produced by a soil Actinomycete', *Exp Biol Med,* 1951, 76: 93–97.
Hazen, E. L. and Brown, R., 'Nystatin', *Ann N Y Acad Sci,* 1960, 27(89): 258–266.
Hazen, E. L. and Brown, R., 'Two antifungal agents produced by a soil actinomycete', *Science,* 1950, 112: 423.
Hempelman, L. H. et al, 'Neoplasms in persons treated with x-rays in infancy: Fourth survey in 20 years', *J Natl Cancer Inst,* 1975, 55: 519–530.
Henrici, A. T., 'Characteristics of fungous diseases', *J Bacteriol,* 1940, 39: 113–138.
Hesseltine, H. C., 'Diabetic and myctoic vulvovaginitis: Preliminary Report', *JAMA,* 1933, 100(3): 177–178.
Hewitt, G., 'Lectures on the diagnosis and treatment of diseases of women', *BMJ,* 1862, i: 54.
Higgins, I. T. T., 'The epidemiology of chronic respiratory disease', *Preventive Medicine,* 1973, 2(1): 14–33.
Higginson, J., 'Epidemiology of cancer', *Proc R Soc Med,* 1968, 61: 724.
Higginson, J., 'The geographic pathology of primary liver cancer', *Cancer Research,* 1963, 23: 1624–1633.
Higham Cooper, R., 'The Supposed risks attending x-ray treatment of ringworm', *BMJ,* 1909, ii: 454–457.
Hillier, T., 'On ringworm and vegetable parasites', *BMJ,* 1861, ii: 552 and 577.
Hinson, K. W. F. et al, 'Broncho-pulmonary aspergillosis: A review and a report of eight new cases', *Thorax,* 1952, 7: 317–333.
Hirschmann, J. V., 'The early history of coccidioidomycosis: 1892–1945', *Clin Infect Dis,* 2007, 44: 1202–1207.
Hirst, H. L. et al, 'Methods of administration of penicillin', *J Lab Clin Med,* 1947, 32: 32.
Hirst, J. D., 'Public health and the public elementary schools, 1870–1907', *History of Education,* 1991, 20: 107–118.
Hischmann, J., 'The early history of coccidioidomycosis: 1892–1945', *Clinical Infectious Diseases,* 2007, 44(9): 1202–1207.
Hitchcock, C. A. et al, 'UK-109,496. 'A novel wide-spectrum triazole derivative for the treatment of fungal infections: Antifungal activity and selectivity in vitro', in *Proceedings and Abstracts of the 35th Intersciences Conference on Antimicrobial Agents and Chemotherapy,* Washington DC: American Society for Microbiology, 1995: 125.
Hodgson, G. A., 'The history of coal miners' skin diseases', in Cule, J. ed, *Wales and Medicine: An Historical Survey from Papers Given at the Ninth British Congress on the History of Medicine,* London: British Society for the History of Medicine, 1975, 59.
Hogg, J., 'The vegetable parasites of the human Skin', *BMJ,* 1859, i: 241.

Holmes, J. G. and Gentles, J. C., 'Diagnosis of foot ringworm', *Lancet*, 1956, ii: 62–63.

Homei, A., 'Specialization and medical mycology in the US, Britain and Japan', *Stud Hist Philos Biol Biomed*, 2008, 39(1): 80–92.

Howard, R. J. et al, 'Fungal infections in renal transplant recipients', *Ann Surg*, 1978, 188: 598–605.

Huppert, M. D. et al, 'Pathogenesis of *C. albicans* infection following antibiotic therapy, I: The effect of antibiotics on the growth of *C. albicans*', *J Bacteriol*, 1953, 65: 171–176.

Hurley R., and de Louvois, J., '*Candida* vaginitis', *Postgrad Med J*, 1979, 55: 645–647.

Hurley, R. and Morris, E. D., 'The pathogenicity of Candida species in the human vagina', *Br J Obstet Gyneacol*, 1964, 71(5): 692–695.

Hurley, R., 'Candidal vaginitis', *Proc R Soc Med*, 1977, 70(Suppl 4): 1–2.

Hurley, R., 'General discussion', *Proc R Soc Med*, 1977, 70(Suppl 4): 30.

Hutt, M. S. R. and Burkitt, D., 'Geographical distribution of cancer in East Africa: A new clinicopathological approach', *BMJ*, 1965, ii: 719–722.

Hyams, K., 'Developing case definitions for symptom-based conditions: The problem of specificity', *Epidemiologic Reviews*, 1998, 20(2): 148–156.

Ikemoto, H. B., 'Treatment of pulmonary aspergilloma with amphotericin B', *Arch Intern Med*, 1965, 115: 598–601.

Infectious Diseases and Immunization Committee of the Canadian Paediatric Society, 'Candidiasis: current misconceptions', *Can Med Assoc J*, 1988, 139: 729.

Jacyna, S., 'Pious pathology: J. L. Alibert's iconography of disease', in Hannaway, C and La Berge, A., eds, *Constructing Paris Medicine*, London, Clio Medica/The Wellcome Series in the History of Medicine, 185–219.

Jawetz, E., 'Infectious diseases: Problems of antimicrobial therapy', *Ann Rev Med*, 1954, 5: 1–26.

Jawetz, E., 'The rational use of antimicrobial agents: Reason versus emotion in chemotherapy', *Oral Surg Oral Med Oral Pathol*, 8(9): 982–987.

Jewkes, J. et al, 'Pulmonary aspergilloma: analysis of prognosis in relation to haemoptysis and survey of treatment', *Thorax*, 1983, 38: 572–578.

Jibson, R. W. et al, 'An outbreak of coccidioidomycosis (Valley Fever) caused by landslides triggered by the 1994 Northridge, California Earthquake', in Welby, C. W., and Gowan, M. E., *A Paradox of Power: Voices of Warning and Reason in the Geosciences*: Geological Society of America, Reviews in Engineering Geology, 1998, 53–61.

Jillson, O. F., 'Mycology', *N Engl J Med*, 1953, 249: 523–530 and 561–566.

Joekes, T. H. and Simpson, R. H., 'Bronchomoniliais', *Lancet*, 1923, ii: 108–111.

Joffe, B., 'An epidemic of coccidioidomycosis probably related to soil', *N Engl J Med*, 1960, 262: 720–722.

Johnson, N. P. A. S. and Mueller, J., 'Updating the accounts: Global mortality of the 1918–1920 "Spanish" Influenza Pandemic', *Bull Hist Med*, 2002, 76(1): 105–115.

Johnson, R. H. et al, 'The great coccidioidomycosis epidemic: Clinical features', in Einstein, H. E., and Catanzaro, A., eds, *Coccidioidomycosis: Proceedings of the 5th International Conference*, Washington, National Foundation for Infectious Diseases, 1996: 77–87.

Kane, R. L., 'Iatrogenesis: Just what the doctor ordered', *Journal of Community Health*, 1980, 5(3): 149–158.

Kay, A. B., 'Alternative allergy and the general medical council', *BMJ*, 1993, i: 122–124, 328–31 and 582.

Kirkland, T. N., and Fierer, J., 'Coccidioidomycosis: a reemerging infectious disease', *Emerg Infect Dis,* 1996, 2(3): 192–199.

Klein, R. S. et al, 'Oral candidiasis in high-risk patients as the initial manifestation of the acquired immunodeficiency syndrome', *N Engl J Med*, 1984, 311: 354–358.

Kligman, A. M., 'The pathogenesis of tinea capitis due to *Microsporum audouini* and *Microsporum canis*', *J Invest Dermatol*, 1952, 18: 231–246.

Kligman, A. M. and Anderson, W. W., 'Evaluation of current methods for the local treatment of tinea capitis', *J Invest Dermatol*, 1951, 16: 155–168.

Kligman, A. M., 'Are fungus infections increasing as a result of antibiotic therapy', *JAMA*, 1952, 149: 979–983.

Knowles, R. B., 'Factors Influencing dermatitis in coal-miners', *BMJ*, 1944, ii: 430–432.

Koerth, C. J. et al, 'Fungus disease of the lung', *Texas State Journal of Medicine*, 1942, 38: 1–58.

Kohn, H., 'Ein fall von pneumonomycosis aspergillina', *Deutsche Medicinische Wochenschrift*, 1893, 50: 1332–1333.

Korobkin, M. and Williams, E. H., 'Hepatoma and groundnuts in the West Nile district of Uganda, *Yale J Biol Med*, 1968, 41(1): 69–78.

Kozinn, P. J. et al, 'Candida albicans: Saprophyte or pathogen? A diagnostic guideline', *JAMA*, 1966, 198(2): 170–172.

Kwon-Chung, K. J. and Campbell, C. C., 'Chester Wilson Emmons', *Medical Mycology*, 1986, 24(1) 89–90.

Lambert, D. R. et al, 'Griseofulvin and ketoconazole in the treatment of dermatophyte infections', *Int J Dermatol,* 1989, 28: 300–304.

Lane, S. L., 'A review of current opinion on the hazards of indiscriminate antibiotic therapy in dental practice', *Oral Surg Oral Med Oral Pathol*, 1956, 9: 952–961.

Lang W. R. et al, 'Nystatin vaginal tablets in the treatment of *Candida*l vulvovaginitis', *Obstet Gynecol*, 1956, 8: 364–367.

Lapham, M. E., 'Aspergillosis of the lungs and its association with tuberculosis', *JAMA*, 1926, 87(13): 1031–1033.

Laufer, P. et al, 'Allergic bronchopulmonary aspergillosis in cystic fibrosis', *J Allergy Clin Immunol*, 1984, 73: 44–48.

Lawrence, C., ' "Incommunicable Knowledge": Science, technology and the clinical "Art" in Britain, 1850–1910', *Journal of Contemporary History*, 1985, 20: 503–520.

Lederberg, J., 'Infectious history', *Science*, 2000, 288: 287–293.

Legge, R. T. et al, 'Incidence of foot ringworm amongst college students: Its relation to gymnasium hygiene', *JAMA*, 1929, 93: 170.

Legge, R. T. et al, 'Ringworm of the foot: Preliminary Report', *JAMA*, 1929, 92: 1507–1508.

Levine, H. B., 'Miconazole in coccidioidomycosis', *Proc R Soc Med*, 1977, 70(Suppl 1): 13–17.

Lewis, D. R. and Lloyd, A. W., 'Treatment of ringworm of the scalp with thallium acetate', *BMJ*, 1933, ii: 99–100.

Li, J. W.-H. and Vederas, J. C., 'Drug discovery and natural products: End of an era or an endless frontier?' *Science*, 2009, 325: 161–165.

Lindemann, E., 'Importing AIDS drugs: Food and drug administration policy and its limitations', *George Washington Journal of International Law and Economics*, 1994, 28: 133–170.

Linker, B., 'Resuscitating the "Great Doctor": The career of biography in medical history', in Söderqvist, T., ed, *Poetics of Biography in Science, Technology, and Medicine*, Aldershot, Ashgate Press, 2007, 221–239.

LiPuma, J. J., 'The changing microbial epidemiology of cystic fibrosis', *Clin Microbiol Rev*, 2010, 23: 299–323.

Liston, G. and Cruickshank, L. G., 'Leucorrhoea in pregnancy: A study of 200 cases', *Brit J Obstet Gynaecol*, 1940, 47: 109–129.

Liston, G. and Cruickshank, L. G., 'On thrush, with special reference to vaginal thrush', *Edin Med J*, 1940, 47: 369–390.

Littman B. et al, 'Coccidioidomycosis and its treatment with amphotericin B', *Am J Med*, 1958, 24(4): 568–592.

Liveing, R., 'Lecture on the peculiarities of ringworm and its treatment', *Lancet*, 1879, ii: 642–644, on 643–644.

Loh, W. P. and Baker, E. E., 'Fecal flora of man after oral administration of chlortetracycline or oxytetracycline', *Arch Intern Med*, 1955, 95(1): 74–82.

Ludlam, G. B. and Henderson, J. L., 'Neonatal thrush in a maternity hospital', *Lancet*, 1942, i: 64–70.

M'Call Anderson, T., 'Introductory lectures to the study of the diseases of the skin', *Lancet*, 1870, i: 149–151.

MacCormac, H., 'Ringworm of the foot', *BMJ*, 1940, i: 739–741.

MacCormac, H., 'Skin-diseases under war conditions', *Brit J Dermatol*, 1917, 29: 113–131.

Macfarlane, J. T. and Worboys, M., 'The changing management of acute bronchitis in Britain, 1940–1970: The impact of antibiotics', *Medical History*, 2008, 52: 47–72.

MacKenna, R. M. B. et al, 'Dermatological practice in war-time', in *Medicine and Pathology: History of the Second World War*, London, Her Majesty's Stationery Office, 1952.

Maclennan, J. G., '*Candida* and "20th-century disease" ', *Can Med Assoc J*, 1986, 134: 1112–1113.

MacLeod, J. H. M., 'The treatment of ringworm of the scalp by X-rays', *BMJ*, 1905, ii: 13–15.

Maertens, J. A., 'History of the development of azole derivatives', *Clin Microbiol Infect*, 2004, 10, Suppl 1: 1–10.

Maertens, J. A., 'History of the development of azole derivatives', *Clin Microbiol Infect*, 2004, 10 Suppl 1: 3–4.

Maggon, K. K. et al, 'Biosynthesis of aflatoxins', *Bacteriol Rev*, 1977, 41: 822–855.

Maibach, H. I. and Klgman, A. M., Short-term treatment of onychomycosis with griseofulvin', *Arch Dermatol*, 1960, 81: 733–734.

Majima, A., 'The invention of "athlete's foot": Lifestyle, cleanliness, and american leisure classes in the early twentieth century', *Seikatsugaku ronsō*, 2010, 17: 3–13.

Malo, J. L. et al, 'Studies in chronic pulmonary aspergillosis', *Thorax*, 1977, 32: 254–261.

Markel, H., ' "The Eyes Have It": Trachoma, the perception of disease, the United States public health service, and the American Jewish immigration experience, 1897–1924', *Bull Hist Med*, 2000, 74: 525–560.

Martin, D. S. and Jones, C. P., 'Further studies on the practical classification of the Monilias', *J Bacteriol*, 1940, 39: 609–630.

Martin, D. S. et al, 'A practical classification of the Monilias', *J Bacteriol,* 1937, 34: 99–129.

Martin, G. W., 'Are fungi plants?', *Mycologia*, 1955, 47(6): 779–792.

Martin, M. V., 'Comparison of voriconazole (UK-109,496) and itraconazole in prevention and treatment of *Aspergillus* fumigatus endocarditis in guinea pigs', *Antimicrob Agent Chemother*, 1997, 41: 13–16.

McCarthy, G. M., 'Host factors associated with HIV-related oral candidiasis: A review', *Oral Surg Oral Med Oral Pathol*, 1992, 73: 181–186.

McGovern, J. J. et al, 'The effect of aureomycin and chloramphenicol on the fungal and bacterial flora of children', *N Engl J Med*, 1953, 248(10): 397–403.

McKee, G. M. et al, 'Treatment of tinea capitis with Roentgen rays', *Arch Derm Syphilol,* 1946, 53: 458–470.

McKeown, T. and Record, R. G., 'Reasons for the decline of mortality in England and Wales during the nineteenth century', *Population Studies*, 1964, 16(2): 94–122.

McMahon, F. G., 'Drug combinations: A critique of proposed new federal regulations', *JAMA*, 1971, 216: 1008–1010.

McNeil, C., 'Death in the first month and the first year', *Lancet*, 1940, i: 819–821.

McNeill, M. et al, 'Mortality in the United States, 1980–1997, due to candidiasis, aspergillosis, and other mycoses in persons infected and persons not infected with HIV Trends in Mortality Due to Invasive Mycotic Diseases in the United States, 1980–1997', *Clin Infect Dis*, 2001, 33(5): 641–647.

Medical Research Council, 'Treatment of pulmonary tuberculosis with streptomycin and para-aminosalicylic acid', *BMJ* 1950, ii: 1073–1085.

Medical Research Council, 'Various combinations of isoniazid with streptomycin or with PAS in the treatment of pulmonary tuberculosis', *BMJ*, 1955, i: 1005–1014.

Meier, F. C. with field notes and material by Lindberg, C. A. 'Collecting microorganisms from the Arctic atmosphere, *Scientific Monthly*, 1935, 40: 5–20.

Meiklejohn, A., 'The development of compensation for occupational diseases of the lungs in Great Britain', *Br J Ind Med*, 1954, 11: 198–212.

Menzies, M. F., 'Hospital or domiciliary confinement?', *Lancet*, 1942, ii: 35–38 and 201.

Mettam, A. E., 'Aspergillosis – Aspergillar mycosis', *Trans R Acad Med Irel*, 1911, 29: 484–494.

Meyer, R. et al, 'Aspergillosis complicating neoplastic disease', *Am J Med*, 1973, 54: 6–15.

Mildenhall, R., '*Candida* views', *Observer*, 26 June 1988, 37.

Miller, F. G., 'Poisoning by phenol', *Can Med Assoc J*, 1942, 46(6): 615–616.
Miller, J. L. et al, 'Local treatment of tinea capitis', *JAMA*, 1946, 132: 67–70.
Mirsky, H. S. and Cuttner, J., 'Fungal infection in acute leukemia', *Cancer*, 1972, 30: 348–352.
Mitchell, J. H., 'Ringworm of the hands and feet: An historical review', *JAMA*, 1951, 146(6): 541–546.
Modan, B. et al, 'Thyroid neoplasms in a population irradiated for scalp tinea in childhood', in De Groot, ed, *Radiation Associated Thyroid Carcinoma*, New York, Grune & Stratton Inc, 1977, 449–459.
Monod, O. et al, 'New form of pulmonary aspergillosis: aspergilloma causing bronchiectasis', *Bull Acad Natl Med*, 1951, 135(29–30): 508–511.
Montgomery, B. J., 'Belgian oral antifungal agent looks promising', *JAMA*, 1980, 243(1): 12.
Morgan, P. P., 'Should scientists study "20th-century disease"?', *Can Med Assoc J*, 1985, 133: 961–962.
Morgan, W. J., ' "The Miners" Welfare Fund in Britain 1920–1952', *Social Policy & Administration*, 1990, 24: 199–211.
Morris, M., 'Ringworm in elementary schools', *Lancet*, 1891, ii: 348.
Morris, M., 'The Harveian lecture on some new therapeutic methods in dermatology', *BMJ*, 1905, i: 699.
Morrow, M. B. et al, 'Mold fungi in the etiology of respiratory allergic diseases, I: A survey of air-borne molds', *J Allergy*, 1942, 13: 215–226 and 231–247.
Mroueh S. and Spock, A., 'Allergic bronchopulmonary aspergillosis in patients with cystic fibrosis', *Chest*, 1994, 105(1): 32–36.
Mumby, K., 'Science or flat earthers? The clinical ecologist replies', *BMJ*, 1993,ii: 1055–1056.
Nailor, M. D. and Sobel, J. D., 'Progress in antifungal therapy: Echinocandins versus azoles', *Drug Discovery Today: Therapeutic Strategies*, 2006, 3(2): 221–226.
Natale, S., 'The invisible made visible: X-rays as Attraction and Visual Medium at the End of the Nineteenth Century', *Media History*, 2011, 17(4): 345–358.
Nelson, L. et al, 'Aspergillosis and atopy in cystic fibrosis', *Am Rev Respir Dis*, 1979, 120: 863.
Neushul, P., 'Science, government and the mass production of penicillin', *J Hist Med Allied Sci*, 1993, 48(4): 371–395.
Newcomer, V. D. et al, 'Current status of amphotericin B in the treatment of the systemic fungus infections', *J Chron Dis*, 1959, 9: 354–374.
Newcomer, V. D. et al, 'The treatment of systemic fungus infections with amphotericin B', *Ann N Y Acad Sci*, 1960, 89: 221–239.
Nickerson, W. J., 'Medical mycology', *Ann Rev of Microbiol*, 1953, 7: 245–272.
Nickerson, J. W. et al, 'Sandals and hygiene and infections of the feet', *Arch Derm Syphilol*, 1945, 52: 365–368.
Novey, H., 'Epidemiology of allergic bronchopulmonary aspergillosis', *Immunol Allergy Clin N Amer*, 1998, 18: 641–653.
Oblath R. W. et al, Pulmonary moniliasis', *Ann Intern Med*, 1951, 35: 97–116.
Odds, F. C., 'Coccidioidomycosis: Flying conidia and severed heads', *Mycologist*, 2003, 17: 37–40.
Odds, F. C., 'Epidemiological shifts in opportunistic and nosocomial *Candida* infections: mycological aspects', *Int J of Antimicrob Agents*, 1996, 6: 141–144.

Odds, F. C., 'Laboratory evaluation of antifungal agents: A comparative study of five imidazole derivatives of clinical importance', *J Antimicrob Chemother*, 1880, 6: 749–761.

Odds, F. C. et al, 'Antifungal effects of fluconazole (UK-49858), a new triazole antifungal, in vitro, *Antimicrob Agents Chemother*, 1986, 18: 473–478.

Ormsby, O. S. and Mitchell, J. H., 'Ringworm of the hands and feet', *JAMA*, 1916, 67: 711–717.

Oura, M. et al, 'A new antifungal antibiotic, Amphotericin B', *Antibiot Annu*, 1955–1956, 3: 566–573.

Oxford, A. E. et al, 'Griseofulvin, $C_{17}H_{17}O_6Cl$, a metabolic product of *Penicillium griseo-fulvum* Dierckx, *Biochem J*, 1939, 33: 240–248.

Pace, H. and Schantz, S., 'Nystatin (Mycostatin) in the treatment of Monilial and NonMonilial vaginitis', *JAMA*, 1956, 162: 268–271.

Paget, G. E., 'The experimental toxicology of griseofulvin', *Arch Dermatol*, 1960, 81: 750–757.

Paget, G. E. and Walpole, A. L., 'Some cytological effects of griseofulvin', *Nature*, 1958, 182: 1320–132.

Pamboukian, S., ' "Looking Radiant": Science, photography and the X-ray craze of 1896', *Victorian Review*, 2001, 27(2): 56–74.

Pappagianis, D., 'Epidemiology of coccidioidomycosis', *Current Topics in Medical Mycology*, 1988, 2: 199–238.

Pappagianis, D., 'Epidemiology of coccidioidomycosis', in McGinnis, M. R., ed, *Current Topics in Medical Mycology, Vol 2*, New York: Springer-Verlag, 1988: 199–238.

Pappagianis, D., 'Epidemiology of coccidioidomycosis', in Stevens, D. A., ed, *Coccidioidomycosis: A Text*, New York: Plenum Book Company, 1980, 63–81.

Pappagianis, D., 'Marked increase in cases of coccidioidomycosis in California: 1991, 1992, and 1993' *Clin Infect Dis*, 1994, 19, Supplement 1: S14–S18.

Pappagianis, D. and Einstein, H., 'Tempest from Tehachapi takes toll or coccidioides conveyed aloft and afar', *West J Med*, 1978, 129: 527–530.

Pappagianis, D. et al, Evaluation of the protective efficacy of the killed *Coccidioides immitis* spherule vaccine in humans', *Am Rev Respir Dis*, 1993, 148: 656–660.

Pappas, P. G., et al, 'Blastomycosis in immunocompromised patients', *Medicine*, 1993, 72: 311–325.

Park, D. L. and Stoloff, 'Aflatoxin control – How a regulatory agency managed risk from an unavoidable natural toxicant in food and feed', *Regulatory Toxicology and Pharmacology*, 1989, 9(2): 109–130.

Patterson, T. F. et al, 'Efficacy of fluconazole in experimental invasive aspergillosis', *Rev Infect Dis*, 1990, 12(Suppl): S281–S285.

Patterson, T. F. et al, 'Invasive aspergillosis: Disease spectrum, treatment practices, and outcomes', *Medicine*, 2000, 79(4): 250–260.

Pauling, L. et al, 'On the orthomolecular environment of the mind: Orthomolecular theory', *Am J Psychiat*, 1974, 131: 1251–1267.

Pauling, L., 'Orthomolecular psychiatry: Varying the concentrations of substances normally present in the human body may control mental disease', *Science*, 1968, 160: 265–271.

Payne, J. F., 'An address on bacteria in diseases of the skin', *Lancet*, 1896, ii: 2–3.

Pepys, J., 'Allergic broncho-pulmonary aspergillosis', *Clinical Allergy*, 1971, 1: 261–286.

Pepys, J. et al, 'Clinical and immunological significance of *Aspergillus fumigatus* in sputum', *Am Rev Resp Dis*, 1959, 80: 167–180.

Percival, G. H., 'The treatment of ringworm of the scalp with Thallium acetate', *Br J Dermatol*, 1930, 42(2): 59–69.

Pesle, G. D. and Monod, O., 'Bronchiectasis due to aspergilloma', *Chest*, 1954, 25(2): 172–183.

Peterkin, G. A. G., 'The diagnosis and treatment of tinea pedis', *Practitioner*, 1957, 180, 543–552.

Peto, R. and Beral, V., 'Doll, Sir (William) Richard Shaboe (1912–2005)', *Oxford Dictionary of National Biography*, Oxford University Press, January 2009, [http://www.oxforddnb.com/view/article/95920, accessed 23 May 2013].

Petrow, V. and Hartley, Sir Frank, 'The rise and fall of British drug houses, Ltd.', *Steroids*, 1996, 61: 476–482.

Pfaller, M. A., 'Nosocomial fungal infections: Epidemiology of candidiasis', *Journal of Hospital Infection*, 1995, 30 (Suppl): 329–338.

Phillips, B., 'The Phenol-Camphor treatment of dermatophytosis', *Br J Dermatol*, 1944, 56(11–12): 219–227.

Pickworth, K. H., 'Farmer's lung', *Lancet*, 1961, ii: 660.

Pignot, M. M., 'Souvenir sur Raimond Jacques Sabouraud 1864–1938', *Mycopathologia*, 1954, 7: 348–364.

Pillsbury, D. M., 'Griseofulvin therapy in dermatophytic infections', *Trans Am Clin Climat Assoc*, 1959, 71: 52–57.

Pillsbury, D. M. and Livingood, C. S., 'Experiences in military dermatology: Their interpretation in plans for improved general medical care', *Arch Derm Syphilol*, 1947, 55: 441–462.

Plass, E. D. et al, 'Monilia vulvovaginitis', *Am J Obstet Gynecol*, 1931, 21: 320.

Plumbe, S., 'History, pathology and treatment of ringworm and scald-head', *Lancet*, 1835, i: 926–928 and ii: 50–51.

Plumbe, S., 'Remarks on the contagious ring-worm of the scalp', *Lancet*, 1835, 858.

Podack, M., 'Zur Kenntniss der Aspergillusmykosen im menschlichen Respirationsapparat', *Virchow's Archiv*, 1895, 139(2): 260–281.

Porter, R., 'Diseases of civilization', in Bynum, W. F. and Porter, R., *Companion Encyclopaedia of the History of Medicine*, London, Routledge, 1993, 585–600.

Porter, R., 'The patient's view: Doing medical history from below', *Theory and Society*, 1985, 14: 175–198.

Power, D'A., 'Wilson, Sir (William James) Erasmus (1809–1884)', revised Geoffrey L Aserton *Oxford Dictionary of National Biography*, Oxford University Press, 2004. Accessed 15 August 2008, http://www.oxforddnb.com/view/article/29702.

Pranatharhti, H. and Molinari, J. A., 'Oral candidiasis: Forerunner of acquired immunodeficiency syndrome (AIDS)?', *Oral Surg Oral Med Oral Pathol*, 1985, 60: 532–534.

Presthus, R. V., 'British public administration: The national coal board', *Public Administration Review*, 1949, 9(3): 200–210.

Prior, J. R., 'X-ray treatment of ringworm', *Public Health*, 1910–1911, 24: 153–154.

Pusey, W. A., 'Roentgen-ray therapy twenty years ago, *JAMA*, 1923, 81(15): 1257–1260.

Quillen, J. H. et al, 'Blastomycosis in North Tennessee', *Chest*, 1998, 114(2): 436–443.

Quinn, J. P. et al, Ketoconazole and the yeast connection, *JAMA*, 1986, 255: 3250.

Quintal, D. and Jackson, R., 'The development of 20th century dermatologic drugs', *Clinics in Dermatology*, 1989, 7(3), 42–43.

Ramires, J., 'Pulmonary aspergilloma: Endobronchial treatment', *N Engl J Med*, 1964, 271: 1281–1285.

Raper, K. B., 'The development of improved penicillin producing molds', *Ann N Y Acad Sci*, 1946, 48: 41–56.

Reiss, F., ed, 'Medical mycology', *Ann N Y Acad Sci*, 1950, 50: 1209–1404.

Renfro, L. et al, 'Yeast connection among 100 patients with chronic fatigue', *Amer J Med*, 1989, 86: 165–168.

'Report of the lancet sanitary commission on the sanitary condition of our public schools', *Lancet*, 1875, i: 795–796, 859–861 and ii: 111–112, 314–315, 422–423, 574–575, 682, and 785–787.

Report, 'Athlete's foot', *Literary Digest*, 22 December 1928, 17.

Report, 'Bears investigate athlete's foot', *Los Angeles Times*, September 27, 1931, F5.

Report, 'Fixed combinations of antimicrobial agents: National academy of sciences – national research council division of medical sciences drug efficacy study, *N Engl J Med*, 1969, 280: 1149–1154.

Report, 'Fluconazole: A major advance for cryptococcal meningitis and other systemic fungal infections?" *AIDS Treatment News*, 1987, 41.

Report, 'Food and drug administration warns of phenol camphor mixture', *JAMA*, 1942, 119: 713.

Report, 'Griseofulvin and dermatomycoses: An international symposium sponsored by university of miami, October 26–27, 1959', *Arch Dermatol*, 1960, 51: 649–789.

Report, 'Histoplasmosis cooperative study. I. frequency of histoplasmosis among adult hospitalized males: Veterans administration cooperation study on histoplasmosis', *Amer Rev Resp Dis*, 1961, 84: 663–668.

Report, 'Mycostatin available for laboratories', *Journal of the Franklin Institute*, 1956, 261: 285.

Restrepo, A. et al, 'Introduction', *Rev Infect Dis*, 1980, 2(4): 519.

Reverby, S. M. and Rosner, D., ' "Beyond the great doctors" revisited: a generation of the "new" social history in medicine', in Huisman F. and Warner J. H., eds, *Locating Medical History: Stories and Their Meanings*, Baltimore, Johns Hopkins University Press, 2004, 167–193.

Richard, J. L., 'Discovery of aflatoxins and significant historical features', *Toxin Reviews*, 2008, 27: 171–201.

Richardson, K. et al, 'Discovery of fluconazole, a novel antifungal agent', *Clin Infect Dis*, 1990, 12: S267–71.

Richardson, K. et al, 'Discovery of fluconazole: A novel antifungal agent', *Rev Infect Dis*, 1990, 12: S267–71.

Richardson, M. D., 'Changing patterns and trends in systemic fungal infections', *J Antimicrob Chemother*, 2005, 56: S1, i5–i11.

Rippon, J. W., 'Forty four years of dermatophytes in a Chicago clinic (1944–1988)', *Mycopathologia, 1992,* 119: 25–28.

Rippon, J. W., 'Symposium on medical mycology', *Mycopathologia*, 1987, 99: 144.

Robbins, W. J., 'Bernard O Dodge, mycologist, plant pathologist', *Science*, 1960, 133: 741–2.
Roberts, L., 'The present position of the question of vegetable hair parasites', *BMJ*, ii: 1894, 685–688.
Robertson, M. H. et al, 'Oral therapy with ketoconazole for dermatophyte infections unresponsive to griseofulvin', *Rev Inf Dis*, 1980, 2(4): 578–581.
Rook, A., 'Dermatology in Britain in the late nineteenth century', *Br J Dermatol*, 1979, 100(1): 3–12.
Rook, A., 'James Stratin, Jonathan Hutchinson and the blackfriars skin hospital', *Br J Dermatol*, 1978, 99: 215–219.
Roper, J., 'Heart graft Briton dies', *Times*, 1 September 1969: 1a.
Rosenberg, C. E., 'Pathologies of progress: The idea of civilization as risk', *Bull Hist Med*, 1998, 72(4): 714–730.
Rosenberg, M. and Paterson, R., 'Allergic bronchopulmonary aspergillosis: An emerging disease', *J Chron Dis*, 1977, 30: 193–194.
Rosenthal, T., 'Perspectives in ringworm of the scalp: Treatment through the ages', *Archives of Dermatology, 1960,* 82(6): 851–856.
Rosenthal, T., 'Samuel Plumbe', *Arch Derm Syphilol*, 1937, 36(2): 348–354.
Rosenthal, T., 'Samuel Plumbe', *Arch Dermatol*, 2008, 16: 36–43.
Rosman, N., 'Infections with *Trichophyton rubrum*', *Br J Dermatol*, 1966, 78(4): 208–212.
Rothstein, N. E. et al, 'Risk factors for severe pulmonary and disseminated coccidioidomycosis: Kern county, California, 1995–1996', *Clin Infect Dis,* 2001, 32(5): 708–714.
Rovner, S., 'HEALTHTALK: The yeast theory', *Washington Post,* March 9, 1984: D5.
Rubin H et al, 'The course and prognosis of histoplasmosis, *Am Med J*, 1959, 27(2): 278–288.
Rudolph, E. D., 'Carroll William Dodge, 1895–1988', *Mycologia*, 1990, 82(2): 160–164.
Russell, B. et al, 'Chronic ringworm infection of the skin and nails treated with griseofulvin: Report of a therapeutic trial', *Lancet*, 1960, i: 1141–1147.
Russell, C. S., 'Leucorrhoea', *BMJ*, 1953, ii: 91–93.
Sabouraud, R., 'La Question des Teignes (Au Congress de Londres)' *Annales de dermatologie et syphiligraph,* 1896, 7: 1333–1357.
Sabouraud, R., 'X-ray Treatment of Tinea tonsurans', *International Clinics*, 1904, 2: 41–49.
Sabouraud, R. and Noiré, H., 'Traitement des teignes tondantes par les rayons X', *La Presse Mèdicale*, 1904, 12: 825–827.
Sabouraud, R. et al, 'La Radiotherapie die teignes a l'ecole Lallier en 1904', *Bulletin de la Société française de dermatologie et de syphiligraphie*, 1905, 16: 10.
Sáez-Gómez JM and Romero-Maroto, M., 'Scientific ideas on muguet (Thrush) in the XVIII century', *Journal of Dental Research*, 2010, 89: 571–574.
Sakewitz, A. B., 'Treatment of genitourinary moniliasis with orally administered nystatin', *Ann Intern Med*, 1955, 42(6): 1187–1189.
Salvin, S. B., 'Public health aspects of fungus infections', *Ann N Y Acad Sci,* 1950, 50: 1217.
Sanderson, P. H. and Sloper, J. C., 'Skin disease in the British Army in SE Asia', *Br J Dermatol*, 1953, 65: 252–264, 300–309 and 362–372.

Sanger, P. et al, '*Candida* infection as a complication of heart surgery: Review of the literature and report of two cases', *JAMA*, 1962, 181: 108.
Sargeant, K. et al, 'Toxicity associated with certain samples of groundnuts', *Nature*, 1961, 192: 1096–1097.
Saubolle, M. and Sutton, J., 'Coccidioidomycosis: Centennial year on the North American continent', *Clinical Microbiology Newsletter*, 1994, 16(18): 137–144.
Scales, I. K. et al, 'Oral fungus infection: Candidiasis albicans', *Oral Surg Oral Med Oral Pathol*, 1956, 9: 970–977.
Scambler, G. and Scambler, A., 'The illness iceberg and aspects of consulting behaviour', in Fitzpatrick, R., ed, *The Experience of Illness*, London, Tavistock, 1984, 35–37.
Schneider, E. et al, 'A coccidioidomycosis outbreak following the Northridge, California, Earthquake', *JAMA*, 1997, 277: 904–908.
Schwartz, H. J. et al, 'A comparison of the prevalence of sensitization to *Aspergillus* antigens among asthmatics in Cleveland and London', *J Allergy Clin Immunol* 1978, 62: 9–14.
Schwartz, L. et al, 'Control of the scalp amongst school children', *JAMA*, 1946, 132: 58–62.
Schwarz, J. and Baum, G. L., 'Histoplasmosis', 1962', *Arch Intern Med*, 1963, 111(6): 710–718.
Schwarz, J. and Baum, G. L., 'A critical review of medical mycology in the United States, 1946–1956', *Mycopatholgia et Mycologia Applicata*, 1957, 8: 271–326.
Seelig, M. S., 'The role of antibiotics in *Candida* infection', *Amer J Med*, 1966, 40: 887–917.
Seidelman, R. D. et al, '"Healing" the bodies and souls of immigrant children: The ringworm and Trachoma Institute, Sha'ar ha-Aliyah, 1952–1960', *Journal of Israeli History*, 2010, 29(2): 191–211.
Seligmann M. et al, 'AIDS – An immunologic reevaluation', *N Engl J Med*, 1984, 311: 1286–1292.
Semon, H. C., 'The non-venereal affections of the genitalia', *Br J Vener Dis*, 1929, 5: 114–127.
Sequeira, J. H., 'The varieties of ringworm and their treatment', *BMJ*, 1906ii: 193–196.
Sharman, A., 'The significance of leucorrhoea', *BMJ*, 1935, ii: 1199–1201.
Sharp, B. B., 'Vulvo-vaginitis', *Br J Vener Dis*, 1930, 6(4): 301–317.
Sharp, J. L., 'The growth of *Candida* ablicans during antibiotic therapy', *Lancet*, 1954, i: 390–392.
Shockman, J. and Urbach, F., 'Tinea Capitis in Philadelphia', *Internat J Dermatol*, 1983, 22(9): 522–523.
Shoemaker, J. V., 'Ringworm in public institutions', *Trans Am Med Assoc*, 1878, 29: 139–147.
Shrand, H., 'Thrush in the newborn', *BMJ*, 1961, ii: 1530–3, and 1962, i: 186 and 567.
Shrewsbury, J. D., 'The genus *Monilia*', *J Path Bact*, 1934, 38: 213–254.
Shurtleff, William and Akiko Aoyagi, 'History of Koji – Grans and/or Soybeans Enrobed with a Mold Culture (300 BCE to 2012)', 17 July 2012, http://www.soyinfocenter.com/books/154, accessed 3 May 2013.
Sichel, G., 'The X-ray treatment of ringworm', *BMJ*, 1906, i: 256–257.

Sidransky, H. and Friedman L., 'The effect of cortisone and antibiotic agents on experimental pulmonary aspergillosis', *Amer J Path*, 1959, 35: 169–183.
Sidransky, H. et al, 'Experimental pulmonary aspergillosis', *Arch Path,* 1965, 79: 299.
Sievers, M. L., 'Coccidioidomycosis and race', *Am Rev Respir Dis,* 1979, 119(5): 839.
Skinner, C. F., 'The yeast-like fungi: *Candida* and Brettanomyces, *Bacteriol Rev*, 1947, 11(4): 227–274.
Slavin, R. G., 'Allergic bronchopulmonary aspergillosis', *Clin Rev Allerg Immu*, 1985, 3(2): 167–182.
Slavin, R. G., 'Allergic bronchopulmonary aspergillosis – A north American rarity', *Am J Med*, 1969, 47: 306–313.
Slavin, R. G., 'What does fungus among us really mean?', *J Allergy Clin Immunol*, 1978, 62: 1–2.
Slavin, R. G. and P Winzenberger, 'Epidemiologic aspects of allergic aspergillosis', *Ann Allergy*, 1977, 38(3): 215–218.
Sloane, M. B. 'New antifungal antibiotic: Mycostatin (Nystatin) of the treatment of Moniliasis: A preliminary report', *J Invest Dermatol*, 1955, 24: 569–571.
Smith, C. E., 'Epidemiology of acute Coccidioidomycosis with *Erythema nodosum* ("San Joaquin" or "Valley Fever")', *Am J Publ Health*, 1940, 40: 600–611.
Smith, D. F., 'Food panics in history: corned beef, typhoid and "risk society" ', *J Epidemiol Community Health*, 2007, 61(7): 566–570.
Smith, D. T. 'The diagnosis and therapy of mycotic infections', *Bull N Y Acad Med*, 1953, 29(10): 778–795.
Smith, G., 'The subway grate scene in tThe seven year itch: The staging of an appearance-as-disappearance', *Cinémas: Journal of Film Studies*, 2004, 14(2–3): 213–244.
Smith, J. H., 'The distribution of power in nationalized industries', *Brit J Sociol*, 1951, 2(4): 275–293.
Smith, R. J., 'Institute of medicine report recommends complete overhaul of food safety laws', *Science*, 1979, 203: 1221–1223.
Smith, T. J., 'Antibiotic-induced disease', in R. H. Moser, ed, *Diseases of Medical Progress*, Springfield, Ill, Charles C Thomas, 1963, 16.
Sobel, J. D. et al, 'Clotrimazole treatment of recurrent and chronic candida vulvovaginitis', *Intern J Gynecol Obstet*, 1989, 29(4): 386.
Solomon, E. and Dockeray, G. C., 'Vaginal discharges', *Irish Journal of Medical Science*, 1936–1937, 11: 548–551.
Souter, J. C., 'A Clinical note on fungus infection of the skin of the feet', *Proc R Soc Med*, 1937, 30: 1107–1116.
Spensley, P. C., 'Aflatoxin, the active principle in turkey 'X' disease', *Endeavour*, 1963, 22: 75–79.
Sproot, N. A., 'Athlete's foot', *BMJ*, 1957, ii: 1064 and 1243.
St Clair Symmers, W., 'Amphotericin pharmacophobia', *BMJ*, 1973, ii: 460–463.
Stearns, S. S., 'Issues in evolutionary medicine: Pearl Memorial Lecture', *Am J of Human Biol*, 2005, 17: 131–140.
Stefan Buczacki, 'Ainsworth, Geoffrey Clough (1905–1998)', *Oxford Dictionary of National Biography*, Oxford University Press, 2004 [http://www.oxforddnb.com/view/article/71235, accessed 3 May 2013].

Stevens, D. A. et al, 'Allergic bronchopulmonary aspergillosis in cystic fibrosis – state of the art': Cystic Fibrosis Foundation Consensus Conference, *Clin Infect Dis,* 2003, 37(Suppl 3): S225–S264.
Stevens, D. A. et al, 'Dermal sensitivity to different doses of spherulin and coccidioidin', *Chest,* 1974, 65: 530–533.
Stevens, D. A. et al, 'Immunotherapy in recurrent coccidioidomycosis', *Cell Immunol,* 1974, 12: 37–48.
Stevens, D. A., 'Coccidioidomycosis', *N Engl J Med,* 1995, 332: 1077.
Stevens, D. A. et al, 'Miconazole in coccidioidomycosis-II: Therapeutic and pharmacologic studies in man', *Am J Med,* 1976, 60: 191–202.
Stevens, R. J. and Lynch, F. W., 'Ringworm of the scalp: A report on the current epidemic', *JAMA,* 1947, 133: 306–309.
Stoloff, L., 'Molds and mycotoxins: What FDA is doing about the mycotoxin problem', *Farm Technol Agri-Fieldman,* 1972, 28: 60a.
Strauss, J. S. and Kligman, A. M., 'An experimental study of tinea pedis and onychomycosis of the foot', *AMA Arch Derm,* 1957, 76(1): 70–79.
Strauss, J. S. and Kligman, A. M., 'Effect of x-rays on sebaceous glands of the human face: radiation therapy of acne', *J Invest Dermatol,* 1959, 33: 347–356.
Stringer, J. R. et al, 'A new name (*Pneumocystis jiroveci*) for pneumocystis from humans', *Emerging Infectious Diseases,* 2002, 8(9): 891–896.
Stuart Wilkinson, J., 'Some remarks upon the development of epiphytes: With the description of a new vegetable formation found in connexion with the human uterus', *Lancet,* 1849, ii: 448–451.
Studdert, T. C., 'Farmer's lung', *BMJ,* 1953, i: 1305–1309.
Study, S., 'Looking for trouble: Medical science and clinical practice in the historiography of modern medicine', *Soc Hist Med,* 2011, 24(3): 739–757.
Sulzberger, M. B. and Kano, A., 'Undecylenic and propionic acids in the prevention and treatment of dermatophytosis', *Arch Derm Syphilo.* 1947, 55: 391–395.
Summers, W. C., 'On the origins of the science in Arrowsmith: Paul De Kruif, Félix d'Hérelle and phage', *J Hist Med Allied Sci,* 1991, 46(3): 315–332.
Swartz, J. H., 'The role of fungi in medicine', *N Engl J Med,* 1936, 215, 322–330.
Swayne, J. G. and Budd, W., 'An account of certain organic cells in the peculiar evacuations of cholera', *Lancet,* 1849, ii: 398–399.
Task Force on Clinical Ecology, 'Clinical ecology – a critical appraisal', *West J Med,* 1986, 144: 239–245.
Taubenberger, J. K. and Morens, D. M. '1918 Influenza: the mother of all pandemics', *Rev Biomed,* 2006, 17: 69–79.
Tenenbaum, M. J. et al, 'Blastomycosis', *Crit Rev Microbiol,* 1982, 9(3): 158–160.
Thomas, H. H., 'Candidal vulvovaginitis: Treatment with mycostatin', *Obstet Gynecol,* 1957, 9(2): 163–166.
Tilbury Fox, G., 'The true nature and meaning of parasitic diseases of the surface', *Lancet,* 1859, ii: 5–7, 31–32, 201, 260–261, 283–284 and 507–508.
Tilbury Fox, W., 'On ringworm of the head and its management', *Lancet,* 1877, ii: 643–644.
Tilbury Fox, W., 'On the identity of parasitic fungi affecting the human surface', *Lancet,* 1880, ii: 260–261.
Tilbury Fox, W., 'Ringworm in schools', *Lancet,* 1872, i: 5–6.

Timmermann, C., 'To treat or not to treat: Drug research and the changing nature of essential hypertension', in Schlich, T and Tröhler, U., eds, *The Risks of Medical Innovation: Risk Perception and Assessment in Historical Context,* London, Routledge, 2006, 133–147.

Tobie, W. C., 'Aspergillin: A name misapplied to several different antibiotics', *Nature*, 1946, 158: 709.

Troke, P. F., 'Efficacy of UK-49,858 (Fluconazole) against *Candida* albicans experimental infections in mice', *Antimicrob Agents Chemother,* 1985, 28(6): 815–818.

Truss, C. O., 'Restoration of immunologic competence to *C. albicans*', *J Orthomol Psychiatr*, 1980, 9: 287–301.

Truss, C. O., 'The role of candida albicans in human illness', *Orthomolecular Psychiatry*, 1981, 8: 228–238.

Truss, C. O., 'Tissue injury induced by *C. albicans*: Mental and neurologic manifestations', *J Orthomol Psychiatr* 1978, 1: 17–37.

Tucker, R. M. et al, 'Adverse events associated with itraconazole in 189 patients on chronic therapy', *J Antimicrob Chemother*, 1990, 26: 561–566.

Tucker, W. B., 'The evolution of the cooperative studies in the chemotherapy of tuberculosis of the Veterans administration and Armed Forces of the U.S.A.: An account of the evolving education of the physician in clinical pharmacology', *Bibl Tuberc*, 1960, 15: 1–68.

Tweedale, G. and Hansen, P., 'Protecting the workers: The medical board and the asbestos industry, 1930s-1960s', *Medical History*, 1998, 42: 439–457.

Underwood, E. A., 'National health and physical fitness', *Public Health*, 1937–1938, 51: 328–333.

Underwood, G. B. et al, 'Overtreatment dermatitis of the feet', *JAMA*, 1946, 130(5): 249–256.

Utz, J. P. and Roberts, W. C. '*Candida* endocardititis', *Ann Intern Med*, 1961, 54: 1058.

Van Cutsem, J. et al, 'Itraconazole, a new triazole in that is orally active in aspergillosis', *Antimicrob Agents Chemother,* 1984, 26: 527–534.

Varkey, H. B. and Rose, H. D., 'Pulmonary aspergilloma: A rational approach to treatment', *Am J Med*, 1976, 61: 626–631.

Vaughan, J. E. and Ramirez, H., 'Coccidioidomycosis as a complication of pregnancy', *Calif Med*, 1951, 74(2): 121–125.

Vickers, H. R., 'Arthur Rupert Hallam', *BMJ*, 1955, ii: 741–751.

Wack, E. E., et al, 'Coccidioidomycosis during pregnancy: An analysis of ten cases among 47, 120 pregnancies', *Chest*, 1988, 94: 376–379.

Wagner, J. M. and Kessel, I., 'Complications of *C. albicans* infection in infancy', *BMJ*, 1958, ii: 362–366.

Wainwright, M., 'Some highlights in the history of fungi in medicine – A personal journey', *Fungal Biology Reviews*, 2008, 22: 97–102.

Waksman, S. A. and Schatz, A., 'Strain specificity and production of antibiotic substances', *PNAS*, 1943, 29(2): 74–79.

Waksman, S. et al, 'Antifungal antibiotics', *Bull World Hlth Org*, 1952, 6: 163–172.

Walker, J., 'The dermatophytoses of Great Britain: Report of a three year survey', *Br J Dermatol*, 1950, 62: 239–251.

Walker, N., 'Fifty years of dermatology', *Lancet*, 1929, ii: 212.

Walker, N., 'X-rays in the treatment of tinea', *BMJ*, 1904, i: 868.
Walker, P. R. and Moorhead, J. F., 'Infection in the renal transplant patient', *J R Soc Med*, 1978, 71: 84–85.
Walsh, D., 'The removal of superfluous hair by a combination of X-ray exposure and electrolysis, *Lancet*, 1901, ii: 1191–1192.
Walsh, T. J., 'Treatment of aspergillosis: Clinical practice guidelines of the infectious diseases society of America', *Clin Infect Dis*, 2008, 46: 327–360.
Wang, J. L. et al, 'The management of allergic bronchopulmonary aspergillosis', *Am Rev Respir Dis*, 1979, 120(1): 87–92.
Warnock, D. W., 'Trends in the epidemiology of invasive fungal infections', *Jpn J Med Mycol*, 2007, 48: 1–12.
Waterson, A., 'Acquired immune deficiency syndrome', BMJ, (Clin Res Ed) 1983, 286: 743–746.
Weig, M. et al, Clinical aspects and pathogenesis of *Candida* infection', *Trends in Microbiology*, 2012, 20(8): 468–470.
Weinstein L. et al, 'Infections occurring during chemotherapy', *N Engl J Med*, 1954, 251: 251–259.
Wells, P. A. and Herrick, H. T., 'Citric Acid Industry', *Ind Eng Chem*, 1938, 30(3): 255–262.
West Walker, J., 'On diphtheria', *BMJ*, 1863, i: 504–508.
Weston Hurst, A., 'Protoporphyrin, cirrhosis and hepatomata in the livers of mice given griseofulvin', Br J Dermatol, 1963, 75(3): 105–112.
Weyers, W., 'Medical experiments on humans and the development of guidelines governing them: the central role of dermatology', *Clinics in Dermatology, 2009,* 27(4): 384–394.
Wheat, J., 'Endemic mycoses in AIDS: A clinical review', *Clin Microbiol Rev* 1995, 8(1): 146–153.
White, C. J., 'Fungus disease of the skin, clinical aspects and treatment, *Arch Derm Syphilol,* 1927, 15: 387–414.
Whitfield, A., 'A note on some unusual cases of trichophytic infection', *Lancet*, 1908, ii: 237–238.
Whittaker, R. H., 'New concepts of kingdoms of organisms', *Science*, 1969, 163: 150–161.
Whorton, J., 'Antibiotic abandon: The resurgence of therapeutic rationalism', in Parascandola, J., ed, *The History of Antibiotics: A Symposium*, Madison, Wis, American Institute of the History of Pharmacy, 1980, 125–136.
Wikler, A. et al, 'Mycotic endocarditis: report of a case', *JAMA*, 1942, 119, 33.
Wilks, S., 'Address in medicine', *BMJ*, 1872, ii: 146–153.
Williams Jr, M. H. and Serff, N. S., 'Chronic obstructive pulmonary disease: An analysis of clinical, physiologic and roentgenologic features', *Am J Med*, 1963, 35: 20–30.
Williams, D. I. et al, 'Griseofulvin', *Br J Dermatol*, 1959, 71: 434.
Williams, D. I. et al, 'Oral treatment of ringworm with Griseofulvin', *Lancet*, 1958, ii: 1212–1213.
Williams, R. D., 'Living with AIDS: New treatments give hope', *FDA Consumer*, January-February 1992, 26.
Wilson, B. J. and Wilson, C. H., 'Toxin from *Aspergillus flavus*: Production on food materials of a substance causing tremors in mice', *Science*, 1964, 144: 177–178.

Wilson, L. G., 'The historical decline of tuberculosis in Europe and America: Its causes and significance', *J Hist Med Allied Sci*, 1990, 45(3): 366–396.
Wogan, G. N., 'Aflatoxin as a human carcinogen', *Hepatology*, 1999, 30: 573–575.
Wogan, G. N., 'Chemical nature and biological effects of the Aflatoxins', *Bacteriol Rev*, 1966, 30: 460–470.
Woodruff, P. and Hesseltine, H. C., 'Relationship of oral thrush to vaginal mycosis and the incidence of each', *Am J Obstet Gynecol*, 1938, 36: 467–471.
Woods, J. W. et al, 'Monilial infections complicating the therapeutic use of antibiotics', *JAMA*, 1951, 145: 207–211.
Worboys, M., 'Unsexing gonorrhoea: Bacteriologists, gynaecologists and suffragists in Britain, 1860–1920', *Soc Hist Med*, 17(1), 31–59.
Worboys, M., 'Delépine, Auguste Sheridan (1855–1921)', *Oxford Dictionary of National Biography*, Oxford University Press, 2004 [http://www.oxforddnb.com/view/article/57113, accessed 5 August 2011].
Wright, D. J. M., 'Obituary: H I Winner', *BMJ*, 1993, 306: 1335.
Wright, E. T. et al, 'Treatment of moniliasis with nystatin', *JAMA*, 1957, 163: 92–94.
Young, R. C., 'Aspergillosis: The spectrum of disease in 98 patients', *Medicine*, 1970, 49(2): 147–173.
Zakon, S. J. and Benedek, T., 'David Gruby and the centenary of medical mycology, 1841–1941', *Bull Hist Med*, 1944, 16: 155–168.
Zimmerman, B. and Weber, E., '*Candida* and "20th-century disease" ', *Can Med Assoc J*, 1985, 133: 965–966.

Permissions

All chapters in this book were first published by Springer by Aya Homei & Michael Worboys; hereby published with permission under the Creative Commons Attribution License or equivalent. Every chapter published in this book has been scrutinized by our experts. Their significance has been extensively debated. The topics covered herein carry significant information for a comprehensive understanding. They may even be implemented as practical applications or may be referred to as a beginning point for further studies.

We would like to thank the editorial team for lending their expertise to make the book truly unique. They have played a crucial role in the development of this book. Without their invaluable contributions this book wouldn't have been possible. They have made vital efforts to compile up to date information on the varied aspects of this subject to make this book a valuable addition to the collection of many professionals and students.

This book was conceptualized with the vision of imparting up-to-date and integrated information in this field. To ensure the same, a matchless editorial board was set up. Every individual on the board went through rigorous rounds of assessment to prove their worth. After which they invested a large part of their time researching and compiling the most relevant data for our readers.

The editorial board has been involved in producing this book since its inception. They have spent rigorous hours researching and exploring the diverse topics which have resulted in the successful publishing of this book. They have passed on their knowledge of decades through this book. To expedite this challenging task, the publisher supported the team at every step. A small team of assistant editors was also appointed to further simplify the editing procedure and attain best results for the readers.

Apart from the editorial board, the designing team has also invested a significant amount of their time in understanding the subject and creating the most relevant covers. They scrutinized every image to scout for the most suitable representation of the subject and create an appropriate cover for the book.

The publishing team has been an ardent support to the editorial, designing and production team. Their endless efforts to recruit the best for this project, has resulted in the accomplishment of this book. They are a veteran in the field of academics and their pool of knowledge is as vast as their experience in printing. Their expertise and guidance has proved useful at every step. Their uncompromising quality standards have made this book an exceptional effort. Their encouragement from time to time has been an inspiration for everyone.

The publisher and the editorial board hope that this book will prove to be a valuable piece of knowledge for students, practitioners and scholars across the globe.

Index

www.ingramcontent.com/pod-product-compliance
Lightning Source LLC
LaVergne TN
LVHW062237200926
848484LV00006B/1560